*Performance-Enhancing Technologies in Sports*

Joseph S. Alper, Catherine Ard, Adrienne Asch, Jon Beckwith, Peter Conrad, and Lisa N. Geller, eds. *The Double-Edged Helix: Social Implications of Genetics in a Diverse Society*

Mary Ann Baily and Thomas H. Murray, eds. *Ethics and Newborn Genetic Screening: New Technologies, New Challenges*

Audrey R. Chapman and Mark S. Frankel, eds. *Designing Our Descendants: The Promises and Perils of Genetic Modifications*

Lori P. Knowles and Gregory E. Kaebnick, eds. *Reprogenetics: Law, Policy, and Ethical Issues*

John D. Lantos and William L. Meadow. *Neonatal Bioethics: The Moral Challenges of Medical Innovation*

Carol Levine and Thomas H. Murray, eds. *The Cultures of Caregiving: Conflict and Common Ground among Families, Health Professionals, and Policy Makers*

Maxwell J. Mehlman. *The Price of Perfection: Individualism and Society in the Era of Biomedical Enhancement*

Erik Parens, ed. *Surgically Shaping Children: Technology, Ethics, and the Pursuit of Normality*

Erik Parens, Audrey R. Chapman, and Nancy Press, eds. *Wrestling with Behavioral Genetics: Science, Ethics, and Public Conversation*

Mark A. Rothstein, Thomas H. Murray, Gregory E. Kaebnick, and Mary Anderlik Majumder, eds. *Genetic Ties and the Family: The Impact of Paternity Testing on Parents and Children*

Thomas H. Murray, Consulting Editor in Bioethics

# Performance-Enhancing Technologies in Sports

Ethical, Conceptual, and Scientific Issues

Edited by

THOMAS H. MURRAY

KAREN J. MASCHKE

ANGELA A. WASUNNA

The Johns Hopkins University Press

*Baltimore*

© 2009 The Johns Hopkins University Press
All rights reserved. Published 2009
Printed in the United States of America on acid-free paper
2 4 6 8 9 7 5 3 1

The Johns Hopkins University Press
2715 North Charles Street
Baltimore, Maryland 21218-4363
www.press.jhu.edu

Library of Congress Cataloging-in-Publication Data

Performance-enhancing technologies in sports : ethical, conceptual, and scientific issues /
edited by Thomas H. Murray . . . [et al.].
p.   cm.
Includes bibliographical references and index.
ISBN-13: 978-0-8018-9361-2 (hardcover : alk. paper)
ISBN-10: 0-8018-9361-5 (hardcover : alk. paper)
1. Doping in sports. 2. Athletic ability. 3. Gene therapy. I. Murray, Thomas H., 1946–
[DNLM: 1. Doping in Sports. 2. Athletic Performance. 3. Genetic Enhancement—ethics.
4. Sports—ethics. QT261 P4385 2009]
RC1230.P478 2009
362.29—dc22      2009002902

A catalog record for this book is available from the British Library.

*Special discounts are available for bulk purchases of this book. For more information,
please contact Special Sales at 410-516-6936 or specialsales@press.jhu.edu.*

The Johns Hopkins University Press uses environmentally friendly book materials,
including recycled text paper that is composed of at least 30 percent post-consumer waste,
whenever possible. All of our book papers are acid-free, and our jackets and covers are
printed on paper with recycled content.

# CONTENTS

LARRY D. BOWERS, PH.D., Senior Managing Director, U.S. Anti-Doping Agency, Colorado Springs, Colorado

ROBERT J. DONOVAN, PH.D., Professor of Behavioural Research, Division of Health Sciences, and Professor of Social Marketing, School of Marketing, Curtin University, Bentley, Perth, Western Australia

THEODORE FRIEDMANN, M.D., Director, Program in Human Gene Therapy, University of California, San Diego, La Jolla, California

GARY A. GREEN, M.D., Clinical Professor, UCLA Division of Sports Medicine, Pacific Palisades Medical Group, Pacific Palisades, California

JOHN HOBERMAN, PH.D., Professor and Chair, Department of Germanic Studies, University of Texas at Austin, Austin, Texas

ERIC P. HOFFMAN, PH.D., Director, Research Center for Genetic Medicine, Children's Research Institute, Children's National Medical Center, Washington, DC

ERIC T. JUENGST, PH.D., Professor of Bioethics, Associate Professor of Oncology, Department of Biomedical Ethics, Case Western Reserve University, Cleveland, Ohio

SIGMUND LOLAND, PH.D., Rector, The Norwegian University for Sport Sciences, Oslo, Norway

KAREN J. MASCHKE, PH.D., Research Scholar, Editor, *IRB: Ethics & Human Research*, The Hastings Center, Garrison, New York

MAXWELL J. MEHLMAN, J.D., Arthur E. Petersilge Professor of Law, Director, Case Western Reserve University School of Law, Professor of Bioethics, Case Western Reserve University, Cleveland, Ohio

THOMAS H. MURRAY, PH.D., President and CEO, The Hastings Center, Garrison, New York

ANGELA J. SCHNEIDER, PH.D., Associate Professor, School of Kinesiology, The University of Western Ontario, London, Ontario, Canada

JAN TODD, PH.D., Professor and Roy J. McLean Fellow in Sport History, Department of Kinesiology and Health Education, College of Education, The University of Texas at Austin, Austin, Texas

TERRY TODD, PH.D., Director, H. J. Lutcher Stark Center for Physical Culture and Sports, College of Education, The University of Texas at Austin, Austin, Texas

Untested ideas, like unchallenged athletes, can become weak and flabby. The best insurance against intellectual flabbiness is to press an idea hard: look at what surrounds it, the context in which it arises and is sustained; turn it over, whack it around a bit, and see how resilient it is when attacked.

That strategy describes the project conducted by The Hastings Center, "Ethics and Endurance-Enhancing Technologies in Sport." The central idea under examination was that certain performance-enhancing technologies that are or might be used in sport are unethical and that a good case can be made to prohibit their use by athletes. The goal of the Working Group was not to reach a consensus but rather to put important ideas about the ethics of performance-enhancing technologies in sport through a rigorous workout. The result of these conversations is this book—a compilation of original essays on the historical and cultural context, ethical and policy implications, and scientific context of using performance-enhancing technologies in sport. It is not possible to do justice in this preface to the full range of issues raised in the meetings of the Working Group or reflected in this volume, but a brief road map to the debate may be useful.

*Doping* is the term used in the sports world to refer to the use of means such as drugs, infusions of red blood cells, or, perhaps in the near future, genetic manipulation to enhance athletes' performance. Of course, all athletes, from neighborhood basketball and soccer players to professionals and Olympians, seek constantly to improve their performance. What justifies calling certain performance aids "doping" and creating an institutional apparatus to deter, detect, and punish those means? To many who participate in or enjoy watching sports, the answer is obvious: doping is cheating, cheating is wrong, end of story. Athletes commonly call for protecting their freedom to compete on a "level playing field." When some competitors get an edge from anabolic steroids, EPO (biosynthetic erythropoietin), or other substances, the clean athlete is at a disadvantage. Fair enough, the skeptic can say, but we could also level the playing field by allowing all competitors to use drugs.

The calls to allow doping in sport rely on a variety of arguments. We mention five here, briefly. First is the libertarian call for athletes (at least all competent adult athletes) to be free to use any and all ways they wish to improve performance. As an autonomous individual, the libertarian argues, each athlete has the moral right to decide what goals to pursue and what risks are worth taking on that path. John Hoberman (chapter 1) provides historical and cultural context on the contingent nature of the "freedom" that elite athletes experience. Thomas Murray (chapter 7) examines the ethical implications of the inherently coercive nature of competitive sport.

Skeptics can take a second route, arguing that the rules of sport ought to reflect what athletes are doing in reality. And, they claim, athletes are doping in large numbers, so sport should acknowledge and accept the practice. (The bioethicist Søren Holm calls this the "conventionalist" view.) This position fails to ask whether even the athletes who are doping want to continue or would rather compete clean. Angela Schneider (chapter 2), a philosopher and former Olympian, offers an athlete's insights. Jan Todd and Terry Todd (chapter 3) describe, in fascinating detail, what happened to the non-Olympic sport of powerlifting when some leaders of the sport opted to abandon the prohibition of doping.

A third line of attack is to claim that all efforts to draw meaningful and defensible lines between doping and the other things athletes do to improve performance are fruitless and misguided. Murray calls this the "line-drawing" critique and responds to it in chapter 7.

The fourth attack, a popular one in recent years, may be called the "harm reduction" approach. It draws an analogy between sports doping and conventional drug addiction; it argues that sports doping is a public health problem that must be managed with decriminalization and by putting physicians in charge of supervising athletes' drug taking. Gary Green (chapter 4), a university sports medicine physician, offers insights into the medical management of college athletes. Hoberman, through his extensive study of the state-sponsored East German doping programs that relied heavily on physicians and scientists, offers, in chapter 1, a sober cautionary note. An often-touted advantage of medically supervised doping is the claim that it would lead quickly to much better scientific knowledge of the effects of the drugs that athletes take. Green and, more directly, Karen Maschke (chapter 5) cast doubt on this happy prospect through a careful examination of the dynamics and ethics of such research on athletes.

The fifth critique is rooted in a particular view of technology and its relationship to people in general and athletes in particular. We can call it the transhumanist or Promethean view. Advocates of this view pop up with increasing frequency. Savulescu and colleagues, for example, say this about Olympic athletes: "Their ideal is superhuman performance at any cost . . . Far from being against the spirit of sport, biological manipulation embodies the human spirit— the capacity to improve ourselves on the basis of reason and judgment. When we exercise our reason, we do what only humans do . . . Olympic performance would be the result of human creativity and choice, not a very expensive horse race."* Maxwell Mehlman (chapter 10) provides a somewhat sympathetic plea for that part of the transhumanist/Promethean program that would promote the use of genetic manipulation to overcome the vast inequalities of talent distributed among us through the natural lottery. Murray describes some of the implications and assumptions of the transhumanist/Promethean view in chapter 7 and gives a more detailed response to Mehlman's arguments in chapter 11.

Interwoven through several of these critiques is a challenge to the meaning— or, as it is sometimes called, the "spirit"—of sport. Some are skeptical that any such meaning or spirit exists. They assert that sport just is what people say it is; if they changed their minds tomorrow and said it was something else, then that's what it would be. Today, baseball; tomorrow, Calvinball (the "Calvin and Hobbes" game in which the only rule is that you cannot use the same rule twice). Others assert that differences across human cultures condemn to failure or unintelligibility all efforts to find a cross-cultural meaning. (We cannot help noting that the ability of the 2008 Beijing Olympic Games to attract athletes from 204 countries is at least prima facie evidence that sport is both valued and, to some extent, understood across a vast array of human cultures.)

This debate about the meaning of sport lies at the core of the ethical and philosophical differences over doping. For some, it goes to the heart of what counts as fairness in sport. Sigmund Loland (chapter 8) defends his "fair opportunity principle" as a foundation for sport and as a reason to worry about what he calls "expert-administered technologies" through which "the welfare of individuals becomes increasingly dependent on the moral standards of their support systems and . . . athletes can be exploited and treated as means toward system survival." By contrast, Eric Juengst (chapter 9) argues that sport reifies genetic hierarchies—at a time when moral progress urges us to turn away from just such genetic sorting criteria. Murray (chapter 11) responds to Loland and Juengst and suggests that the meaning and significance of sport is inextricably interwoven with our relationship to our own embodiment.

The final two chapters include the analyses of leading scientists on the future role of genetic manipulation of athletes (Theodore Friedmann and Eric Hoffman; chapter 12) and on the science of endurance enhancement (Larry Bowers; chapter 13).

With this rough roadmap in mind, a brief description of each chapter may provide further guidance to readers. Part I, "Historical and Cultural Context,"

---

* J. Savalescu, B. Foddy, and M. Clayton, "Why We Should Allow Performance Enhancing Drugs in Sport," *British Journal of Sports Medicine* 38 (2004): 666–70.

opens with chapter 1, "Putting Doping into Context: Historical and Cultural Perspectives," in which John Hoberman continues his distinguished contributions to understanding how and why athletes use drugs to enhance their performance. Hoberman offers what he describes as a functionalist, sociological perspective. Rather than condemning individual athletes, he looks at the properties of the sports system, the demands it makes on athletes, and the rewards it offers to them. The roots of the American aversion to drugs in sport, he argues, are to be found in the "crusade that began with the Opium Exclusion Act of 1909 and was later reformulated as 'a total war against drugs' by President Richard Nixon in 1969." No fan of doping in sport himself, Hoberman urges us to look to the larger sporting system, not merely the individual athlete, if we want to have any genuine success in controlling drug use in sport.

Angela Schneider is, as noted earlier, a philosopher and former Olympic athlete, who won a silver medal in rowing for Canada in the 1984 Games. In chapter 2, "The Context of Performance Enhancement: An Athlete's Perspective," she reminds us that "for too long, athletes have been viewed as a form of replaceable commodity—central to the enterprise, but individually of little importance." She calls for athletes to be enlisted as full and genuine participants in all doping-control efforts. Her diagnosis of our current predicament is severe: "At the moment, from the athlete's perspective, we have the worst of all possible worlds. The belief that many athletes are doping places increased pressure to dope on those who currently do not . . . Few competitions are untainted by suspicion, because there is a widespread belief that some competitors are doping, and just about everyone's reputation and integrity fall into question." What athletes most want, Schneider tells us, is a world in which "they could compete cleanly and fairly, assured that others are doing the same." Schneider asks whether current doping-control methods are effective and ethical, and what place law can and should play. She argues for the usefulness of a human rights framework for understanding the role that athletes themselves can play in doping control.

Jan Todd and Terry Todd are coauthors of chapter 3, "Reflections on the 'Parallel Federation Solution' to the Problem of Drug Use in Sport: The Cautionary Tale of Powerlifting." The Todds write with authority. Jan was an internationally renowned powerlifter and, to our knowledge, the only contributor to a Hastings Center book who has ever been featured in *Sports Illustrated* as the "World's Strongest Woman." Jan was also an organizational leader in women's powerlifting and fought for drug testing in her sport. Terry Todd was the U.S. men's 1965 superheavyweight powerlifting champion. He acknowledges experimenting with anabolic steroids late in his career as a powerlifter. The Todds tell their story about the evolution of powerlifting, and its relationship with drugs, with great insight and flashes of revealing detail. It is, after all, also their own story. Powerlifting is a sort of "natural experiment" that bears on the future of sport. The would-be governing bodies for powerlifting, the "federations" in the Todds' account, are divided by many differences, most tellingly their attitude toward performance-enhancing drugs as well as equipment designed to increase the weights a person can lift. You will never look on a shirt in quite the same way once you've read the Todds' account. Powerlifting tests the boundaries between sport and mere entertainment. As the head of one drug-tolerating federation said: "People need to understand that what we're doing is as much entertainment as it is sport. Fans like to see record lifts and our lifters like to make record lifts, so our rules about equipment, drug-testing and performance of the lifts are all designed to create new American and world records. It's show business." One powerlifter, as reported by another official, lamented that powerlifting was becoming "the Hell's Angels of organized sport."

Gary Green's critique, in chapter 4, is "The Role of Physicians, Scientists, Trainers, Coaches, and Other Nonathletes in Athletes' Drug Use." Green is a sports physician who practices family medicine and has taken care of student-athletes for more than 20 years. He is also the medical director for the UCLA Intercollegiate Drug Testing Program, has served on National Collegiate Athletic Association bodies dealing with drug use by athletes, and is a consultant to Major League Baseball. Green reminds us that athletes exist in an ecosystem that includes physicians, sports scientists, trainers, coaches, and others—including a netherworld of labs, chemists, and hangers-on. Nor should we forget the institutions whose interests depend on athletes' performances, such as universities, team owners, and endorsement-seeking sponsors. Focusing control efforts, including sanctions, solely on athletes is both unfair and unwise. Green's enlightening portrait of the elite athlete's world also underscores how the sports systems we've created lead athletes to become accustomed to allowing other people to be responsible for their well-being.

In chapter 5, "Performance-Enhancing Technologies and the Ethics of Human Subjects Research," Karen Maschke takes up the intriguing but rarely addressed connection between doping and medical research. Maschke, the editor of *IRB: Ethics & Human Research*, notes that foundational texts for international attention to the ethics of research with human beings, such as the Nuremberg Code and the World Medical Association's Declaration of Helsinki, set stringent conditions for research conducted on otherwise healthy people, especially if the research is unconnected with any effort to prevent or treat disease. That athletes use drugs in uncommon patterns and sometimes in doses that may be orders of magnitude larger than would be typical in therapeutic regimens runs up against the usual ethical standards that govern research. It is difficult to imagine an institutional review board approving a study that proposed to give megadoses of anabolic steroids to healthy young athletes. Maschke further notes that too many studies of enhancement technologies are flawed by low power, subjects who may not be good stand-ins for elite athletes, and vague endpoints. On the whole, Maschke's chapter should serve as a warning that much more attention needs to be paid to the ethics of research on performance enhancement.

Robert J. Donovan is an expert on health promotion and behavior research in Australia. In chapter 6, "Toward an Understanding of Factors Influencing Athletes' Attitudes about Performance-Enhancing Technologies: Implications for Ethics Education," Donovan fleshes out the implications of Green's observation that athletes exist not in isolation but in ecosystems. Donovan's review of the evidence reveals that athletes are surrounded by influential reference groups—and that not all members of those reference groups are likely to have the athlete's best interest at heart. The entourages surrounding athletes can be both the source of drugs and the spur to use them. He maps the behavioral evidence on moral development against the typical career path of young athletes, which indicates that moral development is largely complete by age 15. Donovan takes this as a warning that engaging athletes in serious moral deliberation about the use of performance-enhancing drugs in sport must begin early and must go far beyond a simple list of prohibitions: rather, young persons must grapple with the moral arguments underlying bans on performance-enhancing drugs and have the opportunity to debate them.

Part II, "Conceptual Maps and Ethical Implications," begins with chapter 7, "Ethics and Endurance-Enhancing Technologies in Sport." Thomas Murray, who is also the lead editor of the volume, attempts to confront the five main lines of attack against efforts to control the use of performance-enhancing technologies in sport, as mentioned earlier: the claim of incoherency; the arbitrariness of line-drawing; antipaternalism and the presumption in favor of individual liberty; the "resistance is futile" objection; and the heroic/Romantic/Promethean dream. Allowing these objections to prevail would lead to the triumph of the performance principle and the loss of most or all of what is meaningful, beautiful, admirable, and fascinating about sport. After considering three conceptions of human nature, the chapter considers the limits for generalizing from sport to other realms of life.

Sigmund Loland is a philosopher and rector of The Norwegian University for Sport Sciences, and he has taught alpine skiing. Chapter 8, "Fairness in Sport: An Ideal and Its Consequences," documents his search for "an interpretation of fairness in sport in terms of the principle of equality of opportunity to perform and its operationalization: the fair opportunity principle." He develops two principles: the "equal opportunity to perform" principle and the fair opportunity principle. The latter "prescribes the elimination of or compensation for essential inequalities that individuals cannot control or influence in any significant way and for which they cannot be held responsible." Loland draws out the implications of his analysis for a variety of differences in sport—age, sex, body mass, access to cutting-edge equipment and sports science, and money, among them. He also considers a set of performance-enhancing means that he dubs "expert-administered technologies," ranging from noncontroversial nutritional regimens, drawn up by specialists, to hypoxic chambers, drugs, and genetic manipulations. His theoretical account provides a basis for thinking critically and insightfully about performance-enhancing technologies in sport. His account also leaves open at least two important matters. First, in the quest to nullify uncontrollable advantages, how should we regard differences in natural talents? Second, with regard to genetic manipulations, Loland warns that they "may challenge radically the idea of athletes as autonomous moral agents and turn sport into a moral front zone in which general ethical questions on the status of agency, freedom, and responsibility are tested and rethought."

Eric T. Juengst, in chapter 9, "Annotating the Moral Map of Enhancement: Gene Doping, the Limits of Medicine, and the Spirit of Sport," mounts a notable challenge to the underlying ethic of sport itself. Juengst begins by describing three frameworks commonly employed to think about the ethics of enhancement: as enhancement versus treatment, as defined by the boundaries of appropriate professional practice, and as the effort to propel human capacities outside the range of normal species-typical functioning. Juengst warns that the prospect of genetic manipulation poses a fundamental challenge to sport. "What is at stake," he writes, "is the very ethos of sport, nothing less than an epochal confrontation between a model of human identity as spelled out in the Book of Genesis and a science-based libertarian model." He worries that if the ethos of sport is to create hierarchies of accomplishment according to differences in natural talents, then in a world struggling to treat people as moral equals, "a social practice that creates and glorifies hierarchies of genetic endowment seems anachronistic and slightly ominous."

Chapter 10, "Genetic Enhancement in Sport: Ethical, Legal, and Policy Concerns," is contributed by Maxwell Mehlman, Arthur E. Petersilge Professor of Law and director of the Law-Medicine Center at Case Western Reserve University School of Law. Mehlman adopts an expansive definition of "genetic intervention"—broad enough to include genetic testing and reproductive choices—as part of his thoroughgoing critique of the ethics of sport. He is skeptical that the Olympic movement could effectively control such technologies as genetic manipulation or selection, and he describes the future prospects for maintaining current policies and principles as "dismal." He advocates an alternative future for sport, a future in which natural talent would be rejected as a basis for athletic success. In that future, Mehlman writes, "Athletes would be tested before competing and handicapped according to their native ability. This would not be performance testing, because that would conflate talent with effort, thereby handicapping athletes who worked hard at the same level as those with inherited or installed ability. Instead, some method would have to be found to measure pure ability—most likely, a sophisticated combination of phenotypic and genetic markers." If—a rather large if—his proposal could be implemented, what would be left is a world of competition in which only those aspects of a person's performance that are morally praiseworthy would be allowed to sort out winners and losers.

The final chapter in part II (chapter 11), "In Search of an Ethics for Sport: Genetic Hierarchies, Handicappers General, and Embodied Excellence," is Murray's appreciation of and response to the challenges posed by the three authors who confront, especially directly, the ethical case for banning endurance- and other performance-enhancing drugs: Loland, Mehlman, and Juengst. An analysis of Loland's proposed "fair opportunity principle" leads us to ask what role differences in natural talents should be allowed to play among all the factors that enter into determining sports performance. Mehlman's call for genetic interventions to neutralize "inherited or installed ability" so that effort, not talent, determines who wins is a bold idea dogged by several problems. Among them is determining just when those traits we want to admire might be shaped by factors—genetic or otherwise—for which we don't deserve moral credit. Then there is the challenge of devising a fair system of handicapping and enhancement. Finally, Juengst's interesting analysis of sport as a system for selecting genetic hierarchies encounters conceptual and scientific difficulties. It also fails to capture many important features of sport.

Part III, "Current and Future Science," begins with chapter 12, "Genetic Dop-

ing in Sport: Applying the Concepts and Tools of Gene Therapy," by two eminent scientists at the cutting edge of research on gene transfer, the technological
underpinning for genetic manipulation of athletes. Theodore Friedmann is a
world-renowned pioneer in both the science and the ethics of gene transfer, and
Eric P. Hoffman is a leading researcher on muscular dystrophy and on the use
of gene transfer to try to prevent or treat this disease. In their sober and scientifically informed analysis of the prospects for genetically enhanced athletes, they
remind us that gene transfer is still, despite decades of research, in an early stage
as something useful and predictable in humans. They describe the technologies
of gene transfer and its achievements in humans—limited thus far, but with considerable promise. They acknowledge the appeal of genetic manipulation for athletic enhancement for both endurance and muscular strength, as well as its particular allure as a possible way of escaping detection. Finally, they note that there
are good reasons why gene-transfer research is heavily regulated and conclude
that "gene-transfer technology, even in applications to life-threatening disease, is
still immature and potentially hazardous. And the physiological complexities and
still unrecognized immune and other responses of the human body to genetic
modification make the use of such methods in healthy young athletes not only
of unproven efficacy but also, potentially, of far greater risk than benefit."

Larry D. Bowers is a chemist, former chief of an International Olympic Committee–certified laboratory in Indianapolis, and senior managing director of the
U.S. Anti-Doping Agency (USADA). Bowers describes the scientific basis for a
range of biomedical endurance-enhancing strategies in chapter 13, "Technologies to Enhance Oxygen Delivery and Methods to Detect the Use of These Technologies." For endurance enhancement, a few such technologies are well known
and have been widely employed, including EPO and blood doping—infusing red
blood cells before a competition. Other technologies are on the horizon, such as
artificial or manipulated hemoglobin, the molecule that carries oxygen to muscles craving it during physical exertion, and perfluorocarbons. Not all the techniques require infusing the body with drugs or artificial products: some athletes
are attempting to increase their endurance through the use of hypoxic chambers
to simulate a "live high, train low" strategy. Bowers provides a concise, expert
guide to the techniques that athletes use and their likely mechanisms of action.
He also takes a brief look at genetic manipulation and at the challenges these
various methods of technological endurance enhancement pose for detection
and control.

With new performance-enhancing strategies stretching the conceptual
bounds of "doping," new doping methods expressly designed to evade detection,

and new challenges to the fundamental ethical rationale for efforts to control doping in sport, we need ethical and conceptual clarity about doping at least as much as we need accurate and sensitive tests. On behalf of the editors and all the contributors to this volume, and with thanks to all participants in our research group over the life of the project, we offer our hope that this book will help the reader understand the context of doping in sport and to think more clearly about the ethics of doping.

Many individuals, and one funder with exceptional foresight, made this book and the project from which it stems possible. The funder is the research arm of USADA, the United States Anti-Doping Agency. The project's formal title is "Ethical, Conceptual, and Scientific Issues in the Use of Performance Enhancing Technologies in Sports." Special thanks are due to Dr. Larry Bowers and Travis Tygart for their patience and support over the life of this effort.

We are also deeply grateful to our colleagues at The Hastings Center who labored, mostly in anonymity, as research assistants. Their unfailing and cheerful help greatly lightened the editors' burden. Stacy Sanders, Alissa Lyon, Michael Khair, Denise Wong, Sophie Kasimow, Alison Jost, and Polo Black Golde all contributed during the life of the project. Jacob Moses was invaluable in the home stretch, keeping track of wayward authors and ever-shifting chapters and tables of contents.

Finally, we thank Jodi Fernandes, who keeps us from the chaos that would otherwise engulf us all.

# PART I

# HISTORICAL AND CULTURAL CONTEXT

# CHAPTER ONE

# Putting Doping into Context

## Historical and Cultural Perspectives

JOHN HOBERMAN, PH.D.

## Two Interpretations of Doping

The doping practices of elite athletes belong to a broader set of pharmacological enhancements of the human organism that are now a fundamental aspect of modern life.[1] In this sense, doping can be understood from a purely practical standpoint as one pharmacological practice among others that are intended to maximize human capacities and productivity. The athlete who throws the shot 22 meters is more "productive" than his competitor who throws only 20 meters, in three ways. He has demonstrated superior strength and technique, he may earn a considerable sum of money, and he might win a medal that will be credited to his country of origin. Any observer of Olympic sport over the past several decades can verify that many athletes, and the sports systems that created them, have operated in accordance with this model of productivity. From this perspective, doping can appear to be a practical necessity whose productive advantages outweigh its risks and costs.

Doping can also be viewed as practical behavior from a sociological perspective, which unlike the athlete and his or her entourage, has no vested interest in the kinds of productivity that doping can make possible. The sociological interpretation of doping behavior is neutral in that it neither endorses doping nor identifies the doping athlete as a transgressor who has earned the unmitigated censure of his or her athletic community and society at large. The sociological interpretation sees the doping athlete not as a fully autonomous actor but rather as enmeshed in a predicament that exerts pressure on him or her to dope. In the context of this predicament, the motivation to dope originates both inside and outside the individual athlete, so that the individual and society share responsibility for doping behavior. The essential point is that neither the athletic community nor society at large has the right to isolate and condemn the athlete as a solitary transgressor of community norms, because either or both of these communities may have encouraged or tacitly required doping behavior for the preservation of athletic careers.

The opposing view, one that condemns doping unreservedly, is interesting in that it requires restraint from athletes on both ethical and medical grounds and seems to be willing to sacrifice a measure of productivity (performance) so that athletes meet a certain standard of conduct. In this scenario, the athlete is both a moral actor and, secondarily, a potential victim who is vulnerable to organic or psychological harm that may result from the use of doping drugs. The moral and medical arguments against doping are typically presented together for the purpose of achieving a kind of synergistic effect, because the prospect of medical harm is alarming and thus intensifies the ethical transgression that originated as the intention to gain an unfair advantage over one's rivals.[2] In this sense, the antidoping campaign that aims to regulate the drug-taking behavior of elite athletes regards these performers as model citizens whose primary obligation is not only to be productive but also to practice self-restraint for the purpose of regulating themselves on behalf of a larger community.

The historical and cultural analysis of doping involves understanding these opposing interpretations of what doping behavior means and what this suggests about how it should be dealt with.

The moral and ethical critique stigmatizes the doping athlete by emphasizing his or her individual responsibility for what is defined as deviant or even degenerate behavior. It is important to understand that thinking about the doping behavior of athletes has been profoundly influenced by the traditional fear and loathing of narcotic drugs such as opium and heroin and of stimulants such as cocaine and amphetamines. "A drug addict," *Lancet* commented in 1937, "suggests to many a vicious and rather disgusting person who, however wretched his condition may be, has brought it upon his own head."[3] The drug addict is a degenerate who is wholly responsible for his own fate and is thus a perfect incarnation of vice or sin. Such people have often been used as potent symbols of evil by political or religious figures. Olympic officials, too, have adopted this idiom to describe doping as "death" (Juan Antonio Samaranch) and as "the evil of all evils" (Willi Daume).[4]

The elite sports world is not, however, a genuine shame culture that stigmatizes and punishes doping consistently and with conviction. The condemnation and rehabilitation of accused and convicted dopers around the world has never followed a consistent logic. Many athletes who test positive are exonerated on technical or procedural grounds, many federations continue to show little interest in effective testing, and drug-assisted records are defended rather than disqualified on the basis of documented evidence.[5] The relationship to the drug-soaked past (and to the 1980s in particular) thus remains stubbornly unreformed, let alone atoned for. Invoking religious language in the Olympic fashion leads not to virtue but to farce: the commercial requirements of professional cycling, for example, have prompted the Union Cycliste Internationale (UCI) to cite the purging effects of penance for the purpose of getting doped riders back into competition. "The UCI's view," according to its website (www.uci.ch), "is that all humans make mistakes and that even one who commits a serious offence such as an anti-doping violation must have the opportunity to repent and to be reinstated." But rotating athletes in and out of competitions as their hematocrits go up and down is a medical strategy that has little to do with ethics or repentance.[6] The sincere promulgation of ethical standards by the World Anti-Doping Agency (WADA) and others must, therefore, make itself heard amid the din created by a global sports system that has absorbed both the professional ambitions and the resulting amorality and cynicism of the many athletes whose behavior requires regulation.

The sociological interpretation of doping downplays the themes of deviance and degeneration in favor of a functionalist interpretation that offers explanations of why a significant number of athletes succumb to the temptation to dope. The leading practitioner of this method, the German sociologist Karl-Heinrich Bette, points out that it is the functionalist approach that allows us to think of this long parade of doped athletes as something other than moral defectives who should be banned from sport for life. "Doping," he suggests, "is less a case of 'bad' people than of social conditions that produce deviance in predictable ways. As a sociologist, one might well ask, how is it that elite sport has brought together such an assortment of actors, irrespective of discipline or nationality, that collectively demonstrates so many character flaws?"[7] Prof. Dr. Helmut Digel, a sports sociologist and reformist administrator of the German Track and Field Federation (1993–2001), stated flatly in 1998 that "cheating in high-performance sport is inherent in the system."[8] This perspective stands in sharp contrast to the moralizing and shaming approach that focuses exclusively on stigmatizing the athlete. It is significant that this stigmatizing process is carried out by administrative bodies that are not in the habit of examining their own relationship to the doping system.

From a sociological perspective, the doping problem has a great deal to do with the network of interest groups that benefit from the performances of elite athletes. Politicians undermine doping control by encouraging sportive nationalism as a political strategy. Sports federations and professional sports leagues employ administrators, coaches, doctors, and other support personnel whose careers are tied to the international success of the athletes they produce. Vast media operations and a variety of industries are dependent on the entertainment produced by elite athletes. Acknowledging the sheer enormity of this global operation enables us to see the celebrity (or notoriety) of athletes in the much larger context that sustains their careers. The athlete-worker can now be seen to be vulnerable to manipulation in ways that are essentially invisible when he or she is presented to the public as a cheater who has attempted to manipulate the system. Now we can see the economic consequences of the decisions athletes make about doping. The sociological interpretation also makes possible a public health approach to doping that substitutes epidemiological investigation for the emphasis on moral outrage.

Finally, the sociological-historical method does not employ the puritanical approach to "drugs" that has been so influential in the United States over the past century. It is important to understand that the antidoping campaign is an offshoot of the American crusade that began with the Opium Exclusion Act of 1909 and was later reformulated as "a total war against drugs" by President Richard Nixon in 1969.[9] This assault on drug consumption has always been selective, sparing such massively harmful drugs as alcohol and nicotine in favor of targeting drugs associated with social undesirables. Alcohol's exemption from demonization in modern societies reminds us that "drug-free" sport is a variation on the theme of a "drug-free" life that has never existed. "Intoxication," Richard Davenport-Hines points out, "is not unnatural or deviant. Absolute sobriety is not a natural or primary human state."[10] The catastrophic mistake of Prohibition (1920–33) was to legislate a pharmacological standard of virtue that satisfied the puritanical demand for a "drug-free" existence while causing massive social harm that outweighed any possible benefit abstinence had to offer. A similar illusory abstinence is the ideal being promulgated today by the advocates of "drug-free" sport. In fact, the high-performance sports medicine required by modern athletes is unthinkable without a vast array of drugs and other substances that are administered to elite athletes within the rules and without public knowledge.[11]

This gulf between the "drug-free" ideal and the drug- (or "supplement"-) dependent reality continues to haunt the antidoping campaign, because official candor about the medical costs of elite sports careers is not on the public relations agenda of the Société du Tour de France or any other sports organization.

This untenable situation is also sustained by the widely shared conviction that elite athletes are essential role models whose drug consumption should be concealed from the impressionable youth they are supposed to be dissuading from using "drugs." As the past two decades of doping scandals should make clear, this campaign to shield young people from athletes' use of drugs has often failed. Mark McGwire's inadvertent boost to the adolescent market for androstenedione is a well-known case in point. More recently, an academic study reported that most young children in France already accept performance-enhancing drugs as an integral part of sport. "Children of six years find it just as legitimate to take drugs to improve sporting performance as it is to take them to cure a sickness," according to the professor who supervised the survey.[12] Such reports, which are as troubling to me as they are likely to be to many readers of this chapter, suggest that the sporting public will have to find new ways to appreciate athletic performances if anything resembling "drug-free" sport is to survive the new era of enhancements that is already upon us.

## Doping as Enhancement

Over the past century, and coinciding with the rise of high-performance sport, the official and unofficial, legal and illegal pharmacopoeias of modern societies have increasingly been aimed at boosting a variety of human capacities. Such abilities employ the powers of mind and body to promote the fulfillment of human needs and ambitions in ways that include, but are hardly limited to, the kinds of athletic achievement with which this chapter is primarily concerned. The use of amphetamines by all of the major armies during World War II and by U.S. Air Force pilots to this day are cases in point.[13] In recent years, the pharmaceutical industry's promotion of several medications to relieve "erectile dysfunction" in (mostly aging) men has helped establish a presumptive right to lifelong sexual fulfillment that has gone almost unchallenged by critical voices. The use of widely prescribed stimulants such as Ritalin and Adderall by college students, as a kind of "brain doping" to achieve mental focus over many hours of studying, has become commonplace on American campuses. As one lonely skeptic puts it: "Societal opinion, and especially politically correct opinion, is strongly set in favour of accepting almost any demand, based on the autonomy of the demanding person; and against professional assessment of needs, which is seen as paternalistic, and even as a conspiracy against the people."[14] Athletes' sense of entitlement to drugs must be understood in the context of this presumed right to pharmacological support of various kinds.

Indeed, "paternalistic" medical opinion has already lost much of its authority to regulate lifestyle drugs that now include testosterone and human growth hormone (HGH) as well as the by now familiar drugs for erectile dysfunction. This transformation of patients into empowered consumers has been accompanied by the transformation of many doctors into "antiaging" specialists who sell hormone treatments to patients with the blessing of the U.S. Food and Drug Administration (FDA).[15] Testosterone, anabolic steroids, and HGH thus lead parallel lives as legitimate drugs for aging adults and as illegitimate doping drugs for younger athletes and bodybuilders of all ages. The federal law underlying FDA policy defines legitimate hormone use as a medical therapy and illegitimate hormone use as an impermissible enhancement of athletic ability or muscle mass. As the distinction between therapeutic and lifestyle drugs becomes increasingly difficult to define and justify, so does the idea that doping is an illegitimate procedure, because all of this hormone consumption falls under the rubric of performance enhancement of one kind or another. A populist pharmacology that responds to public demand is thus an inherently libertarian pharmacology that will tend to endorse, without bias, the use of drugs to fulfill personal ambitions of various kinds.

Synergistic relationships between marketing strategies and popular demands for enhancements served the pharmaceutical industry well throughout the twentieth century. But this linkage between the industry's ability to create demand and the public's response to marketing initiatives is more powerful today than in the past. The legalization of drug companies' direct-to-consumer marketing in 1997 has exposed the American public to an endless series of advertising messages that proclaim a right to health, physical attractiveness, and improved functioning of mind and body. Endorsements of such products by athletes subvert the antidoping campaign in sport by identifying athletes with a market for enhancements that shows every sign of expanding without limits. As this market grows, its products acquire an aura of legitimacy, and it becomes increasingly difficult for ordinary people to stigmatize any particular enhancement procedure as illegitimate. The new respectability of such enhancement procedures inevitably affects how people judge the doping practices of athletes, because these techniques cannot be distinguished in principle from many nonathletic medication practices that are now a part of everyday life in modern societies.[16] The gradual erosion of this boundary between athletic and nonathletic performance enhancement is confirmed by public opinion data indicating an already substantial and growing acceptance of medically regulated doping by professional athletes.[17]

This trend toward what may be called "libertarian" pharmacology is thus of great importance for understanding the cultural status of athletic doping at the present time. Even a cursory survey of the current markets for a variety of drugs and supplements demonstrates the wide range of therapies and enhancements these markets aim at supplying. To boost energy levels there are energy bars,[18] supercaffeine drinks,[19] a guarana soft drink,[20] the extract of the hoodia cactus of South Africa,[21] and in Japan a drink called Vaam (vespa amino acid mixture) that has been promoted by the Japanese winner of the women's marathon at the 2000 Sydney Olympic Games.[22] There is a pill for attention deficit disorder (Strattera),[23] chocolate for strengthening the heart,[24] drugs that are supposed to improve memory,[25] Provigil (modafinil) to promote vigilance,[26] a new type of sleeping pill to vanquish insomnia,[27] and a hormone nasal spray to curb hunger.[28] Nonpharmacological enhancements include the booming market for sex toys that are defined, according to the Texas law that prohibits them, as items "designed or marketed as useful primarily for the stimulation of human genital organs."[29] Among the unexpected enhancing techniques, we may now include the video games whose cognitive effects include the development of "selective visual attention such as skill in monitoring more than one location simultaneously."[30]

The demand for these and other products that are assumed to boost human capacities and performances has grown directly out of two powerful modern value systems: the related ideologies of individual fulfillment and limitless productivity that have been gaining momentum in all modern societies since the 1960s. Indeed, what we now call the "globalization" of culture and commerce is driven by such aspirations to achieve meaningful lives and by the competitive ethos that demands productivity in a manner analogous to that of high-performance sport. It is not surprising, therefore, that corporate advertising around the world often employs dynamic images of athletes to represent the otherwise invisible power of financial and electronic systems. Frequent use of the term *world-class* in business environments points again to a fusion of sportive and corporate value systems that share an obsession with high performance and the techniques that make it possible.

There are two related observations to be made about the world of competition described above. The first is that in this world, performance enhancement is a self-evident virtue; the second is that self-restraint on the part of the competitor is likely to appear both anomalous and anachronistic. Why should anyone practice self-restraint in the face of a competitive challenge, when winning promises tangible rewards? And why should any competitor renounce an innovation that provides an advantage over his rivals? As the medical ethicist Erik Parens points out, "there is something indeed odd in worrying about aiming technologies at the 'enhancement of human capacities.' What after all is worrisome about improving a human capacity? Because enhancing human capacities is taken to be a fairly self-evident good, worries about it are often dismissed as being a function of unnecessary anxiety or fear about the new."[31]

The "oddness" of counseling restraint in the pursuit of enhancement applies as well to high-performance sport. The modern world has chosen to interpret the Olympic motto, *citius, altius, fortius* (swifter, higher, stronger), as the pursuit of linear progress without any apparent end, and it is this interpretation of Olympic sport that made the doping epidemic of the modern era inevitable. There are practical limits to non-enhanced athletic performance that sports officials have routinely ignored, and it is the rare sports official who counsels athletes to practice restraint in preparing for international competition. The formulation of Olympic qualifying norms, which require certain minimum performances before athletes are eligible for the Games, is one example of how the self-interested ambitions of sports officials have always prevailed over any manifest interest in determining the parameters of drug-free athletic performances. The doping crisis thus points to the subordinate role of ethics and its ideal of self-restraint in some of the major sports cultures that shape public perceptions of what athletes are expected to do. Indeed, the role of self-restraint in elite competitions is so diminished that doping control now serves as the only manifestation of sportive ethics at this level of competition. In today's sports world, the assertion "I have never tested positive for doping drugs" is the functional equivalent of a statement of conscience. During the 1980s and 1990s, "I have a clean conscience" was the formula with which former East German athletes disclaimed any moral responsibility for having competed while using drugs. In neither case does the principle of self-restraint play a meaningful role.

One source of the current doping crisis in sport is that the antidoping code that has been promulgated, and sometimes enforced, by federation and Olympic officials is, in a world of imperfectly regulated competitions, both anomalous and anachronistic. The ideal of drug-free sport has never been achieved, and today there is a growing consensus that, like some other behaviors regarded as antisocial, doping can never be wholly eradicated. This does not mean that the antidoping ideal is wrong in principle or that it cannot serve a worthwhile purpose. The point is rather that it is clearly incompatible with some high-performance sports cultures in which doping practices have become particularly conspicuous over the past several decades. The incompatibility of principled self-restraint with athletic success at the elite level in some sports also raises questions about athletes' commitment to ethical standards and the role-modeling functions they are often assigned to fulfill. The familiar claim in this regard is that athletes combine a single-minded pursuit of high performance with an honorable determination to regulate their own behavior in conformity with rules that include the renunciation of doping. From this perspective, doping in elite sport amounts to a long series of ethical failures by a minority of athletes who have chosen to medicate themselves in an illicit manner and thus violate the norms of the athletic communities to which they belong.

## Athletes' Interest in Doping Drugs

This standard model of doping behavior is flawed, for the reasons examined above. Another essential point is that the history of high-performance athletic effort demonstrates that athletes have far more interest in doping techniques than is generally recognized by those who expect today's elite athletes to adhere to the ideal of drug-free sport. Athletes' interest in doping techniques long antedates the anabolic steroid epidemic that took off during the 1960s. "Virtually all of the training methods of the early sports movement of the second half of the nineteenth century involved the use of substances that today are on the list of banned doping drugs—caffeine, alcohol, nitroglycerine, opium and its derivatives, and strychnine. Above all, those participating in endurance contests (marathon runners and cyclists) were particularly receptive to such performance-enhancing techniques."[32] In 1894, the pioneering French sports physician Phillippe Tissié administered several types of beverage to a cyclist to test their value as performance enhancers. He and other biological scientists of this period regarded the elite athlete as an experimental subject whose exertions and traumas could illuminate some of the mysteries of human physiology. While we associate this era (nostalgically) with the amateur ideal of fair play, this value system was irrelevant both to physicians of the era and to athletes who were attempting to cope with new levels of stress by ingesting stimulants. We must understand that ethical objections to doping did not exist at this time. The use of these drugs was seen instead as a pharmacological antifatigue therapy. Indeed, the idea that professional cyclists are entitled to the analgesic and fortifying effects of drugs persists in the cycling culture to this day, and this view is undoubtedly shared by a large segment of the sporting public that follows their exploits.[33] We will return to the topic of public responses to doping later in this chapter.

Our knowledge of doping practices during the first half of the twentieth century remains limited. There are, however, periodic and credible accounts of a doping culture that closely resembled that of our own era. Although the drugs and other substances used during this period were far less effective than the synthetic hormones that have been in use since the 1960s, the cast of characters, consisting of athletes, coaches, sports officials, physicians, and pharmaceutical companies, is familiar enough. In Germany, for example, the use of drugs by athletes seems to have been widespread and widely known.[34] In 1924, a German doctor noted that he had seen cocaine used at many sports events, and a rumor mill about the efficacy of various drugs flourished in athletic circles.[35]

The idea that the doping behaviors of this era violated the ideals of sportsmanship emerged during the 1920s and 1930s, along with the commercialization of sport and its increasing importance as a mass culture. A revealing critique of contemporary doping practices appears in a lecture delivered at the annual meeting of the German Swimming Association in 1933 by Prof. Dr. Otto Riesser, director of the Pharmacological Institute of the University of Breslau:

> The use of artificial means [to improve performance] has long been considered wholly incompatible with the spirit of sport and has therefore been condemned. Nevertheless, we all know that this rule is continually being broken, and that sportive competitions are often more a matter of doping than of training. It is highly regrettable that those who are in charge of supervising sport seem to lack the energy for the campaign against this evil, and that a lax, and fateful, attitude is spreading. Nor are the physicians without blame for this state of affairs, in part on account of their ignorance, and in part because they are prescribing strong drugs for the purpose of doping which are not available to athletes without prescriptions.[36]

The European doping culture of the 1930s was described by the Danish physiologist Ove Bøje in 1939: "There can be no doubt that stimulants are to-day widely used by athletes participating in competitions; the record-breaking craze and the desire to satisfy an exacting public play a more and more prominent rôle, and take higher rank than the health of the competitors itself." The various substances in use included carbohydrates, glucose, lecithin, calcium, alkalis, ammonium chloride, oxygen, ultraviolet radiation, alcohol, ether, cocaine, caffeine, cola nuts, Benzedrine, digitalis, nitroglycerine, coramine, and gland extracts. Phosphates, in particular, were "in great demand in athletic circles, particularly in Germany, owing to intensive advertising of their beneficial properties."[37] This reference to commercial propaganda points to the (largely neglected) role of the pharmaceutical industry in the doping systems that have developed over the past century. The account cited here suggests that many athletes were receptive to this kind of advertising.

Those who would persuade elite athletes not to use drugs need to understand why the functional view of doping as a coping strategy has been so influential over the past century. Ethical objections, such as the idea that doping is a violation of "the spirit of sport," did not exist at the beginning of the high-performance era, because the entire athletic enterprise was regarded as an exploration of human limits and what could be done to extend them. At a time when scientists were formulating the first physiological explanations of fatigue, the idea of using drugs to combat fatigue seemed like a perfectly natural strategy, because the primary competition was between human beings and their fatigue symptoms. It is, in fact, difficult to determine exactly where and when the idea that doping violates the norms of honorable competition came into existence. Nationalist feeling was one medium in which early antidoping sentiment could grow; as early as 1910, for example, a German scientist accused American athletes of doping themselves with secret concoctions that were not available to athletes of other nationalities.[38] In this case, it is unclear whether the act of doping or the alleged monopoly of a secret formula was more offensive to this German critic of American practices.

The psychological needs of elite athletes have also played a role in legitimizing drug use in the eyes of many athletes and their handlers. During the 1950s, a prominent British commentator on athletes and doping in Britain was Sir Adolphe Abrahams, an Honorary Medical Officer to the International Athletics Board and the British Olympic team. "A trained athlete," he wrote in 1957, "is highly suggestible. He is willing, indeed anxious, to entrust himself to anybody in whom he has confidence, and he will be firmly persuaded that a physical improvement has resulted from the ingestion of anything if the right personality is behind the administration."[39] Like the commentators of the 1920s and 1930s, Abrahams reported "a persistent belief among athletes that there must be something that would create energy or postpone fatigue."[40]

But how should one treat this athlete-patient? The problem for the doctor, Abrahams pointed out, was that "it is not easy . . . to draw the line where legitimate stimulation ends and reprehensible 'doping' begins; the distinction is largely a matter of opinion and of conscience."[41] When the British Association of Sport and Medicine attempted to define doping in 1953, it found itself unable to do so. "A satisfactory definition of 'a drug' in this particular connexion could not be framed, because a comprehensive prohibition was clearly ridiculous. We should have to withhold medicaments that sharpen the appetite, improve digestion, and generally contribute to physical well-being."[42] In the absence of an official definition of what doping was, both athletes and physicians could rationalize the use of various substances to ward off anxiety or fatigue before or during athletic competitions.

We must also recognize that, from a physician's standpoint, objections to "reprehensible 'doping'" in the pre-steroid 1950s focused more on its medical dangers than on the idea that it was a form of cheating. Abrahams wanted to forbid, on medical grounds, any drug that "could stimulate the body to exertion beyond its normal limits of fatigue."[43] His disdain was reserved for any physician who was unwilling to heed this cautionary rule and for overcredulous persons who believed that drugs boosted athletic performance. What he did not do was denounce athletes who doped as moral reprobates. Convinced that they were "highly suggestible" personalities, he was more inclined to see them as the victims of their own foolish ideas about drugs.

Medical attitudes toward doping during the pre-steroid era were also evident in 1957, when the elite milers of that era were accused of having used amphetamine to break the fabled four-minute barrier.[44] The runners dismissed the charge by employing the language of sportsmanship: "Track and field is an amateur sport—a clean sport" (Irish runner Ron Delany); "All the coaches and athletes I know have too much integrity to use drugs" (American Don Bowden).[45] The New York chapter of the American Medical Association took a different approach by denouncing the use of amphetamines as a "vicious practice" on public health grounds. Its statement declared that "the indiscriminate use of such substances is far from harmless in that it may result in effort completely out of proportion to the ability of some athletes, may produce temporary personality changes productive of antisocial behavior, and may produce serious and lasting changes in physical and mental well-being."[46]

The difference between the 1950s and today is that medical assessments of doping at that time were less affected by moral condemnation of athletes who used drugs. Before they were stigmatized as doping drugs during the 1980s, anabolic steroids enjoyed a generally benign reputation that had facilitated their use in medicine since the late 1930s. As late as 1960, testosterone and a new anabolic steroid were being tested as growth stimulants for infants and children.[47] Today, by contrast, media reporting of medical opinion regarding the dangers of anabolic steroids is heavily colored by the climate of moral disapproval that has engulfed these drugs over the past two decades.[48] The current absorption of the antidoping campaign into the federally sponsored "war on drugs" begun by President Nixon in 1969 represents a further step away from the public health approach. Today's campaign against doping combines health warnings with a moral absolutism that condemns doping in sport as a serious, even disgraceful, ethical failure on the part of athletes, who are expected to exercise an appropriate degree of self-restraint.

The functional view of doping was also promoted during the 1950s by a sharp distinction between amateur and professional athletes that has become largely irrelevant in today's elite sports world. While traditional class distinctions still defined the gentleman amateur as the more prestigious (and drug-free) athletic type, the professional athlete of this era was widely seen as inhabiting a different moral universe in which the use of doping drugs was tolerated or even expected. This segregation of athletes by ethical category was openly acknowledged in 1960 by a then-recent president of the American College of Sports Medicine. While this physician used words such as "perversion" and "malignancy" to condemn the use of drugs by amateurs, he calmly viewed the doping of professionals as an inescapable fact of life: "The professional athlete has a job to do which may be his sole livelihood; under such conditions it is an accepted fact that he may employ any means which will permit him to achieve his best possible physical performance."[49] Facing the prospect of unemployment if he fails, the athlete-worker does not feel that he has the moral luxury of adopting "pharmacological Calvinism" as a way of life.

The abolition of Olympic amateurism in 1981 promoted doping by expanding the population of athlete-workers whose performances were now tied to financial incentives. In the 1990s, the International Olympic Committee (IOC) further complicated doping control by pursuing wealthy professional athletes, such as National Basketball Association stars, whose contracts shielded them from drug testing. In 1996, the head of the IOC Medical Commission, Prince Alexandre de Merode, openly acknowledged that doping was inherent in professional sport. Doping penalties, he said, were "excessive" in an era of Olympic professionalism: "Strict sanctions were appropriate when we were dealing with top amateurs, but because sport has become a profession, we are faced with a major social problem. These sanctions have deep repercussions on people and their standard of living."[50] The same right-to-work argument underlay the initial refusal of the UCI to accept WADA's mandatory two-year ban for doping offenses. In the view of the UCI, "a two-year ban is too harsh if, for example, it puts a de facto end to an athlete's career. The UCI's view is that all humans make mistakes and that even one who commits a serious offence such as an antidoping violation must have the opportunity to repent and to be reinstated at a time when he has a chance to compete at a comparable level. The UCI thinks that this is part of civilisation, or at least of the tradition in 'old' Europe." The cultural divide alluded to here appears elsewhere in this document when the authors point out that the World Anti-Doping Code might have "been written in another tradition and language than those of North America."[51] According to this European federation, the fundamental clash between North American moral severity and European compassion for the repentant sinner underlay the split between WADA and the UCI. While it is difficult to take UCI rhetoric at face value, there is a distinction to be made between moral condemnation and the sociological interpretation of doping described at the beginning of this chapter. Let us now take a closer look at how the sociology of doping is influenced by the political world in which it operates.

## Sportive Nationalism and Doping

Both democratic and authoritarian governments exert political pressure on athletes that drives doping practices. The comprehensive athletic doping program of the former East Germany was exceptional in its scope, secrecy, and scientific ambition.[52] A similar doping program existed in the Soviet Union.[53] Both operated under the protection of the secret police establishments of these dictatorships and were coercive in nature.

Performance demands imposed on elite athletes by democratic governments are more interesting in that they require politicians to explain to the public why democratic societies need internationally competitive athletes. In Germany, for example, Chancellor Helmut Kohl declared in 1996 that the country's victorious soccer team set a positive example for the country's malingering workforce.[54] In May 1997, President Roman Herzog called Germany's elite athletes an antidote to "pessimism" and to "a paralysis in our society." "Sport," he proclaimed, "is dynamism. We are optimists."[55] Twenty years earlier, the conservative Bundestag deputy Wolfgang Schäuble had called for the "limited use" of steroids "and only under the complete control of the sports physicians because it is clear that there are [sports] disciplines in which the use of these drugs is necessary to remain competitive at the international level."[56] Fifteen years later, Schäuble was Germany's interior minister and still defending the importance of sportive nationalism as a self-evident requirement of national vitality.[57] In September 2003, a Social Democratic member of the Bundestag responded to Germany's dismal showing at the World Track and Field Championships in Paris by calling for a return to the old East German sports system.[58] In 2007, after two decades of discussion, the Bundestag finally passed an antidoping law that criminalizes drug trafficking but not athletes who dope.[59]

The "national vitality" argument also plays well in other democratic societies.

In 1995, a British government policy statement, endorsing an initiative of Conservative Prime Minister John Major, declared that "the government has greatly increased the importance of competitive sport."[60] In 1999, Labour Prime Minister Tony Blair was promoting a "play-to-win culture" and the importance of sporting victories for boosting British morale.[61] This sort of nationalist cheerleading is an implicit invitation to promote or tolerate doping practices. President Jacques Chirac made a point of appearing with the victorious French national soccer team despite the fact that 90 percent of the French public believed their heroes practiced doping.[62] The Australian Institute for Sport, which is now charged with producing both elite athletes and credible antidoping research, had its own doping scandal in 1989.[63]

Conflicts between doping control and political interests have become commonplace. In 2001, Australian Prime Minister John Howard was indignantly rejecting suspicions directed at his nation's athletes, despite a steroid scandal involving a prominent coach.[64] In 2002, the Russian Duma voted 417 to 3 to protest the "American conspiracy" that had led to the exclusion of three doping-compromised Russian cross-country skiers from the Salt Lake City Winter Olympics.[65] In February 2004, the Greek sports minister, Giorgio Lianos, was defending the reputations of Greece's male and female champion sprinters, Kostas Kenteris and Ekaterina Thanou, who were widely suspected of doping.[66] In 2002, the Spanish Track and Field Federation was selling its coaches a sophisticated doping manual on the use of anabolic steroids and HGH.[67] Prime Minister Silvio Berlusconi has openly sabotaged antidoping efforts in Italy. In 2001, he denounced the 1998 closing of a corrupt antidoping laboratory in Rome as "a plot by the political left" and appointed as his sports minister the disgraced national Olympic committee official Mario Pescante, who is still a member of the IOC and was then financing the corrupt blood doping doctor Francesco Conconi, who happened to be a longtime cycling companion of Romano Prodi, then European Commission president.[68]

## Doping as a System: The Athlete-Worker

The political exploitation of sportive nationalism can coexist with state prosecutions of doping offenses. This has been most evident in Italy, where, despite Prime Minister Berlusconi's obstructionism, state prosecutors have issued indictments, obtained convictions, and conducted investigations of systematic doping in professional cycling and soccer. Raffaele Guariniello, a state prosecutor in Turin who specializes in occupational diseases, has brought athletes, doctors, coaches, and federation officials into his courtroom in the Palace of Justice to conduct what amounts to epidemiological research into the morbidity and mortality rates of professional athletes. He is also concerned that the conduct of these celebrities affects public health by influencing how children regard the use of doping products.[69]

The public health approach to doping behavior differs fundamentally from the test-and-punish model with which it coexists in Italy. The hygienic paternalism of the state prosecutor aims first at promoting health and then at condemning the "sports fraud" that violates Italian law, while the moral paternalism of the sports officials first aims at punishing the guilty and only then invokes health risks as a justification for doping sanctions. "My purpose," Guariniello said in 2001, "is not to drag the greatest number of people into court, but rather to eliminate the offense . . . The trial itself can produce the desired result. I never focus on the condemnation of the accused. The point is that the crime not be committed again."[70] While the public health approach downplays the criminal aspect of doping behaviors, the punitive approach aims at associating doping behaviors with both cheating and the fear and loathing inspired by drug addiction and moral degeneracy.

The most striking aspect of the public health approach is that it treats the athlete not as a celebrity who is empowered by fame, but as a dependent and an employee who is vulnerable to manipulation by economic forces that are beyond his or her control. "There is no difference between a Fiat worker and a player for [soccer team] Juventus," Guariniello argued. "Both have the same employer, but they are paid differently. We must try to protect the health of all employees in an equitable manner, regardless of how much they take home at the end of the month." This prosecutor has found that few of the many professional athletes appearing before him "demonstrate any awareness of the [medical] dangers involved."[71] In the last analysis, he sees doping among the professionals he has surveyed as a result of economic compulsion: "I want to find out if employees of the [soccer] clubs were forced to take drugs against their will in order to keep their jobs."[72]

Equating a sports star with an ordinary worker in this way deflates the athlete's charismatic (and thus commercial) appeal. The sports entertainment industry is, after all, built on satisfying the emotional needs of people whose fantasies about celebrity athletes are based on the idea that they enjoy privileges denied to ordinary people. The elite athlete thus offers an escape from the quotidian by being a special kind of human being. Far better that he be flawed and extraordinary than virtuous and ordinary. The doping sinner who is caught, sanctioned, and forgiven, even perhaps on repeated occasions, is much better tabloid material than the average athlete who never tests positive at all. Hunted down by the doping police, the doper retains his stature as a rebel and as an outlaw who can intrigue a large segment of the sporting public, which is likely to be more tolerant of doping offenses than is commonly assumed. Transforming this romantic figure into a worker whose principal right is to protection under the occupational health and safety laws subverts his heroic stature. For this reason, it is to the advantage of the sports federations to preserve the image of the athlete as someone who is just the opposite of a vulnerable employee who needs the legal system to protect him. On the contrary, he is presented as the master of his own fate and thus wholly responsible for whatever doping he chooses to do.

The illusion of the free and autonomous athlete who bears absolute responsibility for his or her own doping practices displaces the sociological interpretation of doping that offers more realistic explanations of why so many athletes engage in these behaviors in the first place. As noted earlier, those who reject the sociological analysis of doping confront the unhappy task of explaining why so many ostensibly immoral athletes have infiltrated the world of elite sport and have been practicing doping there for so long. The estimates of doping among elite athletes offered by informed observers over many years simply rule out the idea that doping is eccentric behavior among elite athletes.[73] Anyone seeking official confirmation of this conclusion is referred to the chapter "Extent of Use of Banned Substances" in the Dubin Report published in 1990, following the Canadian government's investigation of the Ben Johnson doping scandal.[74]

The idea that doping results from the actions and attitudes of multiple interest groups in the world of elite sport has had a long and unsuccessful public career. We have already considered reports of widespread use of drugs by athletes from the 1920s and 1930s. By the 1960s, the doping issue had taken on a new urgency that has been intensifying ever since. "The use of drugs—legal drugs—by athletes is far from new," *Sports Illustrated* reported in a cover story in 1969, "but the increase in drug usage in the last 10 years is startling. It could, indeed, menace the tradition and structure of sport itself." This comprehensive and prophetic document emphasizes that athletes are not the only protagonists in this drama, because "it is a scandal that involves the medical Establishment as well as the sporting one." It also points out the intimate relationship between elite athletes and drugs, noting that "modern athletes know a lot about drugs, or at least have a lot of opinions about them, and are willing to experiment with drugs about which no one knows very much. There are probably as many cases of athletes demanding drugs from trainers and physicians as physicians and trainers ordering athletes to take them."[75] Four decades later, the leading Italian antidoping activist, the track-and-field coach and Olympic official Sandro Donati, described these relationships somewhat differently. It was in 1984, he said, that he realized "there are no inherently honest or dishonest athletes, but rather the honest and dishonest coaches, honest and dishonest federation leaders, and honest and dishonest doctors who steer athletes in one direction or another."[76] This view was later endorsed by the Russian antidoping official Nikolai Durmanow. The decision to use performance-enhancing drugs, he said in December 2003, is not a voluntary decision undertaken by a petty criminal mentality, but rather the result of the pressures inherent in an athlete's social situation. The nonathlete counterparts of these people are the unemployed chemists whose economic desperation prompts them to offer themselves as doping experts to athletes who share their economic predicament. Russia, he said, "could pose the same sort of doping threat to Europe as Colombia does to the United States with its cocaine."[77] Such accounts present, in abbreviated form, the "sociological" perspective that sports officials have suppressed over many years out of bureaucratic self-interest.

Official knowledge of the systemic doping practices of American athletes was evident in 1986 when Dr. Don Catlin, chair of the U.S. Olympic Committee's Committee on Substance Abuse, Research, and Education, predicted the consequences of drug-testing certain groups of elite athletes. "If you go in with a sickle and scythe, you could put all their athletes out of business. In some sports, you could wipe out the whole team."[78] His recommendations were for advance notice of drug testing programs and the "education" of American athletes. Both of these proposals have been contradicted by subsequent developments. Unannounced testing is now universally recognized as the only effective form of doping control, while the whole idea of "educating" elite athletes out of their doping practices remains a utopian fantasy. Its political function is to create the illusion that reforming the elite athlete population is the key to creating "drug-free" sport, while Olympic committees, sports federations, and media companies remain free to conduct business as usual, all the while assuring the public that something is being done about "drugs." This kind of damage control serves a variety of economic interests and the ideology of the "war on drugs," while perpetuating the test-and-punish routine that one American athlete dismissed as a futile game of "cops and robbers" as far back as 1968.[79]

# Conclusion

In this chapter I have attempted to situate doping in its modern historical and cultural contexts. The principal lessons of this historical excursion are twofold. The first is that modern doping scandals have been profoundly oversimplified and misunderstood as being reducible to ethical lapses committed by autonomous individuals. This skewed perspective has allowed the institutions that benefit from elite athletic performances to arraign and punish athletes as the solitary villains of the piece, thereby evading public scrutiny of their own acts of omission and commission that have encouraged and even required doping practices of their athletes. (The involvement of the U.S. Olympic Committee with two major blood doping scandals during the 1980s offers a well-documented case in point.)[80] The second conclusion to be drawn from this narrative is that the very idea of "drug-free" sport at the elite level is a fraudulent construct. This unreal notion owes its currency to the selectively prohibitionist attitude toward "drugs" that has long been supported by the U.S. government. The "drug-free" ideal disregards both the documented behavior of countless elite athletes over the past half-century and the longtime policies of sports committees and federations bent on providing the best possible "medical support" to their athletes. The pro-doping lobby within the ranks of sports physicians has long been a matter of record.[81] By now it should be obvious that "drug-free" sport is an ideological construct that is incompatible with the demands of modern high-performance sport. Its continued use by the same sports officials who quietly tolerate the practices of the more aggressive forms of high-performance sports medicine is a rhetorical obfuscation rather than an expression of genuine idealism.

Confronting the implications of the analysis presented in this chapter will not be easy for any of the parties who have vested interests in the sports entertainment industry. This includes the doping-control agencies, such as WADA and the U.S. Anti-Doping Agency, which over the past decade have finally begun to establish a credible doping-control regime after decades of failure and neglect in this area. I would add that confronting the implications of evolving public attitudes toward the medically supervised doping of elite athletes is an important issue not addressed here. Finally, I suggest that antidoping officials think about what may be the most fundamental lesson to be learned from the 1998 Tour de France doping scandal. Professional cycling's culture of lying developed primarily because cycling officials and journalists made a point of concealing both the physiological and psychological costs of this ordeal and the nature of the "medical support" that has made it possible to keep the show on the road.[82] The problem for sports officials is that medical and scientific candor about the origins and consequences of some elite performances will compel them to acknowledge (1) the unattractive medical costs of many athletic careers and (2) the political and commercial pressures that have persuaded them to make demands on athletes that the unaltered human organism cannot meet.

## NOTES

1. See, for example, S. B. Nuland, "Medicine Isn't Just for the Sick Anymore," *New York Times*, May 10, 1998.

2. For a critique of the traditional arguments against doping, written by an academic physician and medical ethicist, see N. Fost, "Steroids Are Only Fair," *Newsday*, February 29, 2004; see also D. Walker, "Wisconsin Pediatrician-Ethicist Says Don't Ban Steroids," *Milwaukee Journal-Sentinel*, January 24, 2004.

3. "Review of *Drug Addiction*, by E. W. Adams," *Lancet*, September 11, 1937, 634.

4. M. Janofsky, "President of I.O.C. Condemns Drug Use," *New York Times*, September 13, 1988; "Doping ist wie der Tod," *Süddeutsche Zeitung*, September 13, 1988; "Doping als Übel aller Übel," *Süddeutsche Zeitung*, January 8, 1986. On Samaranch's antidoping rhetoric, see J. Hoberman, "How Drug Testing Fails: The Politics of Doping Control," in *Doping in Elite Sport: The Politics of Drugs in the Olympic Movement*, ed. W. Wilson and E. Derse (Champaign, IL: Human Kinetics, 2001), 242–43.

5. The International Track-and-Field Federation keeps on its books, for example, a 400-meter world record set in 1985 by Marita Koch, of East Germany, whose documented steroid consumption amounted to 2710 milligrams over the period 1982–84. Her world record in 1985 (47.6 seconds) has not been approached in almost 25 years. See B. Berendonk, *Doping: Von der Forschung zum Betrug* (Reinbek bei Hamburg: Rowohlt, 1992), 150.

6. The same point can be made regarding androgenic hormone levels. For example, all three medalists in the shot put at the 1992 Barcelona Olympic Games had already served bans for either anabolic steroids or an elevated testosterone level when they were honored for their Olympic achievements.

7. K.-H. Bette, "Biographical Risks and Doping," in *Doping and Public Policy*, ed. J. Hoberman and V. Møller, 101–12 (Odense: University of Southern Denmark Press, 2005).

8. Quoted in "Das Digel-Konzept," *Süddeutsche Zeitung*, January 26, 1998.

9. R. Davenport-Hines, *The Pursuit of Oblivion: A Global History of Narcotics* (New York: W. W. Norton, 2002), 421.

10. Ibid., 12.

11. According to one report, the doctors attending the Tour de France riders in 2001 were allowed by the UCI to administer as many as 300 drugs and other substances without publishing the list. See "Tour-medicinmænd," *Information* (Copenhagen), June 22, 2001.

12. Associated Press, "French Children Regard Doping as Normal," March 24, 2004.

13. See, for example, "Energy in Pills," *Business Week*, January 15, 1944, 40–41; "Benzedrine Alerts," *Time*, February 21, 1944, 75; B. Knickerbocker, "Military Looks to Drugs for Battle Readiness," *Christian Science Monitor*, August 25, 2002.

14. D. Black, "Medicalised Erections on Demand?" *Journal of Medical Ethics* 25 (1999): 6.

15. An early (1997) and critical commentary on the new "antiaging" therapies argues that "several recent trends in androgen use are alarming. Because a substantial portion of the androgen market is underground, exact estimates of androgen use in the United States are not available. However, audits of direct and indirect sales indicate that the androgen sales in this country are growing 20–30 percent each year. There is reason to believe that a substantial part of the overall androgen market involves the illicit use of testosterone for unapproved indications, particularly for muscle building by athletes and recreational body builders . . . It is distressing that a significant proportion of hypogonadal men continue to be undiagnosed, diagnosed late, or inappropriately treated. Thus a paradoxical situation has developed in which testosterone replacement therapy continues to be underused or inappropriately used for legitimate indications, while its use for unapproved indications continues to expand." S. Bhasin and W. J. Bremer, "Emerging Issues in Androgen Replacement Therapy," *Journal of Clinical Endocrinology and Metabolism* 82 (1997): 3. The publication of an article on HGH therapy in the *New England Journal of Medicine* in 1990 "incited a proliferation of 'antiaging' clinics and lay publications, such as 'Grow Young with HGH,' extolling the benefits of growth hormone in reversing or preventing aging." Also: "It is not known precisely how much growth hormone is prescribed for 'off label' uses, but estimates suggest that one third of prescriptions for growth hormone in the United States are for indications for which it is not approved by the Food and Drug Administration." M. L. Vance, "Can Growth Hormone Prevent Aging?" *New England Journal of Medicine* 348 (2003): 779, 780.

16. See, for example, C. Møldrup, *Den medicinerede normalitet* (Copenhagen: Gyldendal, 1999).

17. See B. Briggs, "Swifter, Higher, Stronger, Dirtier?" *Denver Post*, November 16, 2003; J. Longman and M. Connelly, "Americans Suspect Steroid Use in Sports Is Common, Poll Finds," *New York Times*, December 16, 2003. For additional commentary on the American public's indifference to doping by professional baseball players, see T. Verducci, "Totally Juiced," *Sports Illustrated*, June 3, 2002, 48.

18. C. L. Hays, "From out of the Gym, into the Grocery Store," *New York Times*, November 22, 1997.

19. D. Barboza, "More Hip, Higher Hop," *New York Times*, August 22, 1997.

20. S. Romero, "Industry and Nature Meet along the Amazon," *New York Times*, June 17, 2000.

21. G. Thompson, "Bushmen Squeeze Money from a Humble Cactus," *New York Times*, April 1, 2003.

22. "Sold here [Japan] under the brand name Vaam, the concoction contains a synthetic version of the juice that gives Japan's giant hornets the strength to fly distances of about 60 miles a day at speeds of almost 25 miles an hour." S. Strom, "What's Faster Than a Speeding Hornet?" *New York Times*, January 3, 2001.

23. G. Harris, "Despite Missteps, Lilly Remains a Hard Stock to Bet Against," *New York Times*, February 25, 2004.

24. E. Olson, "Beyond Delicious, Chocolate May Help Pump up Your Heart," *New York Times*, February 17, 2004.

25. S. S. Hall, "Our Memories, Our Selves," *New York Times Magazine*, February 15, 1998, 26–33, 49–57; B. Meier, "Industry's Next Growth Sector: Memory Lapses," *New York Times*, April 4, 1999; "Viagra fürs Gehirn," *Der Spiegel*, April 28, 2003, 150–54.

26. J. Groopman, "Eyes Wide Open," *New Yorker*, December 3, 2001, 52.

27. A. Pollack, "Putting a Price on a Good Night's Sleep," *New York Times*, January 13, 2004.

28. D. Grady, "Study Tests Safety of a Hormone Nasal Spray to Curb Hunger," *New York Times*, November 13, 2003.

29. M. Navarro, "Arrest Startles Saleswomen of Sex Toys," *New York Times*, January 20, 2004.

30. K. Hafner, "On Video Games, the Jury Is out and Confused," *New York Times*, June 5, 2003. See also S. Blakeslee, "Video-Game Killing Builds Visual Skills, Researchers Report," *New York Times*, May 29, 2003.

31. E. Parens, "Is Better Always Good? The Enhancement Project," in *Enhancing Human Traits: Ethical and Social Implications*, ed. E. Parens (Washington, DC: Georgetown University Press, 1993), 12.

32. A. Krüger, "Die Paradoxien des Dopings—ein Überblick," in *Doping: Spitzensport als gesellschaftliches Problem*, ed. M. Gamper, J. Mühlethaler, and F. Reidhaar (Zurich: NZZ Verlag, 2000), 14. Here is a more detailed account of this early doping scene: "Lasting from Monday morning to Saturday evening, these races placed extreme physical and psychological demands on the riders; consequently many of them turned to various stimulant preparations. The French used a mixture known as 'Caffeine Houdes,' while the Belgians sucked on sugar cubes dipped in ether. The riders' black coffee was 'boosted' with extra caffeine and peppermint, and as the race progressed the mixture was spiked with increasing doses of cocaine and strychnine. Brandy was also frequently added to cups of tea. Following the sprint sequences of the race, nitroglycerine capsules were often given to the cyclists to ease breathing difficulties. The individual 6-day races were eventually replaced by two-man races, but the doping continued unabated. Since drugs such as heroin or cocaine were widely taken in these tournaments without supervision, it was perhaps likely that fatalities would occur." T. Donohoe and N. Johnson, *Foul Play: Drug Abuse in Sports* (Oxford: Basil Blackwell, 1986), 2.

33. See J. Hoberman, "A Pharmacy on Wheels: Doping and Community Cohesion among Professional Cyclists following the Tour de France Scandal of 1998," in *The Essence of Sport*, ed. V. Møller and J. Nauright, 107–27 (Odense: University of Southern Denmark Press, 2002).

34. J. Hoberman, *Mortal Engines: The Science of Performance and the Dehumanization of Sport* (New York: Free Press, 1992), 134, 144.

35. Ibid., 136.

36. O. Riesser, "Über Doping und Dopingmittel," *Leibesübungen und körperliche Erziehung*, 1933, 393–94.

37. O. Bøje, "Doping: A Study of the Means Employed to Raise the Level of Performance in Sport," *Bulletin of the Health Organization of the League of Nations* 8 (1939): 439, 446.

38. Hoberman, *Mortal Engines*, 140.

39. A. Abrahams, "Should Athletes Take 'Pep' Drugs?" *Sunday Times*, June 16, 1957.

40. "Athletic Training," *JAMA* 157 (1955): 1430. This text offers a paraphrase of Abrahams's remarks in a lecture given in England in April 1955.

41. Abrahams, "Should Athlete's Take 'Pep' Drugs?"

42. Adolphe Abrahams, " 'Doping' of Athletes" (letter to the editor), *Times* (London), July 10, 1953.

43. "Athletic Training," *JAMA* 157:1430.

44. "A.M.A. to Study Drugs in Sports; Use in Four-Minute Mile Hinted," *New York Times*, June 6, 1957.

45. Both quoted in "Athletes Deny Use of Drugs," *Times* (London), June 7, 1957.

46. "Resolution on Use of Stimulants, Such as Amphetamine, in Sports," *Journal of the American Medical Association* 164 (1957): 1244.

47. "Use of Testosterone in Undeveloped Children," *JAMA* 173 (1960): 1157; "Use of Anabolic Hormones as Growth Stimulants," *Nutrition Reviews* 19 (January 1961): 2–4. The *JAMA* article ends as follows: "Improved development was seen in both girls and boys, and the results were encouraging."

48. I. Waddington pointed out that "it is important to recognize how public attitudes and anxieties towards the use of controlled drugs in society generally have 'spilled over' into the sports arena and have influenced anti-doping policies in sport." I. Waddington, *Sport, Health and Drugs: A Critical Sociological Perspective* (London: E. & F. N. Spon, 2000), 112.

49. Albert Salisbury Hyman, "Use of Drugs in Sports" (letter to the editor), *New York Times*, September 12, 1960.

50. Quoted in "We're Too Hard on Drug Cheats: Olympic Boss," *Weekend Australian*, December 21–22, 1996.

51. Statement from the Union Cycliste International, March 3, 2003, www.uci.ch/english/news/news_2002/20030303_ad_01.htm.

52. See Berendonk, *Doping: Von der Forschung zum Betrug*; G. Spitzer, *Doping in der DDR: Ein historischer Überblick zu einer konspirativen Praxis* (Cologne: Sport und Buch, 2000); W. W. Franke and B. Berendonk, "Hormonal Doping and Androgenization of Athletes: A Secret Program of the German Democratic Republic Government," *Clinical Chemistry* 43 (1997): 1262–79.

53. "Belege für Sowjet-Doping," *Süddeutsche Zeitung*, September 3, 2003.

54. "Experten für schwierige Lebenslagen," *Süddeutsche Zeitung*, July 2, 1996.

55. Quoted in "Langfristig Bindung gesucht," *Süddeutsche Zeitung*, May 27, 1997.

56. Quoted in Berendonk, *Doping: Von der Forschung zum Betrug*, 45.

57. On German sportive nationalism and doping, see Hoberman, "How Drug Testing Fails," 260–62.

58. "Loblied auf DDR-Sport," *Süddeutsche Zeitung*, September 13/14, 2003; T. Kistner, "Vorwärts in die Vergangenheit," *Süddeutsche Zeitung*, September 13/14, 2003.

59. On the politics of doping in Germany, see Hoberman, *Mortal Engines*, 237–52.

60. Quoted in Waddington, *Sport, Health and Drugs*, 40.

61. "Blair fördert 'Killer instinct,'" *Süddeutsche Zeitung*, June 22, 1999.

62. Krüger, "Die Paradoxien des Dopings—ein Überblick," 28.

63. See "Athlete's Urine Sample Poured down Sink," *Sydney Morning Herald*, June 15, 1989; "No Medal for Truth," *Sydney Morning Herald*, January 14, 1989; "Coach's Drug Denial," *Sydney Morning Herald*, December 14, 1988; "AIS Head Knew of Drug Use: Martin," *Sydney Morning Herald*, December 8, 1988.

64. "Australia's Swimming in Scandal," *Guardian* (Manchester), April 16, 2001.

65. "Dopingrepublik Russland," *Süddeutsche Zeitung*, December 27/28, 2003.

66. See, for example, "Pfiffe des Zweifels," *Süddeutsche Zeitung*, August 12, 2002; "Der undurchsichtige Adonis," *Der Spiegel*, August 11, 2003; "Eine E-Mail für 90 Millionen Euro," *Süddeutsche Zeitung*, February 18, 2004.

67. See A. Singler, "Betrug nach Lehrbuch," *Süddeutsche Zeitung*, March 6, 2002.

68. See "Der Vorkämpfer," *Der Spiegel*, March 4, 2002; "Liebesgrüße aus dem Heizungskeller," *Süddeutsche Zeitung*, October 19, 1998; "Klagen über gesellschaftsschädigende Kontrollen," *Süddeutsche Zeitung*, April 24, 2001; "Moralisch schuldig," *Süddeutsche Zeitung*, March 12, 2004.

69. "Dafür sorgen, daß Doping geächtet wird," *Süddeutsche Zeitung*, May 5, 1999.

70. Quoted in "Der leise Herr aus der Abteilung Desaster," *Süddeutsche Zeitung*, November 14, 2001.

71. Ibid.

72. Quoted in "Eine Doppelspitze gegen den Werteverfall," *Süddeutsche Zeitung*, December 19/20, 1998.

73. For example, at the 1968 Mexico City Olympic Games, Dr. Tom Waddell, an American decathlete who finished in sixth place in his event, "estimated a third of the men on the U.S. track-and-field team were using anabolic steroids at the pre-Olympic training camp held at Lake Tahoe." In 1969, Dr. H. Kay Dooley, a physician for the U.S. Olympic Committee, stated: "I don't think it's possible for a man to compete internationally without using anabolic steroids. All the weight men on the Olympic team had to take steroids. Otherwise they would not have been in the running." In 1972, the American discus-thrower Jay Silvester carried out an informal survey of male track-and-field athletes at the Munich Olympic Games and found that 68 percent had used anabolic steroids in the course of training. In November 1988, the *New York Times* reported that "at least half of the 9000 athletes who competed at the Olympics in Seoul used performance-enhancing drugs in training, according to estimates by medical and legal experts as well as traffickers in these drugs. These experts also contend that the drug testing programs of the IOC and other sports associations have had no impact in reducing the use of such drugs." In July 1996, the British physician Michael Turner told the BBC that at least 75 percent of the track-and-field athletes competing at the Atlanta Olympic Games "will have taken some kind of performance-enhancing drug." J. Todd and T. Todd, "Significant Events in the History of Drug Testing and the Olympic Movement, 1960–1999," in *Doping in Elite Sport: The Politics of Drugs in the Olympic Movement*, ed. W. Wilson and E. Derse (Champaign, IL: Human Kinetics, 2001), 69, 69, 71, 91, 103.

74. Canadian Government, *Commission of Inquiry into the Use of Drugs and Banned Practices Intended to Increase Athletic Performance* (Ottawa: Canadian Government Publishing Centre, 1990), 335–54.

75. B. Gilbert, "Problems in a Turned-on World," *Sports Illustrated*, June 23, 1969; B. Gilbert, "Something Extra on the Ball," *Sports Illustrated*, June 30, 1969.

76. Quoted in "Doping—ein kollektiver Wahnsinn," *Neue Zürcher Zeitun*, March 25, 2000.

77. Quoted in "Der Sport hat verloren," *Süddeutsche Zeitung*, December 27/28, 2003; "Dopingrepublik Russland," *Süddeutsche Zeitung*, December 27/28, 2003.

78. Quoted in Virginia Cowart, "State-of-Art Drug Identification Laboratories Play Increasing Role in Major Athletic Events," *JAMA* 256 (1986): 3069.

79. Todd and Todd, "Significant Events in the History of Drug Testing," 69.

80. On the 1984 blood doping scandal involving seven American athletes at the Los Angeles Olympic Games, see B. Rostaing and R. Sullivan, "Triumphs Tainted with Blood," *Sports Illustrated*, January 21, 1985; R. Ben Cramer, "Olympic Cheating: The Inside Story of Illicit Doping and the U.S. Cycling Team," *Rolling Stone*, February 14, 1985; H. G. Klein, "Blood Transfusions and Athletics," *New England Journal of Medicine* 312 (1985): 854–56. On the 1987 blood doping scandal involving the Nordic skier Kerry Lynch and the future U.S. Olympic Committee executive Jim Page, see P. Hersh, "U.S. Nordic Medalist Admits to Blood Packing," *Chicago Tribune*, December 29, 1987; "Ban Is Almost Certain for U.S. Skier Lynch," *Chicago Tribune*, January 13, 1988; "Olympic Ban Likely for U.S. Skier Lynch," *Chicago Tribune*, January 13, 1988; "Skier Lynch Voted out of Games," *Chicago Tribune*, January 20, 1988; "U.S. Skier Suspended for Two Years," *Chicago Tribune*, June 9, 1988. This incident was mentioned briefly many years later in a mass-circulation sports magazine in the United States. "The Inside Dope," *Sports Illustrated*, October 4, 1999.

81. J. Hoberman, "Sports Physicians and the Doping Crisis in Elite Sport," *Clinical Journal of Sport Medicine* 12 (2002): 203–8.

82. See Hoberman, "'Pharmacy on Wheels.'"

# CHAPTER TWO

# The Context of Performance Enhancement

## An Athlete's Perspective

ANGELA J. SCHNEIDER, PH.D.

## The Desire to Win: Sports Values and the Athlete

At the heart of sport is the athlete. Sport is about athletes—competing, trying, striving, performing, and pushing themselves to their limits. This centrality of the athlete means that sports administrators and leaders need to think from the point of view of the athlete and evaluate doping-control programs and proposals on the basis of how well they promote the growth of athletes as athletes and as people. Many athletes feel that in the current environment they are assumed "guilty until proven innocent," as opposed to the way they think it should be: "innocent until proven guilty."[1]

In this chapter, I review some of the reasons for this current environment and the effect it is having on athletes and their decisions about their health and their participation in sport.[2] I review some of the arguments that athletes might have for their seemingly strong support for the bans on doping in sport, and also address counterarguments, against the bans, from an athlete's perspective. These counterarguments are often tied to civil liberties and the violation of individual rights. The chapter concludes with a look at building a consensus among athletes to help them better express and support their perspective on this issue, which plays such an important role in their lives.

Despite serious societal concerns about doping, first and foremost, doping is an athletes' issue. Athletes' bodies are on the "front lines," so to speak. Doping affects all athletes, those who are clean and those who are not. At the personal level, those who dope not only are taking additional risks with their health but also are destroying the integrity of their own participation in sport. A "win" that comes from cheating is no win at all. Of course, before doping was banned it was not a form of cheating, but it did give an unfair advantage.[3] The athlete who dopes will never have the satisfaction that comes from testing himself or herself in fair competition against others. (In sport, it is best to use the term *fair* rather than *equal*, because any form of mathematical reference is difficult to apply, given the great range of variables involved in competition.) More important, doping undermines the reputation and integrity of the vast majority of athletes who do not dope. The existence of athletes who dope, and the fear that many more are doping than those who are caught, places huge pressure on other "clean athletes" to keep up.

Doping can destroy an athlete's experience in sport and the public's perception of both the athlete and the sport. Public support for sport rests in large measure on the belief that it embodies a good set of values.[4] An athlete's experience in sport can transcend everyday life because it can represent the pinnacle of human aspirations. If athletes and the public come to believe that sport is systemically tainted and that no one has the power or the will to do anything about it, or if there is widespread acceptance of the idea that it is no longer real people competing but doped athletic machines, the outcome will be an utter disaffection that will send the moral value of sport into terminal decline.[5] There may come a point when parents no longer feel that sport is a good thing for their children to participate in, because of the negative impact of doping, cheating, and violence.[6]

At the moment, from the athlete's perspective, we have the worst of all possible worlds. The belief that many athletes are doping places increased pressure to dope on those who currently do not. The problem is not just about belief but about real advantages.[7] Few competitions are untainted by suspicion, because there is a widespread belief that some competitors are doping, and just about everyone's reputation and integrity fall into question. Athletes would prefer a situation in which they could compete cleanly and fairly, assured that others are doing the same.

Athletes tend to rely on their medical support staff and on science for guidance and direction in their sports experience. But doping is not, in the first instance, a crisis of medicine or science, but rather is a crisis of sports ethics and values that affects the athlete. The judgment that a particular substance or activity is "doping" is a moral judgment. Although it should be based on sound scientific evidence and clear reasoning, it is not a scientific judgment. If an activity is considered to be doping, then it is forbidden. Actions that are forbidden enter the moral realm and are not the realm of science. Athletes cannot look to science or medicine to make moral judgments; ethics is not dictated by science and medicine. The relationship is such that ethics has application to science and medicine, and science and medicine provide evidence from which sound ethical judgments can be made. In the case of doping, science and medicine can tell us what substance or practice is performance-enhancing. Science and medicine can also tell us what can be harmful to an athlete's health and what is not harmful—for not all performance enhancement is harmful. However, science and medicine do not define cheating in sport or what should be prohibited.

When athletes believe that they can win by cheating, the avoidance of detection will be seen as just "part of the game." The solution is not simply ever-tougher punishment and control (although, often, both are needed) but rather a shift in attitudes: an agreement that the tainted win is not really a win. New doping-control measures must be rooted in sports ethics and values; they must flow from athletes' agreement; they must respect athletes' rights to privacy; and they must be independently, accountably, and fairly administered.

The International Olympic Committee (IOC) and the World Anti-Doping Agency (WADA) have made some moves forward in the fight against doping, but progress is painfully slow for athletes waiting to be helped with this pervasive problem. Many of the world conferences on doping have finished far short of athletes' expectations, but at least they have made some ground in identifying key issues and working toward a consensus for the agreement on the new World Anti-Doping Code reached in Copenhagen in 2003.[8] However, this ground seems to get lost because the approaches used are not athlete-centered, which makes them inadequate in key areas.

## Doping Control through an Athlete's Lens

There is a great deal of agreement on the ethical status of doping—that it is a bad thing—but far less agreement on what doping is and why it should be banned. Unless athletes clearly know what the enemy is, and why we are fighting it, our battles will be doomed to failure. Part of the problem is that the IOC and WADA have looked to science and medicine to answer an ethical question: What should we prohibit? No scientific or medical criteria allow us to determine whether or not some new substance or practice is doping and thus falls within or outside sports ethics. This is a values-based philosophical question. When the science is determined, the hard questions about permissibility still remain. The choice of whether to permit or prohibit a substance or practice is a decision about the rules and values of sport—especially for the people who have to live with such decisions: the athletes. These decisions are similar to decisions about the permissibility of any technological development in sport. But they are not arbitrary, as some decisions in sport seem to be to outsiders (e.g., the height of the basketball net, the number of players on the court, the length of the game). Of crucial importance is who will be empowered to make the decisions and on what grounds.

Decisions about the permissibility of various substances and methods of doping and decisions about the enforceability of the resultant rules are ultimately decisions about athletes and their bodies, conduct, and privacy. Doping is fundamentally an issue for athletes, so decisions about what constitutes doping and how rules can be fairly enforced must be generated with, and from, athletes.

Until now, the conceptual structure of antidoping efforts has been the creation of rules based on ill-defined criteria, which are then imposed on athletes from above. Antidoping efforts are often seen as heavy-handed, police-like intrusions rather than attempts to facilitate and educate about fair competition. Unless the IOC and WADA seek active and informed agreement and consensus from the community of athletes (not just from the token high-profile athlete), the fight against doping is doomed to the same fate as the IOC's war to preserve amateurism.[9]

The practical implementation of the World Anti-Doping Code, which includes the list of prohibited substances and practices, is also deficient in other crucial areas.[10] Doping control can be accomplished only by effective out-of-competition, no-notice testing. This is because some substances (e.g., anabolic steroids) can be discontinued before competition and retain their effects, and also because of the prevalence of the use of masking agents and the method of urine substitution with catheters. The antidoping code refers to this type of testing but offers no clear practical indication of how such testing would be carried out to ensure informed consent, fairness, effectiveness, and respect for the privacy and dignity of athletes. There are many stories of athletes not understanding the implications of the new code and not having access to education about it.[11] Doping, as well as antidoping programs, raise a variety of issues for athletes, some of which involve human rights. Antidoping rules are part of the rules governing any particular sport. Doping affects the rights of all athletes.

While doping rules are part of an overall set of rules for the governance of a sport, doping also goes beyond the rules of sport—unlike receiving a penalty during a game, doping has implications beyond the sports arena. The referees on the field do not observe doping, and doping may involve criminal behavior for athletes: an incident of doping may be both against the rules of the sport and contrary to specific antidoping legislation or general domestic laws. Doping may have consequences for an athlete's future eligibility to participate in a sport, and it may have civil, professional, or even criminal consequences off the playing field. As a result, doping is a special breach of sporting rules—and other social rules—that have, over time, developed some complicated characteristics.

For example, the terms *banned* and *prohibited* are often used interchangeably in relation to antidoping in sport. In antidoping circles, these terms are usually used to describe the substances and practices that athletes are not allowed to use, as described by antidoping rules and regulations in sport (i.e., included in the World Anti-Doping Code, which was developed primarily by WADA from the IOC's List of Prohibited Substances and Methods and lists compiled by other relevant antidoping authorities).

For the athlete, doping-control testing can have serious moral implications, related primarily to three things. The first is the content of the "banned list," which is the list of all the substances and practices athletes are not allowed to use. For example, some substances on the banned list are accessible over the counter in pharmacies—substances that everyone else in society can use. Other substances on the banned list are required for medical treatment of an illness when prescribed by a physician. These are just two examples that complicate the ethical analysis of the methods used in doping control. The second aspect of doping control that has some serious moral implications is the management of results of the testing process. For the system to have fair and due process, the management of results must be tightly controlled. The athlete should be informed early in the process if he or she tests positive, and the media should be the last to know. This has not always been the case. The third element is the ability, or lack thereof, for athletes to contribute to the process. Athletes need to be part of the decision-making process at all levels, and this also does not always happen.

In other words, the critical concerns are what it is, exactly, that athletes are being tested for; the methods used for testing; and the process for levying penalties against athletes in the event of a positive test result and a doping infraction. It is politically incorrect for athletes to question the moral implications these aspects of doping control will have on them as athletes. The result is that they are afraid of being accused of doping even if they just ask questions about their basic rights as people. Privately, athletes do raise questions about the potential human rights violations and resulting harms that may be caused by the bans and enforcement, because effective antidoping measures cause a serious invasion of privacy. Although most athletes want doping-free sport, some also understand that this violation may not be justified solely by the good those antidoping measures seek to attain. This situation can lead to some mixed feelings for athletes and, from an ethics perspective, may even lead to an impasse: Does the end justify the means? For doping-free sport, which many athletes want, we need effective enforcement. But the steps required for effective enforcement can be invasive of athletes' rights, particularly the personal right to privacy and confidentiality. Further, the culture of sport itself, in many cases, is not one that fosters protection of an athlete's human rights.

To understand the ethical aspects and implications of doping controls for athletes, it is important to understand some central terms or concepts. First, we need to distinguish between (1) *in-competition testing*—drug testing that occurs at a sporting event (usually involving elite athletes) such as a regional, national, or international competition; and (2) *out-of-competition testing*—drug testing that occurs at any time of the year and in any location, such as at the athlete's home, at a training venue, or even while overseas.[12] Out-of-competition testing is usually conducted on a short-notice or no-notice (unannounced) basis.

The most effective way to test for banned substances and practices is random, unannounced, out-of-competition testing. This is because some substances (e.g., anabolic steroids) can be discontinued before competition and still retain their effects and because of the wide use of masking agents and urine substitution with catheters.[13] Athletes could reasonably argue that requiring them to be prepared to submit to urine and/or blood testing at any time is a serious breach of their civil and human rights (this is particularly so in North American countries). This sort of intrusive intervention in athletes' lives (or any people's lives for that matter) could be warranted, from most ethics perspectives, only by the need to protect others from serious harm. It would be fair for athletes to question whether the depth of harm warranting such extreme interference with personal liberty can be established in the case of doping in sport and, in particular, in elite sports.[14] One need only follow all of the recent press releases on the "whereabouts" issue.[15] The debate is centered around athletes' right to privacy and the requirement that they notify the doping control agencies of their whereabouts at all times when preparing for competition.[16]

Athletes have to be aware of some finer points with the problem of doping in sport, particularly with regard to the types of drugs and practices for which testing is required. Broadly speaking, a banned substance or practice may be one intended either to enhance performance on the day of competition or to enhance training in preparation for a major competition. Although the vast majority of performance-enhancing substances, such as stimulants, depressants, and narcotics, can be tested for, with a fair degree of reliability, at the competition site, not all banned substances and practices can be detected with accuracy at the time of the athlete's performance (e.g., human growth hormone). In addition, some performance enhancers work not by directly improving performance on the day of competition, but by enhancing recovery from prior training (e.g., steroids).[17] The upshot is that immediate performance enhancers are more readily detectable by in-competition testing than are the longer-term training enhancers by out-of-competition testing.

In-competition testing used to be the primary form of testing, but it was deemed to be of limited value in detecting training enhancers.[18] In-competition testing was thus seen to be not a completely effective deterrent, but still necessary. Out-of-competition testing was deemed essential, and to prevent athletes' use of masking techniques to hide their doping, the testing had to be unannounced or on short notice. These considerations formed the basis for introducing random, unannounced, out-of-competition testing, which became an essential part of doping control and remains so. Randomness was considered necessary because the expense of testing all athletes is too great. It should be noted that not all out-of-competition tests are random; some are targeted to sports and athletes that have had a history of doping.

The question of targeting specific athletes is still open, because the selection criteria for this activity (i.e., how the people who do the testing choose whom to target for testing) are often not transparent, thus leading to athletes' concerns about the role of hearsay. This state of affairs can lead to the perception by some athletes that the testing is not fair and that athletes are being selected for testing on the basis of unjustified suspicion. Suspicion colors the culture of sport, and it is important to note the potential difficulties. If some athletes believe that testing is targeted toward them on the basis of rumor, the scene could be ripe for vindictive campaigns of harassment. If an athlete's primary rival starts a rumor that there is a suspicion of doping, the accused athlete's life could be made more difficult. But if the testing agency does not follow up on accusations and test accordingly, it runs the risk of being accused of turning a blind eye to "known" abuses and abusers, as has occurred in sports such as cycling, weightlifting, and athletics in which there have been known abuses.[19]

## The Role of Law

Athletes are effectively faced with the enforcement of doping bans potentially requiring that they be prepared to submit to a doping-control test at any time of the day or night, without warning. This also means that athletes are required to give information regarding their whereabouts at all times. Further, not only will the athlete be tested for a wide range of banned substances, but the testing may also include so-called recreational drugs, such as marijuana and cocaine. These drugs are not taken as enhancers and have little proven training-enhancement effect (although cocaine may affect performance if used during competition and thus needs to be tested for by in-competition testing), but, depending on the laws of the country in which the testing takes place, such drugs can carry criminal penalties for ownership or possession.[20]

The degree of legal control varies, depending on the substance. Some substances are "legal" only if dispensed by prescription by a professionally qualified and government-certified person. Some (such as cocaine) are "illegal" under any circumstances, and mere possession can lead to a criminal conviction and imprisonment. The consequences of a positive test can be enormous, even if there is no doping infraction.[21]

## The Human Rights Framework

As a vast and powerful social institution, sport has an obligation to uphold and respect athletes' basic human rights. These rights involve both the fundamental right of athletes to choose how they will live their lives (providing that they do not harm others) and respect for the worth and dignity of each human being. Athletes also have a basic right to privacy. The system can go wrong for athletes when it intrudes into something that is beyond its jurisdiction. It is unfair to athletes to test and penalize beyond what is required to ensure fair competition. Drug testing in sport is an intrusion into an athlete's privacy. That intrusion requires an athlete's consent, something that is, and should be, freely given when the test is conducted to ensure fair competition. However, the demand for consent to test for something that is irrelevant to sport is unfair and coercive. The demand for consent to test for substances not scientifically proven to enhance performance,[22] given the current penalties and lack of education, is unfair because these substances have no proven relevance to sport, and it is coercive because unless the athlete consents to the testing, he or she is prohibited from competition.

John Hoberman, in chapter 1 of this volume (and in other works), gives rich explanations of the environment in which some athletes live. These accounts give us good information on which to base a look at arguments or tensions regarding the moral responsibility of individual athletes. The arguments I am attempting to defend in this chapter may seem to conflict with some of Hoberman's implied conclusions about such responsibility. I am attempting not only to emphasize

different pressures that affect the exercise of that responsibility, but also to miti-
gate that responsibility. The culture in which athletes live would be much more
supportive and trustworthy if there were a history of consistently supporting athletes' rights in these and other areas. There is no such history.[23] Athletes tend
to be viewed as interchangeable commodities (i.e., there is always another new
athlete to replace the last one) that are subject to the control of those who run
the sport. Athletes deserve support for and commitment to their personal rights,
but they need it not just at major events such as the Olympic Games and not just
when a gold medal is at stake. The stakes are high all the time, because even a
two-year ban for drug use can spell the end of a competitive athletic career. This
means the loss not only of sporting opportunity but also, for some athletes in
high-profile sports, of enormous commercial possibilities.

Further, the concept of *strict liability* gives athletes much to be concerned about.
Strict liability is "the responsibility for a state of affairs or for an act regardless of
intent, motive or will."[24] Although WADA is not a legal entity, this is a legalistic
kind of definition (from the *WADA Athlete Guide*) that was developed to prevent
athletes from appealing to "intentionality," which, of course, is important for any
moral blameworthiness. Antidoping rules that define doping as the presence of a
banned substance in an athlete's system make that athlete responsible or "strictly
liable" for the presence of the banned substance—even if the individual had no
knowledge of how the substance came to be in his or her system or did not intend
it to be there. From the point of view of other athletes, how a banned substance
came to be in an individual's system may be irrelevant. It is the advantage the
banned substance may have given that individual—whether known or intended
or not—that matters in the competitive context. In other words, an individual's
competitors will suffer (loss of opportunities to train or compete, loss of top plac-
ings in events, loss of associated endorsements or other opportunities) just as
much from an unintended advantage as one that is planned. However, in some
cases, an athlete may seek early reinstatement or a reduction of the sanction if
he can demonstrate that the positive test was the result of inadvertence, reli-
ance on another person (such as a team doctor) in a position of responsibility, or
even sabotage. But this early reinstatement or reduced sanction certainly doesn't
happen all the time, even when the unintended use is proven (one just needs
to review the Andreea Raducan case from the 2000 Sydney Olympic Games).[25]
The point about unfairness without culpability is important, and the practice of
strict liability without proper educational programs highlights the imbalance in
this area.

In these situations, according to the *WADA Athlete Guide*, the burden or onus of proof is on the athlete. The burden and onus of proof come into play when an athlete is exercising his or her right to challenge a positive test result. Because challenges to doping decisions take place in different languages and different legal traditions, the terms used to describe the burden and onus of proof vary, but the basic principles are common to most procedures that govern challenges. The *burden of proof* describes the quality of the evidence and arguments that an individual must submit to prove the case. Different levels of proof are required from a legal perspective. The burden of proof is sometimes described as the "civil" burden (something that is proven on a balance of probabilities) or "criminal" burden (something that is proven beyond a reasonable doubt). There is also a standard in between these two that is sometimes used in doping matters: clear and convincing evidence. The *onus of proof* relates to who must prove a case. Doping-control authorities generally have the onus (responsibility) to show a positive test result is valid and accurate (by sample collection, chain of custody, and laboratory analysis to an accepted standard), while the athlete then has the onus (responsibility) of showing that there was some departure from the standard or some other error that calls the validity or integrity of the positive test result into question.[26]

In their struggle to be the best they can be, athletes must understand and cope with some serious and complicated matters. Effective antidoping measures require a clear agreement on what is being fought and why, a strong commitment of resources and energy to complete the job, and a willingness to be, and to be seen as, open, fair, and accountable. From an athlete's perspective, all antidoping measures and agencies should be rooted in sports ethics and values and should be driven by athletes' agreement. Athletes should be more involved in these matters than they have been to date, and there should be an improved, more formal process for them to shape the antidoping measures (e.g., code, list, testing procedures, results management, penalties). For this to happen at a practical level, athletes should be represented at all levels of antidoping agencies. The mandate for these agencies should be the preservation of sporting integrity and ethics, which is what athletes want. The antidoping agencies should be independent, open to athletes, and accountable to an independent governing council. They should conduct doping-control measures to the highest international, independent standards, with due respect for the athlete's personal rights and the fairness of due process. To help ensure that this happens, the agencies should conduct ongoing, independent, legal and ethical reviews of their operations and make the results publicly available. Further, the agencies should lead in the development of educational and consensus-building programs to pursue ethics and integrity in sport. All doping-detection research should meet the highest standards of medical and research ethics. In particular, research should not be conducted without the express, written, informed, and noncoerced consent of the athletes whose bodies or samples are being studied.

Many claim that the benefits of sport include the development of the athlete. The concept of development covers a great deal of territory. A good model of athlete-centered sport is found in the International Paralympics Committee.[27] At all levels of sport, sports systems should be designed to promote growth and to ensure fairness, accountability, and the protection of athletes' rights. These goals would entail a fundamental shift in attitude in the way athletes are viewed and treated. One of the first priorities in this matter would be to ensure respect for the athlete as a person, and not as a mere body or performance machine. Athletes are at the center of sport. Persons have autonomy—the general right to have their own interests and make their own decisions. Persons live complete lives—that is, private lives outside their sport and lives that extend beyond their years of active sporting competition. Persons are entitled to respect. In particular, respect entails that athletes should not be caused unnecessary harm (physical, mental, psychological, or moral).

## Building Consensus with the Athlete at the Core

Sport is a great international symbol and festival. The guardians of sport have an obligation to explain and defend what sport represents. Sports administrators control which athletes can compete, and they have a great responsibility to ensure that the rules are open, fair, and effective and that the sport is publicly accountable for its decisions. One way of looking at this responsibility is as a duty of care. A fundamental aspect of sport should be the development of humanity. This means not only that sport should allow humankind, in general, to develop, but also that sport should play a role in the personal development of everyone who participates. One might ask: Would we hold the same views about other jobs? If sport is special, why is that so? After all, elite athletes are paid quite a lot. Why should we insist that their efforts "develop them mentally and morally" too? One important reason is that the Olympic Games, for example, are not just multisport world championships. When asked, the world public identifies Olympic values of excellence, dedication, fair play, and international peace as key ingredients of the Games. The Olympic rings connote a higher set of ethics and values, and this is the basis for public support.[28] We should ensure that participation in sport allows athletes to develop physically, mentally, and morally.

How do we make this happen? Sport and doping-control programs should adopt a principle of athlete-centered decision making. In practical terms, we need to ask: Does the proposal respect the athlete as a complete person? We also need to ask: Does the proposal promote sporting values and principles with integrity? Can the proposal be explained or justified? What are the reasons for adopting the proposal? What is the justification? Does the proposal facilitate or enhance the personal development of the athlete?

Although athletes are at the heart of sport, their voices are not heard clearly, consistently, or authoritatively enough. Athletes tend to be young, geographically dispersed, and mobile, and they have relatively short careers. For the handful of athletes who are recognized nationally and/or internationally, there are thousands more who commit their energies and attention to their sport without recognition or external reward. Athletes can be vulnerable to the vagaries and whims of coaching methods and selection processes, subject to injuries, and victims of abuse. Many athletes labor in poverty.

Sports and antidoping agencies should be driven by concern and care for the safety, well-being, and development of athletes. The existing athletes' representation needs to be strengthened. Athlete-representatives are still too few in number, and they exercise relatively little direct power within the relevant organizations. Sport needs to hear the voices of all athletes, and it needs to hear those voices in their diversity. To achieve this end, athletes need to be more formally organized and strengthened by having independent, democratically based, grassroots associations. It is challenging to create a democratic constituency of athletes. For instance, at the Olympic Games, selection of athlete-representatives to the IOC Athletes' Commission occurs when the athletes are focused on competition and precludes the possibility of offering meaningful platforms. But the challenge must be faced or, as important as it is, "democratically elected" becomes a meaningless veneer. Athletes need a forum in which to talk to other athletes, to share common concerns, and to look for solutions. The athlete-members of the IOC and athletes that sit on other committees and commissions should be the visible tip of an organization that has an ongoing and close connection with athletes around the world. The IOC Athletes' Commission needs links with regional and national athletes' groups, and it needs to campaign actively to defend athletes' rights. This does not now happen in a formal and systematic way.

For too long, athletes have been viewed as a form of replaceable commodity—

central to the enterprise, but individually of little importance. Athletes' associations should be the independent voices of athletes; working associations of active athletes; defenders of athletes' rights, responsibilities, and reputations; creators of common cause and consensus among current athletes; working on athletes' issues; and having democratic voices in governance. For this kind of change to happen, athletes need adequate funding for an association of athletes; year-round regional activities; a representative presence at major games and world championships; national and regional chapters; and regular formal and informal communication.

We must hold firm to our vision for sport. Sport has gone astray in the commercialization process and has fallen short of this vision. Yet the vision itself retains all the vitality and truth necessary to guide us. Sport has a unique position within international society. Sports administrators are the guardians of the ideals of modern sport, and athletes look to them for help. The obligations that such a position imposes are enormous; more importantly, the opportunities for leadership, especially on the doping issue, are unparalleled. Doping, as one of the most serious moral crises facing sport today, has the potential to destroy the vision entirely. The problems are both systemic and personal. These forms of corruption do not occur in isolation. The primary moral agents, however, are the guardians and the athletes. They need to work together closely for change, renewal, and a renaissance of sport. All those who love and follow sport, all those who still believe in the vision, for themselves and for their children, are watching and waiting in the hope that someone will deal with the problem of doping.

Reform of an institution as crucial and special as sport is not a simple matter of applying an existing model or formula to generate "right" answers. Rather, what is essential is a process for reaching justifiable recommendations and fair decisions. This process requires an openness to review and criticism and a willingness to hear a diverse array of voices. It requires a careful balance between the actions required to protect the sport and those required to nurture the athlete. There has already been a contribution to the process from many experts. However, there is an enormous amount of expertise from the athletes that remains untapped. Athletes, if treated with respect, would be willing to share their expertise and eager to express their ideas about doping and how it affects the sport that means a great deal to them. The focus for reform must be on ethics and values, derived from athlete-centeredness and sports ideals.

In one capacity, sport is a business, and it needs to manage its business with prudence and due diligence. But that management can never be the complete story, because the guardians of sport are the guardians of a public trust. Sport should be based on a set of ideals—the ideals of Olympism, a way of life. While the guardians of sport can never own those ideals, they can certainly nurture, protect, and promote them. Developing new antidoping agencies can be only a part of the answer. A genuine cultural and ethical shift must occur. Within sport, there must be a transition from a destructive lust to win at all costs to a constructive desire to enjoy the process of competing and testing oneself fairly against others who are doing the same. Athletes, and all who love and support them, must remember that one cannot win without competition, that competition without fairness is not a meaningful competition, and that a win without fairness is no victory at all. Herein lies our greatest hope, in the pure joy of sport.

## NOTES

1. Canadian Centre for Ethics in Sport, *Canadian Study on the Athletes' Anti-Doping Passport* (Ottawa: Canadian Centre for Ethics in Sport, 2001).

2. Many of the arguments that I try to defend throughout this chapter are based on my experiences as a representative at the meetings leading up to creation of the Canadian Centre for Ethics in Sport and the World Anti-Doping Agency and as a member of working committees in these organizations.

3. For a full discussion of the distinction between cheating and unfair advantages, see A. J. Schneider and R. B. Butcher, "Fair Play as Respect for the Game," *Journal of the Philosophy of Sport* 25 (1998): 1–22.

4. Canadian Centre for Ethics in Sport, "Foundations in Excellence: Annual Report, 2004–5," www.cces.ca/pdfs/CCES-AR-2004-2005-E.pdf.

5. Witness the recent coverage of the U.S. Senate hearings on steroid use in professional baseball. See J. Hoberman, *Mortal Engines: The Science of Performance and the Dehumanization of Sport* (New York: Free Press, 1992).

6. Canadian Centre for Ethics in Sport, "Foundations in Excellence."

7. There are important similarities, for athletes, to the "prisoner's dilemma." See A. J. Schneider and R. B. Butcher, "Why Olympic Athletes Should Avoid the Use and Seek the Elimination of Performance-Enhancing Substances and Practices in the Olympic Games," *Journal of the Philosophy of Sport* 20–21 (1994): 64–81.

8. World Anti-Doping Agency, *World Anti-Doping Code* (Quebec: World Anti-Doping Agency, 2003).

9. The IOC fought to preserve amateurism with a relentless focus on monetary payment and financial rewards for many years, especially under the leadership of Avery Brundage. The fight was given up in 1987. For a detailed argument as to why the war to preserve amateurism was misplaced and that, at the heart of amateurism, there is a concept and a value well worth defending, see A. J. Schneider and R. B. Butcher, "For the Love of the Game: A Philosophical Defense of Amateurism," *Quest* 45 (1993): 460–69.

10. Ibid.

11. Canadian Centre for Ethics in Sport, *Canadian Study on the Athletes' Anti-Doping Passport*.

12. World Anti-Doping Agency, *WADA Athlete Guide*, 4th ed. (Quebec: World Anti-Doping Agency, 2006).

13. The game of testing and masking is constantly evolving. If athletes know when they are to be tested, they have a far greater opportunity to seek to thwart the test.

14. W. Brown, "Ethics, Drugs, and Sport," *Journal of the Philosophy of Sport* 7 (1980): 15-23; P. Thompson, "Privacy and the Urinalysis Testing of Athletes," in *Philosophic Inquiry in Sport*, ed. W. J. Morgan and K. V. Meier (Champaign, IL: Human Kinetics, 1988); A. J. Schneider and R. B. Butcher, "Harm, Athletes' Rights and Doping Control," in *Center for Olympic Studies 1992 Symposium Proceedings*, ed. R. K. Barney, 164–75 (London, ON: University of Western Ontario, 1992).

15. For example, see J. Haskell, "New Testing Policy on Drugs Is Like Big Brother: UK Sport's Latest Drug Regulations Are a Step Too Far Even If Rugby Players Don't Mind Being Tested," *Guardian* (Manchester), March 14, 2009.

16. For an example of a whereabouts program, see the Canadian Centre for Ethics in Sport, "Athlete Whereabouts Program," www.cces.ca/whereabouts.

17. D. Moorcroft, "Doping: The Athlete's View, Dilemmas and Choices," *Lausanne: Olympic Review* 216, no. 10 (1985): 634–35.

18. For example, athletes may use a training-enhancing substances such as anabolic steroids and discontinue use before competition, rendering the detection of these compounds extremely difficult at the time of competition, particularly if masking agents are also used. This is so despite the contemporary use of endocrine profiles that allow us to track endocrine changes in an athlete's body. The logical problem is that endocrine profiles are useful as a testing criterion only for those with a long history of previous tests.

19. Canadian Centre for Ethics in Sport, "Foundations in Excellence"; World Anti-Doping Agency, *WADA Athlete Guide*.

20. Canadian Centre for Ethics in Sport, "Foundations in Excellence."

21. Some of these drugs (e.g., marijuana) are permitted in some nations (the Netherlands, say), but not many. Not all positive test results have led to a charge of a doping infraction (e.g., some therapeutic exemptions).

22. It may be argued that the problem is not enhancement per se but that some athletes are coerced to take harmful steps because of beliefs about what might be effective. A good example of this kind of problem is seen in the Tour de France. For an extensive analysis of the problem, see A. J. Schneider, "Cultural Nuances: Doping, Cycling and the Tour de France," in *Doping in Sport: Global Ethical Issues*, ed. A. J. Schneider and F. Hong, 36–50 (New York: Routledge, 2007).

23. When WADA was set up, this historical lack of support for athletes' rights was one of the issues it had to address.

24. World Anti-Doping Agency, *WADA Athlete Guide*.

25. For example, see articles from the *New York Times* on the injustice of Radican's positive doping infraction and resulting loss of her Olympic medal from the Sydney Olympic Games in 2000, http://topics.nytimes.com/top/reference/timestopics/people/r/

andreea_raducan/index.html. See also "Justice for Andreea Raducan," a petition for the reinstatement of her Olympic medal, www.petitiononline.com/radu2004/petition.html.

26. World Anti-Doping Agency, *WADA Athlete Guide*.

27. International Paralympic Committee, "IPC Strategic Congress Defines Future Policies," www.paralympic.org/release/Main_Sections_Menu/News/Press Releases/2001 _04_29_a. html; International Paralympic Committee, "IPC Athletes' Committee: Objectives, Philosophy, and Activities," www.paralympic.org/paralympian/20001/06.htm.

28. See A. J. Schneider and R. B. Butcher, *Towards the Ethical Foundation for Olympic Reform: The OATH Report* (Toronto: Olympic Advocates Together Honourably, 1999).

# CHAPTER THREE

# Reflections on the "Parallel Federation Solution" to the Problem of Drug Use in Sport

## The Cautionary Tale of Powerlifting

JAN TODD, PH.D., AND TERRY TODD, PH.D.

Although both authors have now retired from competition, our experiences as competitors and as officials in powerlifting inform the analysis that follows. We have tried to be as objective as possible in this chapter, but the reader should know that this is a sporting landscape that we know from the insider's perspective as well as that of the scholarly observer. Terry Todd was a weightlifter in the 1960s who switched to powerlifting and became the first U.S. men's superheavyweight champion in 1965. He used small amounts of methandrostenalone (Dianabol) during his later competitive years; he stopped all use when he retired from competition. Jan Todd, who never used anabolic drugs, was a pioneer in the sport of women's powerlifting, setting numerous world and American records during her 11-year career in the sport, and being featured in *Sports Illustrated* and other publications as the "World's Strongest Woman." She served as the head of both the international and national women's powerlifting subcommittees in the early 1980s and fought for drug testing in powerlifting during her years as an administrator. Since our retirement as competitors, we have remained somewhat active in the sport as collegiate coaches, journalists, referees, and officials.

## Introduction

Sports ethicists, struggling mightily with the issue of drug testing, have produced a surprisingly complex literature on the subject. Ethicists have considered whether testing is justified based on such philosophical precepts as the "coercion factor"—the idea that an athlete would be forced to take drugs to remain competitive; the "unfair advantage argument"—the idea that drugs create a nonlevel playing field; and "paternalism"—the need to protect athletes from harm.[1] Some scholars have also suggested that testing is necessary because the doped body is "not natural."[2] A simplified version of this school of thought is that ergogenic drugs have such power to change the fundamental nature of athletes that the "contest" becomes more about a competitor's level of pharmacological enhancement than about training, will, and genetic gifts. As Michael Burke and Terence Roberts suggest, almost all ethicists who argue in favor of testing do so based on a belief in the essential concepts of fairness and the preservation of good sports contests as sufficient conditions to justify testing for ergogenic drugs.[3]

While there is a strong sentiment in favor of testing within the sports philosophy community, support for testing is by no means unanimous. Some sports ethicists have pointed to the inherent problems of testing in their articles examining privacy and personal liberty, the difficulty in drawing a meaningful line between illegal drugs and other forms of enhancement (such as vitamins, food supplements, or high-altitude sleeping chambers), and the inequitable nature of the penalties imposed for testing positive on a drug test.[4] As Robert Albrecht and colleagues put it: "We have suggested it is: hypocritical to imply that only drugs, among all categories of ergogenic aids, are a threat to 'natural' competition; impossible for drug testing to ensure fair and equal athletic competition; illogical and inconsistent with empirical evidence to test; . . . unethical to coerce athletes to consent to drug testing; unrealistic to believe the results of positive drug tests will remain confidential; and inefficient to spend millions of dollars each year to detect a handful of positive drug tests."[5]

Similarly, Angela Schneider and Robert B. Butcher argue that "the invasion of privacy caused by effective antidoping measures cannot be justified solely by the good those measures seek to attain."[6] And Norman Fost summarized the reservations of more than a few scholars in an article in the *Hastings Center Report* in 1986:

> The widespread alarm about use and abuse of drugs in sports probably arises from some genuine and perhaps rational concern; but it is difficult to discern the basis for that concern in present policies and discussions. If it is based on unfairness, it is irrational, for there are far greater sources of unfairness and whatever is due to drugs can be neutralized by a system that allows all athletes equal access to drugs. If it is based on paternalism, it is disingenuous and misplaced for the risks of sport itself far exceed the demonstrated risks of those drugs that arouse the greatest concern. If it is based on some notion of naturalness, we need more conceptual work

to tell us why synthetic vitamins are considered natural and naturally occurring hormones are considered unnatural. We are not even clear on the moral difference, if any, between a food and a drug, nor is there a clear understanding of those terms.[7]

Terry Black goes even further, arguing that "removal of the ban on drugs will result in fairer contests and greatly reduced health risks."[8]

If the skeptics are right and there are morally defensible reasons *not* to implement doping controls for adults in sport, what happens to those athletes who don't want to use drugs? Where does the drug-free athlete play? One solution would be for sports to have parallel federations—one for drug users and another for those who choose to prepare for competition without the use of ergogenic drugs. By having two federations, it would seem that no one's personal freedom would be unjustly limited and that, in the case of powerlifting, drug-free lifters would not be as likely to leave their sport in the belief that they cannot be competitive. Just such a suggestion was made in 1980 by Mike Lambert, publisher and editor of *Powerlifting USA* magazine, when he urged those who wanted drug testing in powerlifting to leave the dominant organization, the United States Powerlifting Federation (USPF), and create a new federation so that there would be separate national governing bodies, separate national championships, and separate sets of American records.[9] It seemed like such a simple—and obvious—solution. Let's just create two "level playing fields" in the same ballpark.

The "parallel federation solution" does seem logical at first glance. However, as this chapter demonstrates, the creation of parallel federations in powerlifting did not solve the sport's doping problem. Rather, as in a line of falling dominoes, the creation of the first parallel federation touched off a sequence of events that eventually undermined the nature and meaning of this, admittedly minor, sport. In exploring the history and social dynamics of the parallel federation solution, we argue that the attempt to solve the ethical problems of drug use by creating parallel forms of powerlifting failed on several levels. It failed because of athletes' overwhelming desire for recognition and glory; it failed because of the attitudes and the lack of moral authority of the sport's officials; and, in particular, it failed because of an entirely unforeseen consequence—that there would be no way to stop the proliferation of new federations once the idea of multiple federations took root. As we demonstrate, once people realized how easy it was to create a new federation, lifters and officials who didn't care for some aspect of an association's rules saw no reason not to just break away, write new rules, and start their own federation. Just how widespread this attitude has become can be seen in the fact that by January 2008, there were at least 17 "international" federations and 18 "American" organizations advertising their meets in the "Coming Events" column of *Powerlifting USA* magazine. These federations differ on matters of banned drugs, whether and how to test, legal attire on the platform, and even the sport's constitutive rules. One recently formed federation—the Syndicated Strength Alliance—for example, keeps separate sets of records for lifts made while the athlete is wearing a single-ply lifting suit and those made while wearing a suit made of multiple layers of supportive material, which improves a lifter's leverage and thus allows the lifter to achieve higher results. Several other federations keep separate records for those lifters who compete "raw" (without any supportive lifting suits) and those who choose to avail themselves of the advantages offered by the heavy suits and shirts now common in the sport. Several federations also keep both drug-tested and non-drug-tested lifts records. Interestingly, many of these federations designate meets with drug testing as "amateur" meets, even when no prize money is offered in the non-drug-tested divisions of the same federation. In any case, the unforeseen consequence of the decision to have parallel forms of powerlifting is a fractured "sport" whose rules now vary significantly from association to association and whose various sets of national and world records cannot be compared because of those differences. In a nutshell, powerlifting is no longer *one* sport.

## Powerlifting before the Parallel Federation Solution

Powerlifting, which is not an Olympic sport, began informally in the 1940s when a few promoters hosted "odd-lift" contests or exhibitions to hype the gate at their Amateur Athletic Union (AAU) weightlifting meets.[10] Sometimes promoters sponsored odd-lift contests consisting of squats, curls, and deadlifts. At other times, the "press on floor" or the bench press—sometimes called, incorrectly, the "prone" press—was included. By the 1960s, odd lifts were commonly referred to as "power lifts" and had become popular with audiences because the slower nature of the squat and deadlift meant that the audience could see what was happening during the lifts and because much heavier weights were used than in any of weightlifting's quick overhead movements. One person interested in the new sport's possibilities was Bob Hoffman, founder and owner of the York Barbell Company and the leading figure in AAU weightlifting in the first half of the twentieth century.[11] Hoffman owned and edited what was probably the largest-circulation magazine on weight training in the world at the time, *Strength & Health*, and in it he had relied primarily on a succession of world-champion American weightlifters and bodybuilders as a source of inspiration for his readers. However, by 1963, the Eastern Bloc nations had overwhelmed American weightlifting, so Hoffman decided to get behind powerlifting, in which, he realized, Americans could again dominate the world stage. In 1964, Hoffman launched a new magazine, *Muscular Development*, which aimed to cover bodybuilding in depth and to be the "powerlifter's organ." In AAU Weightlifting Committee meetings, he also began discussions about the need to get powerlifting organized as a separate sport.[12] After hosting an unofficial national championship in 1964, at which the sport's first written rules were hammered out, Hoffman got approval from the AAU to host a sanctioned national contest in 1965, and then promoted subsequent national meets for men in 1966, 1967, and 1968.

In its earliest days as an organized sport, then, powerlifting did not have its own national governing body. Instead, it was controlled by the AAU Weightlifting Committee, a group that was more than a bit ambivalent about powerlifting's growing popularity. And it *was* growing. By the end of the 1960s, for example, more powerlifting meet sanctions were issued than weightlifting sanctions, a matter that concerned many weightlifting officials, who realized that the new sport was drawing men away from "Olympic" weightlifting. As Peary Rader, editor of *Iron Man* magazine, put it, "POWER lifting is sweeping the country by storm. For a while we thought that Olympic lifting was holding its own . . . [but] it is not growing . . . All you have to do is announce a power lifting contest anywhere . . . and you soon have a lot of competitors."[13]

Until the passage of the Amateur Sports Act in 1978, the AAU operated as a clearinghouse for nearly all amateur sports in the United States. Most sports under the AAU's umbrella had their own organizing committee to sanction contests, keep records, and create rules. However, some sports, including powerlifting and bodybuilding, were not autonomous but operated under the auspices of a parent sport—in their case, AAU Weightlifting. In 1968, the AAU agreed that powerlifting would be designated as an official subcommittee of AAU Weightlifting, and long-time official Bob Crist began building the first powerlifting organization. Crist drew up a rudimentary constitution for the sport, appointed regional chairmen, and began holding separate powerlifting meetings at the AAU convention each year.[14]

Under Crist's able leadership, American powerlifting entered a golden era. In 1971, the first World Powerlifting Championships were held in York, Pennsylvania, and Americans won nearly every weight class, vindicating Hoffman's earlier belief. Two years later, in a group sitting around a table late one night at a Howard Johnson restaurant in Harrisburg, Pennsylvania, Crist agreed to take on the task of building an international organization as well. According to Crist, the idea to form the International Powerlifting Federation (IPF) came from Jack Kelly, the national AAU president and an old friend of Bob Hoffman's. "We'd been talking about our concerns to control the sport," Crist said, "and Kelly, who was Princess Grace's brother, turned over his placemat and began sketching out a chart. 'What you need, if you want control,' Kelly told us, 'is an international organization just for powerlifting.'" And so, according to Crist, looking around the table where Hoffman, Crist, and weightlifting officials Rudy Sablo, John Terpak, Jim Stephens, and Morris Weisbrott sat, Kelly suggested that Crist be the new group's president, that Clarence Johnson, another long-time AAU official, should be vice president, and that national representatives should be found for as many foreign countries as possible.[15] By 1976, the IPF had grown to 25 member-nations and the AAU had approximately 5000 registered American powerlifters.[16] In 1975, the year the IPF published its first rule book, Americans held 30 of the 40 world records in men's powerlifting, and at the world championships that year, held in Birmingham, England, the United States won 8 of the 10 weight classes and took the team title for the fifth straight year.[17]

Hoffman told Crist that the 1975 victory made him prouder to be an American than anything he'd seen in sports since the 1956 Olympics in Melbourne.[18] By the late 1970s, the National AAU Powerlifting Committee—as it was then known—had grown to more than 8000 members, and both the men's and women's national and world championships were regularly covered by shows such as CBS's *Sports Spectacular* and NBC's *Sports World*.[19] By every possible indicator, American and international powerlifting was a great success. In little more than a decade, the sport had gone from being a simple exhibition oddity to a fully realized international activity with thousands of members, television contracts, and a seemingly limitless future. However, the "gremlins of sport," as Terry Todd later called anabolic steroids, were preparing to throw an ethical monkey wrench into this smoothly running machine.[20]

## The Introduction of Steroids to Powerlifting

Unlike those sports that can look back to a golden age before anabolic steroids became available, powerlifting evolved at exactly the same time that anabolic steroids infiltrated the world of sport. In 1987, Terry Todd documented the first systematic use of anabolic steroids by American athletes, which occurred among a group of three weightlifters, two of whom were members of Bob Hoffman's York Barbell team.[21] The weightlifters agreed to be part of an experiment organized by Hoffman's team physician, John Ziegler. Because powerlifting developed under the organizational umbrella of weightlifting, and because weightlifters and powerlifters often trained together in the early days, it did not take long for word of the success of Ziegler's experimentation with the anabolic drug methandrostenalone (Dianabol) to spread throughout the lifting community. Nor did it take long for powerlifters to begin their own, unsupervised steroid experiments. That powerlifters embraced the new drugs so quickly is not surprising, given the attitude of most Americans to drugs and technology in the 1960s. The average American home of that era contained 30 different medicines, vitamins, and assorted nostrums, so the idea of using drugs to enhance performance seemed acceptable.[22] Furthermore, most powerlifters (then and now) viewed science as the handmaiden of sport and embraced drugs and new equipment innovations simply as a means to the end of better performance. And there was also the lure of the lean, muscular, sexually attractive bodies produced by the combination of drugs and powerlifting. We believe that one reason so many men abandoned weightlifting and began powerlifting—especially after 1972—was that the new sport included the bench press as one of its competitive lifts. Before 1972, weightlifting contests included three lifts—the snatch, the clean and jerk, and the press. Because of judging problems, however, the International Weightlifting Federation dropped the press (a test of arm and shoulder strength) from competition, leaving only the snatch and the clean and jerk (primarily tests of legs, back, and hips). The loss of the press resulted in a new type of weightlifting physique, as the shoulder and arm muscles of weightlifters diminished because those muscles were no longer trained intensely. Powerlifting, however, included the bench press, perhaps the most effective of all exercises for producing heavy muscling in the chest and arms, and a young powerlifter—especially one using steroids—could pursue his dreams of being a national lifting champion and, in so doing, build the thick-chested, bull-shouldered, big-armed physique of a comic book superhero. We believe this had a profound effect, as young men drawn to the weight sports want to *look* strong as well as *be* strong.

Finally, using anabolic drugs fit many of these early powerlifters' notions of themselves as "outlaws." In a sport still operating as a subcommittee under AAU Weightlifting, many men drawn to powerlifting were openly contemptuous of the traditions and the more staid approach to sport exemplified by the old-line weightlifting officials. Powerlifters liked to do things their way, and they wanted to control their own personal and administrative destiny. And, because the IPF was not affiliated with the Olympic Games and had no rules against drug use, most men felt no ethical obligation not to use them. Nine-time world powerlifting champion Larry Pacifico, for example, told *Powerlifting USA* in 1988 that he still felt no guilt over his use of steroids, even though that use eventually led to two felony counts for drug smuggling and distribution and a public admission under oath that he had used steroids to win most of his world championships. Pacifico claimed that he considered steroids to be simply "advanced vitamins" and that he'd started using the drugs when he felt the need to stay ahead of his competitors.[23]

Lest we paint with too broad a brush, however, we should say that many lifters—probably the majority of those involved in powerlifting in the 1960s and early 1970s—were not using anabolic steroids.[24] On what was happening at the elite, national-championship level, however, our personal knowledge reinforces what Peary Rader of *Iron Man* magazine wrote in an editorial in 1969:

> While at the Senior Nationals, I had a chance to discuss the use of drugs with a number of lifters. They all admitted to using them (some of these men are record holders). They did not think them to be dangerous if taken under a doctor's care and not used excessively. They did not feel they had suffered any bad side effects . . . they felt it was worth the chance. They reported they did not know any top lifter who was not taking pills, usually Dianabol. It was their opinion that a man could not reach the top without taking them . . . We know a lot of coaches who encourage their athletes to take the drugs. Anything to win . . . All of you know our opinion of these drugs. We certainly cannot approve them in any way.[25]

## The Powerlifting Drug Subculture

As powerlifting grew in popularity during the 1970s, drug use became increasingly common among American competitors at all levels, resulting in a subculture of users who believed that the drugs were necessary to their performance on the platform and who further believed that there was nothing wrong with using these nonbanned drugs to enhance their performance. By the late 1970s, in fact, the role of androgenic drugs in powerlifting was much the same as that of recreational drugs among the counterculture of the 1960s. Using anabolic steroids identified one as being part of the hip, inner circle of the sport. Taking drugs meant you deserved to be taken seriously as an athlete, for you were willing to pay an extra price for your sport. Some people, like *Iron Man* editor Peary Rader, continued to express concerns about the use of drugs, but most elite male lifters felt little concern for their mortality or their morals. Terry Todd, for example, in the first book written about the sport, *Inside Powerlifting* (1977), openly discussed his own steroid use and suggested that many—if not most—of the nine elite lifters he profiled probably used ergogenic drugs.[26] Larry Pacifico, whose position as a top-level competitor and as a dealer of steroids gave him a good vantage point for observation, claimed that 90 percent of the top male lifters used anabolic drugs by the early 1980s.[27] We personally observed male powerlifters with steroids in their gym bags at contests; saw men inject themselves with adrenaline, steroids, and various stimulants; and saw men taking drugs backstage at meets. Powerlifter Joe Nickele spoke for many male powerlifters in 1977 when he wrote an "Open Letter to All Officials of the IPF" for inclusion in *Powerlifting USA*. "Eventually," Nickele wrote, "the IPF will have to decide whether or not to test for steroids at national and international championships." However, rather than recommend testing for the sport, Nickele asked the IPF to take a stand *against* testing. If the IPF decides not to test, he wrote, "Criticism will come from all directions, of course . . . However, the IPF should be responsive to the desire of the majority of the lifters." And those lifters, Nickele explained, didn't want testing. "If you ask around, you will probably find that the majority of lifters agree that what counts in powerlifting is the lifter's *strength*, not HOW he got strong."[28]

One of the best expressions of the mindset of the drug users of this era appeared in a "how-to" book written by powerlifting champion and outspoken drug proponent Fred Hatfield in 1982. In *Anabolic Steroids: What Kind and How Many*, Hatfield argued that powerlifters believed in a "new ethic." "New ethic athletes are pioneers," Hatfield wrote. "Implicit in their philosophy is the notion that no amount of legislation has ever been able to halt the progress of science. As pioneers, these athletes carefully weigh the risk-to-benefit ratio and proceed with caution and with open minds." Hatfield saw no reason not to use drugs, explaining to his readers that drug use may seem unethical "by your moral code, but not by OURS!"[29]

The idea of the drug-using athlete as a manly individualist / scientific innovator resonated across the strength sports during this era. One dealer who sold to both bodybuilders and powerlifters claimed that steroids were "needed by people who wished to set themselves apart from the rest of our weakling society . . . they're adventurers who think for themselves and want to accomplish something noble before they are buried and become worm food."[30] Sociologist Jay Coakley's work on overconformity and deviance provides a good model for understanding the dynamics of drug-using elite powerlifters.[31] Coakley writes: "As high performance athletes endure the challenges of maintaining their membership in select groups and teams at the highest level of accomplishment in their sport, they develop not only extremely strong feelings of unity with other athletes but also the sense that they are unique and extraordinary people." These feelings of superiority, Coakley argues, lead many athletes to fall prey to hubris—the idea that one is separate from and superior to others. As Coakley goes on to note, elite sports encourage and even normalize behaviors that the general public would find deviant.[32] Patrick Mignon's study of doping in the Tour de France reveals many parallels. Mignon writes: "The sportsman using doping belongs to the category of innovative deviant who accepts the general aims but rejects the legal means in favor of illegal means." But the athlete is not alone, Mignon explains, for doping is supported by a cooperative subculture of officials, physicians, and coaches.[33] This certainly proved to be the case in powerlifting, where many elite lifters believed themselves to be unique, special, and above the rules.

## The Struggle for Testing and the First Parallel Federation Solution

Through most of the 1970s, powerlifters didn't have to worry about being "above the rules," because there were no rules banning drug use. Drug testing entered the sport's discourse only in the late 1970s. The debate began in response to the decision by the International Olympic Committee (IOC) to test for anabolic steroids at the 1976 Montreal Olympic Games—a move that prompted many amateur sports organizations to adopt similar testing programs. Rather than powerlifting quickly adopting a program of testing similar to the IOC's, however, a heated debate broke out among American powerlifters and officials about whether the sport should test at all. In the United States, the introduction of women's powerlifting in 1977 and the influx of a new group of mostly non-drug-using athletes to the sport changed the constituency of powerlifting and created a vocal group that wanted the USPF to test.[34] Internationally, there was also strong support for testing among some European teams and, in 1979, the IPF adopted Regulation 5.02, which called for drug testing at world championships beginning in 1979 and at national championships beginning in 1980. Although recorded in the minutes, the rule had little immediate impact.[35] No testing occurred at either the men's or women's world championships in 1979 or 1980, and in 1981 the IPF tested only for amphetamines at the men's world championships.[36]

The IPF's passage of Regulation 5.02 did not cause the U.S. administrators to adopt a similar rule for American lifters. In national committee meetings in 1978, 1979, and 1980, a request for drug testing at the national championships was proposed by the members of the women's subcommittee (USPF Women's Committee). Each year, the proposal failed to pass on a simple majority vote. The arguments put forward by those opposed to testing ranged from nationalistic outrage that the IPF should dictate policy to Americans, to funding concerns, to fears that the tests would not be accurate, to fears that the tests would go too far back in time and catch those who hadn't had time to properly prepare for being tested. Some committee members even claimed testing would kill the sport because there would be no new world records and that the USPF would lose its national TV contracts as a result. Others took the libertarian position that no one should dictate to an individual lifter what that lifter could do to his or her own body. Attempts to separate testing for men and women also failed, as the overwhelmingly male national committee realized that if drug testing was allowed for women and worked smoothly, then testing for men would not be far behind. As might be expected, the public (and private) debate over the topic was frequently personal, often heated, and resulted in a sport split into rival camps. Those in favor of testing lost faith in administrators who continued to put up roadblocks. The pro-testing group also felt less respect for those athletes whose records and performances were now suspect. Likewise, those opposed to testing questioned the motivations of those wanting it, claiming the pro-testing faction was motivated by jealousy and self-interest and that it could not be trusted to handle the testing program fairly.[37]

As to why a group of sport administrators would *not* be in favor of drug testing, this was largely due to the organizational culture of the sport. Powerlifting had always been run by unpaid volunteers, most of whom, at the end of the 1970s, were still active competitors. During the years that powerlifting existed as a subcommittee of AAU Weightlifting, the sport's administration included older, retired weightlifters who had been associated with the Olympic movement and who viewed issues from the more objective perspective of the noncompetitor. However, as noted earlier, following the passage of the Amateur Sports Act in 1978, powerlifting left the AAU and formed an independent organization—the U.S. Powerlifting Federation. After that point, the USPF stood alone as an autonomous body.[38] As such, it had no affiliation with the AAU, the U.S. Olympic Committee, or any multisport agency advocating or conducting drug testing in sport. There was no code of ethics in the early USPF rulebooks; there were no discussions about what constitutes good sportsmanship. What mattered to the majority of these lifter-administrators was lifting more and more weight, watching the federation grow, and enjoying the United States' domination of the world record lists. Some of these early administrators also had commercial interests in powerlifting, and nearly all of them were deciding policy matters that would affect either their own competitive careers or their livelihoods. Such an arrangement does not promote objectivity. Because elections were held in conjunction with the men's national championships each year, many of the USPF's new administrators were elite-level male athletes openly opposed to any form of drug testing. And, because only state chairmen (appointed by the president) and executive committee members could vote in the national committee meetings, the USPF president could directly influence policy decisions through the people he appointed.[39]

Things finally came to a head in 1981 when, after lengthy debate and compromise, the USPF national committee voted by a narrow margin to test at the 1982 men's national championships *if* the IPF announced it would do a full IOC drug screen at the world championships in 1982. Several months later, when the IPF sent word to its national affiliates that there would definitely be testing at the 1982 world meets for men and women, the USPF executive committee overruled the previous summer's vote and announced that there would be no national testing program in 1982.[40] As frustration mounted among those who'd fought for testing since 1978, Edmund Martin Bishop—Brother Bennet of the Catholic order of the Brothers of the Sacred Heart—decided to abandon the USPF and give "drug-free" lifters another venue in which to compete.[41] The idea, as noted earlier, was not totally new.

Mike Lambert, editor of *Powerlifting USA*, had suggested a similar sort of organization in 1980 when he wrote in an editorial about the growing schism in the sport: "How does this sound? Let's form an organization . . . open only to powerlifters who will sign their name to a document stating that they will not take drugs as long as they hold membership. And let's keep track of the performances of the members of this organization . . . keep records of their clean lifts, perhaps even run local, regional and national contests for the members of the organization. With enough members and proper preparation, such an organization could exert significant political and even ethical influence on the sport eventually."[42]

In November 1981, at a meeting in Arlington, Virginia, Bennet and a group of like-minded friends adopted by-laws, elected an executive committee, and set up testing policies for the American Drug Free Powerlifting Association (ADFPA).[43] Bennet's approach to sport was based on his Christian belief in the goodness of humanity and the need for ethics and values in sport. "Drugs offend the concept of fairness," Bennet argued in a speech in 1982. "Athletic competitions are becoming more and more chemical competitions. Does this sound right?? Moral?? Ethical?? . . . If we are to have respect for others, we must first have respect for ourselves. A different world cannot be made by indifferent people."[44]

Trusting and honest, Bennet asked each new member of his organization to sign an oath swearing that "I hereby give my word of honor as an athlete that I have not used any strength-inducing drugs (i.e., any anabolic steroids or natural hormones) as part of my training during the past twelve months." Although Bennet hoped he would attract only those athletes whose word meant something, there were many instances of steroid-using athletes signing the oath to enter meets in which they thought they would have a better chance of winning a trophy.[45] Bennet caught some of these less-than-honorable offenders, but many fell through the cracks in his polygraph-based testing program. Because the ADFPA promised to test 10 percent of the lifters in every meet, the only economically feasible way to do that in the early days of the association was through the use of the polygraph, perhaps the least satisfying method of testing. Meet promoters were welcome to do urinalysis testing if they could afford it, but few ADFPA meets made enough money to offset the cost of this more reliable method.[46]

Despite many people's (including our own) reservations about the ADFPA's testing program, the organization grew considerably in 1982 and 1983 as large numbers of women and men abandoned the USPF in favor of "drug-free" competitions. Judy Gedney, longtime ADFPA lifter and administrator, explained her conversion: "If it hadn't been for the development of the ADFPA, I'm sure that the frustration of dealing with drug use within the USPF and the IPF would have discouraged me from continuing to participate in this sport . . . Drug testing motions were placed on the annual agendas regularly; sadly the sporting administrators had no interest in allowing drug testing within the sport of powerlifting. The organization of the USPF Women's Committee helped to promote drug-testing within the sport. Still, with the exception of select leaders with character, the USPF as a body did not want to establish a drug testing program."[47]

Yet, despite the new federation's rapid growth—the ADFPA held national championships for both men and women in 1983, and the first men's nationals attracted 120 lifters—there was still one big problem.[48] The USPF remained the officially recognized member of the IPF and so ADFPA athletes could not enter the now drug-tested IPF world championships, while the nontested USPF champions were free to go. Consequently, many drug-free athletes maintained memberships in both federations because they wanted the chance to attend the "worlds." (There was no parallel international federation at this time.)

As it grew, the ADFPA began to pose a threat to the growth of the USPF. In an attempt to gain control of the drug-free organization, USPF president Dr. Conrad Cotter proposed that the two groups co-sanction meets and thus, in effect, become truly parallel forms of the same sport. Although the ADFPA and the USPF jointly sanctioned a few meets in that first year, including the 1982 women's nationals, Brother Bennet soon realized that most of his lifters and administrative supporters wanted nothing to do with the USPF. Like Gedney, they'd lost confidence that the USPF would ever recognize the need for testing, and they'd lost respect for the people running the organization. *Ironman* publisher Peary Rader and his wife, Mabel, resigned from the USPF in 1982 for precisely those reasons. So did drug-testing advocate Nate Foster, a senior member of the USPF executive committee. In a letter to Rader on September 11, 1982, Bennet wrote: "It was a sad day indeed when you resigned from the USPF, but I can fully understand your disgust. So did Nate Foster. Then, perhaps, on the other hand, these are good signs because the people of integrity are beginning to show a greater interest in the ADFPA."[49]

## The Second Parallel Federation Solution

While "people of integrity" gravitated to the ADFPA over the next few years, the USPF, with even fewer members pushing for testing, became much more intransigent on the drug issue. When the IPF passed legislation in 1982 requiring all world record applications to include a negative drug-test report from an official IOC lab, Cotter and the USPF executive committee responded by announcing that they would begin keeping "USPF-Recognized World Records," which would follow IPF regulations in all respects except that no drug test would be required.[50] Cotter admitted that this would soon mean that many USPF records would probably exceed the IPF world records. However, he and some USPF leaders viewed the new IPF regulation as specifically anti-American as well as antidrug, and so decided to defy the IPF and start their own record list.[51]

The IPF rule regarding the testing of world records infuriated many of the top USPF lifters, whose primary reason for participating in powerlifting was to set records. In response, Ernie Frantz, a master (age group) lifter from Chicago, and his friend, nine-time world powerlifting champion Larry Pacifico, decided they would form a third national powerlifting organization, which they named the American Powerlifting Federation / American Masters Powerlifting Federation (APF/AMPF; also referred to simply as the APF). In a full-page ad in the January 1983 issue of *Powerlifting USA*, Frantz wrote: "Don't be dictated to—Lift the way you want to lift . . . Don't want testing? We won't have any." As Frantz went on to explain in the ad, "We want to run our own organization the way we, the lifters see fit . . . There are more powerlifters in the US than any other country in the world, yet we are dictated to by a small minority of foreign lifters. The . . . APF will bring the power back where it belongs—to you, the American lifter."[52]

The APF held its first organizational meeting on January 28, 1983, on the same weekend and in the same place as the USPF women's national championships. From the beginning, Frantz wanted there to be no confusion about the drug stance of his group. In the promotional materials he circulated that weekend, trying to get members to join with him, "Item One" on his "Proposal for APF/AMPF Meeting" reads: "I don't believe in any testing whatsoever at any time." Frantz's reason for starting the new federation was more complicated than simply a desire to use drugs and lift big weights. He was not happy, he told Jan Todd, about being a rule breaker. In a conversation that weekend, Frantz explained that he was tired of the hypocrisy of the USPF's position on drug testing and he didn't like the idea that he was using drugs in a federation that supposedly banned them. He felt that a more ethical choice would be to have a federation in which everyone knew that drug use was a permitted option and in which drug-using lifters weren't taking a trophy from some clean lifter who didn't want to use drugs.[53] Although Frantz's position sounds admirable, the reality was that most lifters who joined the APF did not give up their USPF membership, because that was still the only avenue to the IPF world championships.

So, while some top lifters joined the APF, many stayed with the USPF, especially after the IPF announced that any lifter participating in an APF meet (with its open drug policy) would face a two-year suspension from the world championships.[54] As things stood, however, antitesting lifters in the United States had little reason to leave the USPF with President Cotter at the helm. At the 1984 women's nationals held in Austin, for instance, urine samples from the winners, record breakers, and other, randomly selected lifters were sent to the new IOC testing lab at the University of California, Los Angeles. However, Cotter imposed no sanctions against those women who tested positive, nor did he publicly announce who they were.[55] Writing in *Powerlifting USA*, Cotter—with tortured logic—claimed that even though the USPF had voted to test, the vote did not mean that it also had to impose sanctions: "It will, of course, be argued that the pro testing people, especially members of the Women's Committee, feel very strongly that sanctions must be applied, however belatedly, in order to preserve the integrity of the US team and the sport. It will be argued that failure to impose sanctions will make a mockery of drug testing and will unfairly nullify the victory of those who fought so hard for testing at Austin last July. It will be argued that sanctions may legitimately be implied from this contract." However, Cotter continued, "Strong feelings confer no legal right," and he saw no need to impose sanctions, because the legislation had not specifically included such directions.[56] That the legislation specifically required that IOC protocol be followed, in all respects, did, of course, imply sanctions.[57] However, no sanctions were ever imposed.[58] Why the IPF did not drop the USPF at this juncture and offer membership to the ADFPA remains a mystery. However, despite the USPF's intransigence on the drug question—in July 1984, for instance, its national committee again voted not to have mandatory testing at either the men's or women's nationals in 1985—the IPF did not sever its relationship.[59]

And so, by 1984, American powerlifting had three distinct federations with three sets of records and three different philosophies on the drug question. And, within a couple of years—when it became clear that the IPF intended to continue its alliance with the USPF—there were three international federations as well.[60] The APF's world championships were scheduled for Chicago on September 17, 1984.[61] However, among those who responded to Frantz's invitation was a small group of South African lifters who'd been banned from participation in the IPF because of apartheid.[62] Although that meet attracted only 20 lifters, it proved to be a pivotal event in the history of powerlifting. Following the contest, the IPF suspended Ernie Frantz; Maris Sternberg, the APF's secretary; lifter Felicia Johnson; and Ernie's wife, Diane Frantz, also a top U.S. lifter. For Sternberg and Johnson, this meant they were also off the USPF world team, a position they'd earned by their victory in the USPF nationals. They decided to sue. According to Sternberg, "We ended up serving court papers to the USPF and IPF officials at Men's Senior Nationals in June 1985 in Chicago. The lawsuit included Ernie, Diane, Frantz Sports, and me. There were a number of charges, including restriction of trade and violation of civil rights . . . Eventually, we wound up in court . . . We sued under the Clayton Act which simply stated that you can't ban an amateur athlete from competing any place they choose."[63]

The Frantz lawsuit named the IPF, the USPF, and Conrad Cotter as an individual.[64] The legal battle stretched on for four years, ending at the Seventh U.S. District Court in the spring of 1988. In the end, the court found that Frantz and the IPF were both at fault. Some of Frantz's antitrust charges were clearly frivolous. However, the court also found that the IPF could not limit the participation of an amateur athlete to only one federation if it operated in the United States. The lawsuit's impact reverberated throughout the powerlifting community as lifters realized that powerlifting membership could not be controlled by any one federation. Now, anyone, anywhere in the United States could begin a new federation, write rules that fit his or her notion of what the sport should be, and begin sponsoring meets with impunity. What no one could have predicted as an outcome of the Frantz lawsuit, however, was that powerlifting would attract *so many* adherents to the Frank Sinatra ("I did it my way") school of ethics.

## Parallel Federations for Everyone

Even before the Frantz lawsuit finished its passage through the U.S. courts, disagreement about what constituted a "drug-free" lifter had prompted the formation of several new powerlifting federations. At issue was the ADFPA's policy that lifters had only to swear that they hadn't taken any anabolic drugs in the past 12 months. Some lifters who had never used anabolic drugs felt they were at a disadvantage against the athlete who had used drugs in the past. So, the Natural Powerlifting Federation formed, and by 1986 it was holding meets for "lifetime drug-free" lifters whose status was theoretically verified by polygraph testing. Although the ADFPA increased its "clean period" to 18, 24, and finally 36 months over the next decade, another group, the International Powerlifting Alliance, also formed, requiring lifters to have abstained from drug use for a period of at least 5 years. In 1988, the American Natural Physique and Powerlifting Committee offered yet another alternative by hosting 5-year, 10-year, and lifetime drug-free divisions.

The proliferation of powerlifting federations was inadvertently accelerated by the USPF. In 1985, the USPF sent what it assumed would be winning teams to the IPF world championships for men and juniors. In both instances, the American teams won the championships and then had to forfeit the team trophy when postcompetition drug tests found American lifters positive for banned substances. Two American women were also found positive at the 1985 women's world championships, prompting Mike Lambert of *Powerlifting USA* to write: "This is the greatest drug testing scandal in American powerlifting annals and many lifters are appalled at what has taken place." One lifter told him that powerlifting had degenerated into the "the Hell's Angels of organized sport."[65]

The USPF responded to this public humiliation by—at long last—agreeing to follow IPF testing guidelines at its 1986 national championships. USPF president Conrad Cotter softened the blow for his constituents, however, by recommending a popular drug guidebook that would help lifters calculate their chances of being caught by the test.[66] Rather than attracting "drug-free" users back to the USPF, as Cotter had hoped, the new testing program was viewed with distrust by most in the ADFPA. An informal poll of ADFPA lifters revealed that they felt more comfortable lifting in a federation in which every meet was tested by polygraph than they did lifting in a federation in which testing occurred only at the national championships.[67]

It was clear that because most of the USPF's top administrators had for years been recalcitrant on the question of testing, "drug-free" lifters of any affiliation had little faith in the integrity of the officials administering the new testing program. It was no secret that Cotter and the USPF voted to test only when they'd been publicly humiliated and threatened with expulsion from the IPF after the 1985 world championship results. Still, rather than promising his constituents that he and his administrators planned to clean up the sport, Cotter subtly let it be known that the testing program the USPF planned to put in place would not stop drug use. In an editorial in *Powerlifting USA*, Cotter chastised ADFPA lifters for not rejoining the USPF, while at the same time making fun of their preference for a more holistic testing program. Cotter described ADFPA members as "bitter" and wrote: "They are angry when they learn with state-of-the-art drug testing the millennium has not arrived." Cotter added: "They cannot cope with the fact that one may test negative by tapering wisely and by turning to other, legal anabolic agents."[68]

What's more, some drug-using lifters who didn't want to learn how to beat the test and were tired of the hypocrisy abandoned the USPF in favor of Frantz's APF, bolstering its numbers considerably. Other lifters, however, fell into what *Powerlifting USA* author Ted Kurlowicz described as the "grey area between the drug free lifters and those who openly use such substances." Kurlowicz claimed that these lifters, who he believed constituted the majority of American powerlifters, would simply continue taking their drugs, learn how to beat the USPF urinalysis tests (or avoid the USPF nationals when testing occurred), or gamble that they could beat an ADFPA polygraph exam.[69] If this assessment is correct, which seems likely, having parallel federations simply gave the drug-using athlete more venues in which to strive for trophies, while the nonuser was still not guaranteed a drug-free playing field.

Another lifter, in a letter to the editor printed two months after Cotter's announcement of the new testing program, undoubtedly expressed what many drug-using athletes felt at this moment in time:

> Perhaps it is the end of an era in powerlifting, but I don't think so, not unless the competitors are all gone. You see, so long as there are real competitors in our sport or, for that matter, in any sport, there will be some sort of drug use. A competitor just can't draw a line between what to do and what not to do to win . . . it's a very simple decision. You do anything & everything . . . Just winning a contest is not enough, not unless the performance was absolutely perfect. Only when there is perfection can there be no improvement, and we all know that perfection does not exist in our mortal world. There is always room for improvement, always another goal to attain, always another level of achievement to be reached. Competitors will

drive themselves to these goals using all means available. It has been instilled in us as far back as Little League . . . It's a tough path to follow, but it's the path that many of us have chosen.[70]

In an attempt to regain some of its members and to clean up its image, the USPF gave permission for Oklahoma meet promoter Rich Peters to begin sponsoring USPF "drug-free" contests in 1986. Using polygraph testing of the participants, Peters gave trophies in three divisions: 1 to 3 months clean, 2 to 6 months clean, and 1 year clean.[71] Peters claimed that he started these new meets to "offer everyone an opportunity to clean up and go natural."[72] However, a powerful incentive for many was the chance to win one of the five- to six-foot-tall trophies Peters regularly gave to his winners and the chance to set a new kind of American record.

The desire to take home a trophy or be a record holder is undoubtedly at the heart of many of powerlifting's problems. Unlike marathon running, cycling, tennis, and other forms of adult sport in which large numbers of athletes compete but only a few receive medals or trophies, powerlifting promoters give away dozens of trophies in a variety of age and weight divisions at each meet. A 19-year-old woman, for instance, could conceivably take home the open trophy for her weight class, the collegiate trophy for her weight class, the junior trophy for her weight class, and, if it was her first meet, perhaps a novice trophy, too—even if she was the only lifter in her weight class. Because powerlifting has 11 weight classes for men and 10 for women, and it is normal to give awards through the first five places in a variety of age and experience groups, it is not uncommon for every lifter who enters a meet to leave with some sort of trophy. At the 2004 Longhorn Open Powerlifting Championships, in Austin, Texas, for example, 109 trophies were awarded to the 98 lifters in the meet. In 2007, the Longhorn Open had 129 lifters and awarded 111 trophies.[73] In fact, most meet directors order trophies based on the number of entries received.

Records work in much the same way. World, national, state, age-group, and experience-group records are kept for each weight class, in all three lifts, and in the combined total, for both men and women. Before the parallel federation solution, powerlifting had one set of world records and one set of American records, and the men and women who held those records felt a considerable sense of achievement. By early 2008, however, there were approximately 18 federations keeping American records and at least 17 "international" associations keeping world records. To talk about records these days, one has to first identify the federation in which the record was set and then specify both the rules for the performance of the lift (which now vary widely from federation to federation) and the kind of supportive equipment the federation allows. A 600-pound bench press for a superheavyweight in the 100 percent Raw Powerlifting Federation, for example—in which a normal T-shirt must be worn—would be a phenomenal achievement. The same lift made by a superheavyweight at a World Powerlifting Organization (WPO) meet would be laughed off the stage. This is so because the WPO allows lifters to wear specially made, highly supportive bench-press shirts with multiple layers of fabric (canvas and denim preferred, with bungee cords or Kevlar often sewn in as reinforcement to provide a springlike effect), which are generally thought to add several hundred pounds of mechanical advantage to the lift. Former American powerlifting champion Joe Ladnier, for example, told us in October 2004 that he decided to return to lifting after a 10-year retirement when he realized that the 350-pound benches he performed regularly in training would allow him to lift more than 600 pounds when wearing one of these remarkable shirts.[74]

Beyond records and trophies, however, the most common reason for the proliferation of federations in powerlifting has been a personal desire to control the drug testing programs and other constitutive rules of the sport. Rich Peters, for example, wasn't content to just run the "natural nationals" program for the USPF. After an unsuccessful campaign to become the new USPF president in 1990, Peters left the USPF to focus his energies on building a new organization—the Natural Athletes Strength Association. This association, which still sanctions meets and keeps both national and "world" records, has a lengthy list of banned drugs on its website, but implementation of testing is now left solely to the discretion of the individual meet director. At some of its meets, as many as 10 lifters are tested; at other meets, only one lifter will be called on for testing, which saves Peters hundreds of dollars in testing fees.[75] Further, Peters has deviated from other organizations' rules by creating "power sport" divisions in which lifters do the curl, bench press, and deadlift—as they did in early odd-lift meets—and by allowing lifters to wear squat suits and bench-press shirts that aren't permitted in other organizations.[76]

Most of the other federations on the powerlifting landscape over the past two decades were started by individuals who wanted the sport to move in a particular direction or who felt that they had no power within the existing associations. L. B. Baker, for example, began his career in the USPF, moved to the APF, and now runs the American Powerlifting Committee (APC). Baker said in a telephone interview: "When Ernie Frantz decided to sell his federations to Kieran Kidder, it made many of us angry. We didn't like Kieran's vision for the sport and so a group of us got together and formed the APC and WPC [World Powerlifting Congress]. What Kieran's running is like a wrestling circuit . . . He just wants the stars to break records and everyone knows that—especially the judges . . . It just didn't sit well with me, so I decided to go my own way." Former APF member Jesse Rogers began the small Southern Powerlifting Federation for similar reasons. "I just wanted to lift with the rules I was used to. When I couldn't do that, I started my own federation. I'm not planning to make this into a national federation. I just want to do things my way, so the local lifters here in my area know their lifts will be judged fairly." Similarly, Dr. Darrell Latch began the Son Light Power Federation (SLP) in 2000 in "reaction to the frustration I was feeling with certain federations, which I had worked with in the past, and which I felt I had been severely taken advantage of." Latch, who had previously worked with the American Natural Physique and Powerlifting Committee, an organization that prided itself on testing *every* lifter at its meets, has no clear-cut testing program for his own SLP. His reason for not testing, he explained, was that "any half-smart lifter knows how to get by any test. Plus most of the organizations that claim to test are not doing so, or at least not nearly as many tests as they claim to do." And Sonny Runyon of Muncie, Indiana, decided he'd begin his own federation because he came to believe that "my opinion didn't count." "I work with a lot of kids," Runyon said, "and I kept telling the USAPL [USA Powerlifting] that they needed to change the rules so kids wouldn't have to buy the expensive suits and wraps now required for competition. But they didn't listen so I figured I'd just do things on my own. I've had as many as 800 members in my Indiana State Powerlifting Association and I don't plan to grow. I just want to work with my state, my kids, and to get things going in the right direction."[77]

With such a variety of federations to choose from, some federations, like Latch's SLP, openly compete for members by giving larger and larger trophies and by making things easier on lifters during competition. "I have gotten to the point," Latch said, "where I encourage lifters to just come and do their best, compete mostly against yourself (because there are now so many divisions and weight classes, every lifter will receive a nice award). I allow any kind of equipment . . . I figure if a person spends the money they should be able to use it."[78]

The APF led the way in deviating from the existing IPF rules (on matters other than drug testing) by instructing its referees to ease up on small infractions. "The lifters have come here today to find out who's best and that's the important thing," Frantz told a reporter at the APF world championships in 1987. "If we've got to switch a bar to help a person out in the middle of a meet, we're going to do it; if they need extra time for warmup we're going to do that also

. . . you have to be able to bend with the majority of lifters . . . we better pay attention to these top lifters or there isn't going to be any organization."[79] Kieran Kidder, who purchased Frantz's APF and WPC holdings and began the professional WPO in 2003, put it even more bluntly. "I find it puzzling to think that so many lifters still insist on lifting in overbearing, domineering federations that brainwash them," Kidder wrote on his WPO website in 2003.[80] On another occasion, Kidder explained that "people need to understand that what we're doing is as much entertainment as it is sport. Fans like to see record lifts and our lifters like to make record lifts, so our rules about equipment, drug-testing and performance of the lifts are all designed to create new American and world records. It's show business."[81]

Whatever their motivations for joining, lifters have had plenty of federations to choose from over the past two decades. An examination of the "Coming Events" column in *Powerlifting USA* over the past 25 years reveals more than a dozen additional federations that are no longer in existence. Throughout this era there have been numerous calls for reunification of the sport, and in 1996, after lengthy and painful negotiations, the ADFPA merged with part of the membership of the USPF; the new association was named USA Powerlifting (USAPL) and was finally admitted as the official American representative to the IPF.[82] Since that time, USAPL has risen to prominence in the United States as the largest and most influential of all federations. USAPL does urinalysis testing at all contests and also runs an out-of-competition testing program. However, USAPL is still just one of many federations sanctioning meets and keeping records in the United States.

Table 3.1, compiled primarily from web documents, shows all federations known to be in existence in January 2008. A similar list, compiled in 2003 for presentation at The Hastings Center's Conference on Ethical, Conceptual and Scientific Issues in the Use of Performance Enhancing Technologies in Sport, included 16 American federations and 11 international organizations. As can be seen, there is still considerable diversity among these groups.

## Is There a Future for the Parallel Federation Solution?

When we began our study of parallel federations as a possible solution to the problem of doping in sport, we looked for other sports that had experience with this. However, although we asked many academic friends, as well as the members of the Sport History List Serve, the only other sport we found with parallel federations was bodybuilding. Bodybuilding also has both drug-tested and non-

TABLE 3.1

The Drug-Testing Policies and Equipment Rules of National and International Powerlifting Associations, January 2008

| Powerlifting Associations | Details | Drug-Testing Policy | Equipment Rules |
|---|---|---|---|
| **NATIONAL** | | | |
| AAU Powerlifting Committee (AAUPC) | Keeps world and U.S. records | Urinalysis by independent group; out-of-competition testing | Permits denim and Velcro on bench-press shirts; only 1-ply for lifting suits |
| Amateur American Powerlifting Federation (AAPF) | Partner organization to APF; formed by Ernie Frantz | Uses non-IOC-level labs to test for shortened list of drugs; not comparable with USAPL or IPF testing programs | No limit on number of layers of fabric; Velcro, canvas, and denim OK |
| American Drug Free Powerlifting Federation (ADFPF) | Formed after unification of ADFPA with USPF by group of former drug-free lifters, so U.S. lifters could continue to compete in WDFPF | Same testing program as WDFPF, which includes IOC-type and out-of competition testing | Follows WDFPF rules that allow for only 1-ply fabric in shirts and suits; no Velcro, canvas, or denim |
| American Frantz Powerlifting Federation and Amateur Frantz Powerlifting Federation (AFPF/AAPF) | Announced by Ernie Frantz in December 2007; inaugural meet in March 2008 | No testing | Permits unlimited layers of material in suits and shirts; canvas, denim, and Velcro OK |
| American Powerlifting Alliance (APA) | Runs "standard" and "unlimited gear" divisions, drug-tested and nontested divisions | Testing at meet director's discretion; no list of banned substances; Aegis Lab, Inc., is designated testing facility; if testing, 10% of top 3 lifters in each division are tested | "Standard" division: canvas and denim not permitted; "unlimited gear" division: canvas gear with any number of layers |
| American Powerlifting Committee (APC) | Formed by L. B. Baker after sale of APF in May 2003; U.S. affiliate to GPC | Amateur division tested; no list of drugs or methods on website; no testing at pro level | Permits suit and shirt with any number of layers as long as just 1 suit or 1 shirt; denim OK, canvas not permitted |

| Federation | Description | Testing | Equipment rules |
|---|---|---|---|
| American Powerlifting Federation (APF) | Formed by Ernie Frantz in 1983; now affiliated with WPC | No testing | No limit on number of layers of fabric; Velcro, canvas, and denim OK |
| Anti-Drug Athletes United (ADAU) | Begun by Al Siegel; keeps U.S. records only and runs only "raw" meets | Urinalysis and polygraph testing; publishes urinalysis results on website | No supportive gear of any kind permitted, except knee wraps and belt |
| Iron Boy Powerlifting (IBP) | Offers both "equipped" and "raw" divisions | Website claims there is substance abuse program, but no details of drug testing found | "Raw" division: no supportive equipment permitted; "equipped" division: only 1-ply fabric in suits and shirts |
| National Alliance of Powerlifters (NAP) | Aim is to give "all powerlifters the opportunity to compete in a drug-free environment without unreasonable parameters" | Urinalysis | No rules on website; mission statement suggests more supportive gear permitted than in other drug-free federations |
| Natural Athletes Strength Association (NASA) | Keeps U.S. and world records; begun by Rich Peters, formerly of USPF | Lengthy drug list, including androstenedione; testing at discretion of officials, who determine who and how many are tested | Permits only 1-ply suits and shirts; uniforms must be sanctioned by NASA |
| Python Powerlifting League | Local federation started by T. Meyers in Augusta, GA | Drug-free; no explanation of testing | Permits shin guards in deadlift; shorts OK for all lifts; hats and head gear OK |
| Southern Powerlifting Federation (SPF) | Began as regional organization in 2000, then formed WBPA in 2004; now also offers world records | No testing | "Equipped" division: suits or shirts of any thickness permitted |
| Syndicated Strength Alliance (SSA) | Motto: "No Idols, No Heroes, No Leaders; Just Pure Inner Strength"; runs two divisions of contests based on type of equipment | No testing | Requires suits and bench shirts for all meets. "A maximum of 'if you got it, bring it' layers are allowed." No restriction on thickness or type of material or mix of material; no restriction on plies as long as only 1 component. |

continued

TABLE 3.1 *continued*

| Powerlifting Associations | Details | Drug-Testing Policy | Equipment Rules |
|---|---|---|---|
| United Powerlifting Association (UPA) | Formed in 2007 | Short list of banned drugs on website; no discussion on how testing works | Permits suits and shirts with 2 layers of fabric of any type |
| United States Powerlifting Federation (USPF) | Splinter group that kept USPF name after ADFPA and old USPF unified | Website: "Nothing in the rule book about testing; no test for a World Record" | Permits 1-ply polyester squat suits only, 1-ply poly or denim in bench shirts |
| USA Powerlifting (USAPL) | Largest federation in U.S.; formed from unification of ADFPA and USPF in 1996; U.S. affiliate to IPF | Rigorous testing program; includes out-of-competition testing; uses WADA list of banned substances | Permits only 1-ply suits and shirts; no canvas, denim, or Velcro |
| USA Raw Bench Press Federation | Formed by Darrel Latch, founder of Son Light Power Federation | No testing | Permits only T-shirts and other nonsupportive shirts |
| **INTERNATIONAL** | | | |
| Amateur World Powerlifting Congress (AWPC) | Division of WPC that sponsors drug-tested competitions; many federations use *amateur* to denote athletes who do not use drugs | Uses own list of banned drugs; shorter list than IOC | Permits multiple-ply suits and shirts; canvas, denim, and Velcro OK |
| Global Powerlifting Committee (GPC) | Formerly known as World Powerlifting Committee; U.S. affiliate is APC | No testing | Permits up to 2-ply bench shirts, polyester or denim; Velcro OK, but no canvas; unlimited-ply lifting suits allowed, polyester, denim, or canvas |
| 100% RAW Powerlifting Federation | Founded in 1999; keeps world and U.S. records | Urinalysis and polygraph testing | No gear allowed except T-shirts, belts, and 1-layer, lightweight, nonsupportive lifting suits (singlets) |
| International Powerlifting Association (IPA); Amateur IPA (AIPA) | | Tests only in amateur division; very short list of banned drugs | Simple rule book; few regulations; only 2-ply fabric; any fabric; no thickness limit on belt |

| Federation | Description | Testing | Equipment |
|---|---|---|---|
| International Powerlifting Federation (IPF) | Oldest, most prestigious international federation; USAPL is U.S. affiliate | Follows WADA/IOC rules, including out-of-competition testing | Permits only 1-ply fabric; no canvas or denim. IPF still sets the standards in rules and equipment from which all other federations deviate. |
| International Strength Association (ISA) | Established in 2000; very lax rules on uniform | No testing mentioned on website | Permits 2 shirts, each of multiple layers, for bench press; suits with no more than 2 thicknesses of fabric; no mention of illegal fabrics |
| Son Light Power International Powerlifting Federation | Run by Dr. Darrell Latch to make meets more friendly to lifters; holds meets in "raw" and "open" divisions | No testing | "Open" division: no restrictions; no limit on layers or material |
| United World Powerlifting Federation (UWPF) | Formed in 2002 by Dr. Mauro Di Pasquali of Canada, in attempt to unify various international federations | IOC/IPF drug list on website; no clarification of how testing is done | Uses IPF equipment list on website |
| World Association of Benchers and Deadlifters (WABDL) | Sponsors single-lift meets in bench press and deadlift | Website: "tests for steroids, clenbuterol, and speed . . . abnormally high testosterone levels and TE ratios. It does not test for anything that is available over the counter such as Norandrosterone or the various 19 norandros . . . Ephedrine or any legal, over the counter stimulant is allowed but not recommended because of the harmful side effects." | Permits shirts with up to 2-ply material for bench press; specifies manufacturers, types of seams, and types of stitching considered legal in contests; uses different rules for bench press than IPF and many other federations |
| World Bench and Powerlifting Association (WBPA) | Established in 2004; governing body for SPF in the U.S. | No testing | Permits up to 3 layers of fabric, any type, in suits and shirts; Velcro OK |

*continued*

TABLE 3.1 *continued*

| Powerlifting Associations | Details | Drug-Testing Policy | Equipment Rules |
|---|---|---|---|
| World Drug Free Powerlifting Federation (WDFPF) | ADFPF is U.S. affiliate; has "equipped" and "raw" divisions | Out-of-competition testing; uses WADA/IOC list; at least 20% of lifters must be tested; designates drug-free lifter as one who has not used anabolic drugs for 5 years | Permits only 1-ply lifting suits and shirts; no canvas, Velcro, or denim |
| World Natural Powerlifting Federation (WNPF) | Formerly part of WDFPF, which didn't want to do IOC drug tests; wanted to test back in time using polygraph; offers "lifetime" drug-free divisions; recently announced "unlimited" division, meaning athletes can wear some supportive gear | Combination of urinalysis and polygraph testing; if positive test, 3-year ban | "Single-ply" division: only polyester, 1-ply suits and bench shirts permitted; in new "unlimited" division: 2-ply shirts of poly or denim, squat suits of poly or canvas with up to 3 layers of fabric |
| World Powerlifting Association (WPA) | Affiliated with APA | All contests above local level must offer drug-tested division in which 20% of lifters tested; open-division lifters not tested | Permits bike pants for bench; no denim or canvas in squat suits; denim bench shirts, 2-ply shirts OK; Velcro OK on back; Kevlar equipment not allowed |
| World Powerlifting Congress (WPC) | Established by Ernie Frantz in 1986; now has 30 member-nations | No testing | No limit on number of fabric layers; Velcro, canvas, and denim OK |
| World Powerlifting Federation (WPF) | Formed after Kieran Kidder bought WPA and turned it into WPO | No mention of testing on website | Permits only 1-ply; denim OK; no canvas; Velcro OK on bench shirts |
| World Powerlifting Organization (WPO) | Professional federation formed after purchase of APF/WPC from Frantz | No testing | No rules on supportive gear |

*Source:* Compiled by Jan Todd, mainly from website information, January 2008.

*Abbreviations:* ADFPA, American Drug Free Powerlifting Association; IOC, International Olympic Committee; TE, testosterone/epitestosterone ratio; WADA, World Anti-Doping Agency.

drug-tested federations, and, much like powerlifting, some athletes or administrators who are unhappy with one version of the sport simply stepped away and started their own federation. By January 2008, 19 different bodybuilding organizations had web pages (table 3.2). And like the smorgasbord of federations available in powerlifting, bodybuilding federations also vary dramatically in their lists of banned drugs, methods of testing, and definition of "drug-free."

The finding that bodybuilding's experience with the parallel federation solution seems to have replicated the impact felt by powerlifting prompts us to counsel sports administrators looking for solutions to the problem of drug use in sport to be wary of this "solution." As we've tried to document in this chapter, the implementation of the parallel federation solution in powerlifting has been a classic example of what sociologist Robert Merton called "the law of unintended consequences."[83] While the idea of creating a drug-free federation sounded, at first, like an easy, ethically defensible solution, the lesson from powerlifting's history is that once the idea of parallel federations takes root, there is no way to stop an endless succession of additional federations from forming and interpreting powerlifting on their own—and different—terms. Who could have foreseen, for example, that it would have been so difficult to find general agreement among powerlifters about what it means to be "drug-free." Who could have predicted that more than one nontesting federation would be seen as desirable? For powerlifting, the parallel federation solution has acted like kudzu—a vine imported into the southern United States in the first half of the twentieth century to control erosion and provide food for cattle. Kudzu didn't control erosion, however, and cattle didn't like it. It didn't solve any of the southern farmer's problems and, in fact, added to them when it was discovered that kudzu could grow so rapidly in the warm southern climate that it would completely cover and obscure a house in one summer. In powerlifting, the parallel federation solution is also choking out the very thing it was supposed to save. Underneath these many federations are the remnants of a unified sport, but the growth of vines on top will soon reduce it to just a memory.

Perhaps there is nothing wrong with this. Perhaps we are too wedded to our own memories of the halcyon years of powerlifting when it had national television contracts and mainstream media attention, and when its membership shared a belief that the sport was "going somewhere." The historian Allen Guttmann suggests that sports become "modern" by creating bureaucracies, keeping records, and becoming systematically organized.[84] Powerlifting certainly embraced "modernity" in the 1960s and 1970s as the fledgling sport moved from an exhibition oddity to a rationally ordered sport with a hierarchical international government.

TABLE 3.2

*The Drug-Testing Policies of National and International Bodybuilding Federations*

| Bodybuilding Federations | Details | Drug-Testing Policies |
|---|---|---|
| **NATIONAL** | | |
| Amateur Bodybuilding Association (ABA) | Affiliated with INBA | Urinalysis and polygraph used. "Drug-free" defined as 5-year period of no drug use. Out-of-competition tests on athletes on national team (polygraph and urinalysis). |
| Musclemania | Professional; began in 1991; more a sponsored tour than a true federation | Urinalysis at discretion of meet director; short list of drugs; no growth hormone listed or drugs other than various anabolic agents. |
| National Gym Association (NGA) | Professional and amateur divisions; began in 1979 as means to certify gym employees | Requires 7-year clean period for professional contestants; 5 years for amateurs. Polygraph testing before contests, followed by urinalysis of top 7 competitors in each class. Modified list of drugs, not full WADA or IOC list. |
| National Physique Committee (NPC) | Professional and amateur; U.S. affiliate of IFBB; began in 1982 | Although U.S. affiliate of IFBB, no mention of drug use or drug testing on website. |
| Natural Physique Association (NPA) | Promotes amateur and professional contests; began in 2002 | No testing details available on website. |
| North American Natural Bodybuilding Federation (NANBF) | Affiliated with WNBF and INBF; began in 1989 | Tests at every meet, using combination of polygraph and urinalysis. Athlete must be clean for 7 years. Uses its own list of drugs, not IOC drug list. |
| Organization of Competitive Bodybuilders (OCB) | Founded in 2003; U.S. affiliate of IFPA | Combination of urinalysis and polygraph testing, at discretion of meet director. Like IFPA, certain drugs banned for different time limits. |
| Supernatural Bodybuilding and Fitness Organization (SNBF) | Amateur; contestants must be drug-free for at least 5 years | Uses list of banned substances comparable to WADA/IOC list; both polygraph and urinalysis testing. All competitors must take test each November to stay eligible in the organization. |
| United States Bodybuilding Federation (USBF) | Professional and amateur divisions; began in 1999 when AAU dropped bodybuilding | Uses IOC list of drugs; urinalysis testing only. Tests top finishers in each contest and at least 10% of all competitors. Also some out-of-competition testing. |

## INTERNATIONAL

|  | |  |
|---|---|---|
| International Drug Free Athletics (IDFA) | Founded in 2005 | Uses polygraph, voice stress tests, and urinalysis testing. Organizer (promoter) has option to use more than one method of testing (i.e., polygraph and urinalysis) at an event. Testing based on WADA list of banned substances. |
| International Federation of Bodybuilding and Fitness (IFBB) | Professional; largest, oldest, most prestigious federation; runs Mr. and Ms. Olympia | In 2003, signed an agreement accepting WADA antidoping code. In 2005, adopted rules permitting testing at meets and out of competition. No mention on website of positive drug tests or implementation of testing. |
| International Fitness and Physique Association (IFPA) | Professional; affiliated with OCB | Uses polygraph test for each competitor; after contests, also does urinalysis on winners and top placers. Uses its own drug list and sets time frames for last use of drugs; e.g., androstendione cannot have been used since 2005; Dianabol cannot have been used since 2002. |
| International Natural Bodybuilding and Fitness Federation (INBF) | Amateur; affiliated with WNBF and NANBF | Tests at every meet, using combination of polygraph and urinalysis. Athlete must be clean for 7 years. Uses own, shorter list of drugs, not IOC list. |
| International Natural Bodybuilding Association (INBA) | Affiliated with PNBA | Advertises that it is now affiliated with WADA, although it also continues to do polygraph tests. "Drug-free" defined as 5-year period of no drug use. Out-of-competition tests on athletes on national team (polygraph and urinalysis). |
| National Amateur Body Builders Association International (NABBA) and NABBAUSA | Second oldest professional organization; sponsors Mr. Universe contest; 50 member-countries; offers drug-tested and nontested contests | At "natural" contests, tests for short list of "anabolic" agents derived from WADA/IOC list. Also does polygraph testing. Positive urinalysis results in 3-year ban. No testing at other contests. |
| Professional Natural Bodybuilding Association (PNBA) | Affiliated with INBA; sponsors Natural Mr. and Ms. Olympia | INBA advertises that it is now affiliated with WADA, although continues to do polygraph tests. "Drug-free" defined as 5-year period of no drug use. Out-of-competition tests on athletes on national team (polygraph and urinalysis). |

continued

TABLE 3.2 *continued*

| Bodybuilding Federations | Details | Drug-Testing Policies |
|---|---|---|
| World Bodybuilding and Fitness Association (WBFA) | Began in 2000; sponsors Mr. and Ms. America contests | No mention of drug testing on website. |
| World Natural Bodybuilding Federation (WNBF) | Professional; runs Pro Natural Mr. Universe; started in 1989 | Each athlete tested by long-method polygraph by certified examiners before admittance to event. Men and women must then submit to urinalysis testing conducted by the California lab that performed urine tests for 1984 Los Angeles Olympics. To win prize money, athletes must pass both tests, verifying that no steroids, diuretics, growth hormones, or other illegal drugs have been used in the past 7 years. |
| World Natural Sport Organization (WNSO) | Aims to promote "natural-looking" physiques and connect athletes with modeling and TV opportunities; sponsors bodybuilding, figure, fitness, and modeling contests | At sanctioned events, athletes screened by a "physique screening panel" the day before contest or during first round of competition on show day. If panel determines athlete does not fit "natural look" and/or it has reason to conclude that athlete has used banned substances, athlete must provide immediate urine sample to be eligible to compete in contest. Overall champions and winners *may* also be flagged for urine testing after contest. Also, random testing out of competition. |

*Source:* Compiled by Jan Todd, mainly from website information, January 2008.

*Abbreviations:* IOC, International Olympic Committee; WADA, World Anti-Doping Agency.

Perhaps our unease comes from the fact that powerlifting is no longer a "modern" sport, as Guttmann defined the concept. Perhaps a better framework for the present powerlifting landscape is postmodernism. Although postmodernism began as a theoretical approach to architecture and art in the 1970s, the concept has great applicability to the study of modern sport.[85] Certainly, powerlifting's many federations are a rejection of the notion that sport must be logically organized and represent a single value system. Postmodernists would ask: Why shouldn't powerlifting turn away from order and bureaucracy in favor of creative interpretations of the rules? Why shouldn't everyone be able to do sport on their own terms?

We would argue that "postmodern" powerlifting is wrong because it is, at its center, egoistic. It rejects any consideration of the integrity of the sport itself and reduces excellence and achievement in powerlifting to a race to get one's name on as many record lists as possible, even though most of those record lists and world and national titles now have little meaning—the sporting equivalent of the Tower of Babel. A good example of this is the story Larry Pacifico told an on-line reporter when he was asked about his funniest memory in powerlifting. Pacifico's remembrance wasn't of some lift he missed because of equipment failure or something that might have happened on one of his many international trips. What he recalled was meeting a young lifter earlier that year who claimed "as many world titles as I have." But, said Larry (who won nine world championships in the old IPF), "he won three in one year," and "for two of them he was the only lifter in his class."[86]

Beyond our concerns about the egoistic nature of modern powerlifting, the parallel federation solution has also resulted in a breakdown of the moral authority of many sports administrators. When athletes are faced with a cornucopia of choices for competition, sports organizations lose their ability to restrict or sanction certain forms of behavior. As the sociologist John MacAloon points out, when "society withdraws its gift of moral legitimation, the organization necessarily falls into a crisis marked by the progressive decline of its moral authority into factionalized assertions of mere power and interest." When there are many federations to choose from, including some whose existence can be attributed solely to the self-interest of the founder, moral authority weakens further. Fearful of taking hard-line stances on rules and doping, many administrators look the other way and concentrate on boosterism. They have become what MacAloon fears most for the future of sport: "mere utilitarians." They are people who have "surrendered any legitimate claim to wider social and moral legitimacy." Finally, just as MacAloon has documented in the IOC on the issue of doping, many pow-

erlifting officials—with their multiplicity of approaches to the doping problem—
"are now resigned at some deep level to the continued presence of what they
recognize, refuse, and morally despise, but cannot any longer imagine how to
stop. In a nutshell, the authorities know they have lost against doping and have
lost permanently."[87]

The concern we have about other applications of the parallel federation solution is that once federations split—and those who want testing leave the dominant organization to form a new drug-free federation—then the game is over. To
quote MacAloon a final time:

> Incompetence can always be rooted out, official co-conspirators can be found, em-
> barrassed, and exiled (if rarely convicted), and ways can at least be sought to raise
> the voices of true authority above the legalists, public relations specialists and mar-
> keting managers. But if there no longer are any such voices and convictions in these
> organizations, if the public and the rest of the international sport community come
> to believe that their leaderships and their organizational culture have thrown in the
> towel in defeat over drugging in sport, then the effect on the overall legitimacy, pres-
> tige and deference afforded these bodies will surely be devastating.[88]

We must be wary that the helping hand does not strike again.

NOTES

1. W. M. Brown, "Paternalism, Drugs and the Nature of Sports," *Journal of the Phi-
losophy of Sport* 4 (1984): 14–22; W. P. Fraleigh, "Performance Enhancing Drugs in Sport:
The Ethical Issues," *Journal of the Philosophy of Sport* 11 (1985): 23–29; R. Gardner, "On
Performance Enhancing Substances and the Unfair Advantage Argument," *Journal of the
Philosophy of Sport* 16 (1989): 59–73; J. Hoberman, "Sport Physicians and the Doping Cri-
sis in Elite Sport," *Clinical Journal of Sport Medicine* 12, no. 4 (2002): 203–10; T. H. Murray,
"The Coercive Power of Drugs in Sport," *Hastings Center Report* 13, no. 4 (1983): 24–30;
S. Olivier, "Drugs in Sport: Justifying Paternalism on the Grounds of Harm," *American
Journal of Sports Medicine* 24 (1996): S343; R. Simon, "Good Competition and Drug En-
hanced Performance," *Journal of the Philosophy of Sport* 11 (1984): 6–13; C. E. Thomas,
*Sport in a Philosophic Context* (Philadelphia: Lea & Febiger, 1983).

2. J. Hoberman, *Mortal Engines: The Science of Performance and the Dehumanization
of Sport* (New York: Free Press, 1992); T. D. Noakes, "Tainted Glory: Doping and Athletic
Performance," *New England Journal of Medicine* 351, no. 9 (2004): 847–49.

3. M. D. Burke and T. J. Roberts, "Drugs in Sport: An Issue of Morality or Sentimentality?" *Journal of the Philosophy of Sport* 24 (1997): 99.

4. R. R. Albrecht, W. A. Anderson, and D. B. McKeag, "Drug Testing of College Ath-

letes: The Issues," in *Ethics in Sport*, ed. W. J. Morgan, K. V. Meier, and A. Schneider, 181–87 (Champaign, IL: Human Kinetics, 2001); T. Black, "Does the Ban on Drugs in Sport Improve Societal Welfare?" *International Review for Sociology of Sport* 31, no. 4 (1996): 367–77; W. M. Brown, "As American as Gatorade and Apple Pie: Performance, Drugs and Sport," in Morgan, Meier, and Schneider, *Ethics in Sport*, 142–68; W. M. Brown, "Practices and Prudence. Presidential Address: Philosophic Society for the Study of Sport," *Journal of the Philosophy of Sport* 17 (1990): 71–84; N. Fost, "Banning Drugs in Sports: A Skeptical View," *Hastings Center Report* 16, no. 4 (1986): 5–10; M. A. Holowchak, "Ergogenic Aids and the Limits of Human Performance in Sport: Ethical Issues, Aesthetic Considerations," *Journal of the Philosophy of Sport* 29 (2002): 75–76; M. Lavin, "Sports and Drugs: Are the Current Bans Justified?" *Journal of the Philosophy of Sport* 14 (1987): 34–43; A. J. Schneider and R. B. Butcher, "An Ethical Analysis of Drug Testing," in *Doping in Elite Sport*, ed. W. Wilson and E. Derse, 129–52 (Champaign, IL: Human Kinetics, 2001); P. B. Thompson, "Privacy and the Urinalysis Testing of Athletes," *Journal of the Philosophy of Sport* 9 (1982): 60–65; M. H. Williams, "The Use of Nutritional Ergogenic Aids in Sports: Is It an Ethical Issue?" *International Journal of Sports Nutrition* 4 (1994): 120–31.

5. Albrecht, Anderson, and McKeag, "Drug Testing of College Athletes," 185.

6. Schneider and Butcher, "Ethical Analysis of Drug Testing," 129.

7. Fost, "Banning Drugs in Sports," 9.

8. Black, "Does the Ban Improve Societal Welfare?" 377.

9. M. Lambert, "Editor's Note," *Powerlifting USA* 4, no. 5 (1980): 21.

10. T. Todd, "The History of Resistance Exercise and Its Role in United States Education" (Ph.D. diss., University of Texas at Austin, 1966); J. D. Fair, "George Jowett, Ottley Coulter, David P. Willoughby and the Formation of American Weightlifting, 1911–1924," *Iron Game History: The Journal of Physical Culture* 2, no. 6 (1993): 3–19; D. P. Webster, *The Iron Game* (Irvine, Scotland: D. P. Webster, 1976), 147–51.

11. J. D. Fair, *Muscletown USA: Bob Hoffman and the Manly Culture of York Barbell* (State College: Pennsylvania State Press, 1999).

12. R. Crist, telephone interview with J. Todd, November 16, 2004.

13. P. Rader, "Grunt and Groan," *Iron Man* (1969), and P. Rader, "Untitled," *Iron Man* (1969), www.americanpowerliftevolution.net/New%20Folder%201969/drugcommentary .html; quotation from "Grunt and Groan."

14. Crist, telephone interview, November 16, 2004; J. Todd, "Chaos Can Have Gentle Beginnings: The Early History of the Quest for Drug Testing in American Powerlifting: 1964–1984," *Iron Game History: The Journal of Physical Culture* 8, no. 3 (2004): 3–22.

15. Crist, telephone interview, November 16, 2004.

16. C. Patterson, message from the National AAU Powerlifting Chairman, 1975, manuscript, Rader, IPF rulebook files, H. J. Lutcher Stark Center for Physical Culture and Sports, University of Texas at Austin (hereafter, H. J. Lutcher Stark Center).

17. International Powerlifting Federation, "World Record List," in *International Powerlifting Handbook*, 1975, Rader files, H. J. Lutcher Stark Center; B. Hoffman and T. Todd, "The 1975 World Power Championships," *Muscular Development* 13 (1976): 9–14.

18. Crist, telephone interview, November 16, 2004.

19. T. Fitton, "World Championships, Perth '77," *Powerlifting USA* 1, no. 6 (1977): 2.

20. T. Todd, "Anabolic Steroids: The Gremlins of Sport," *Journal of Sport History* 14, no. 1 (1987): 87–107.

21. Ibid., 93–94.

22. Ibid., 95.

23. M. Lambert, "Pacifico: The Nine Time World Champ Speaks," *Powerlifting USA* 11, no. 19 (1988): 7–10.

24. Todd, "Anabolic Steroids," 94.

25. Rader, "Untitled."

26. T. Todd, *Inside Powerlifting* (Chicago: Contemporary Books, 1977), 6.

27. Lambert, "Pacifico," 9.

28. J. Nickele, "An Open Letter to All Officials of the IPF," *Powerlifting USA* 1, no. 3 (1977): 20.

29. F. Hatfield, *Anabolic Steroids: What Kind and How Many* (Madison, WI: Fitness System, 1982), 3.

30. D. Nassif, "Steroid Underground," *Muscle and Fitness* 27 (1983): 244.

31. R. Hughes and J. Coakley, "Positive Deviance among Athletes: The Implications of over Conformity to the Sport Ethic," *Sociology of Sport Journal* 8, no. 4 (1991): 307–25; J. Coakley, "Deviance in Sports: Is It out of Control?" in *Sport in Society*, 7th ed., 137–72 (New York: McGraw Hill, 2001).

32. Coakley, "Deviance in Sports," 151.

33. P. Mignon, "The Tour de France and the Doping Issue," *International Journal of the History of Sport* 20, no. 2 (2003): 227–45, 279.

34. Todd, "Chaos Can Have Gentle Beginnings," 7.

35. International Powerlifting Federation, "By-Laws of the International Powerlifting Federation," as amended November 6, 1979, Todd Powerlifting files, binder 1, H. J. Lutcher Stark Center.

36. Todd, "Chaos Can Have Gentle Beginnings," 8.

37. Ibid.

38. Minutes of the National AAU Powerlifting Committee, November 26, 1979, Todd Powerlifting files, H. J. Lutcher Stark Center.

39. Todd, "Chaos Can Have Gentle Beginnings," 11.

40. Ibid., 11–12; J. Todd, minutes of the USPFWC [USPF Women's Committee], Auburn, Alabama, 1982, Todd Powerlifting files, H. J. Lutcher Stark Center.

41. B. Gaynor, "ADFPA Founder Dies," *American Drug Free Powerlifting News* 1, no. 4 (1994): 1–2; A. Gauthier, "Brother Bennet Bishop (1931–1994)," 1994, obituary written for St. Stanislaus College Archives, St. Stanislaus, Mississippi; Todd, "Chaos Can Have Gentle Beginnings," 14.

42. Lambert, "Editor's Note."

43. M. Lambert, "American Drug Free Powerlifting Association," *Powerlifting USA* 5, no. 7 (1982): 40; J. Biasotto and A. Ferrando, "Brother Bennet: The Man behind the ADFPA," *Powerlifting USA* 10, no. 10 (1987): 16–17.

44. Brother Bennet, "Morals and Ethics in Powerlifting: A Speech Given at the Women's Nationals," *Powerlifting USA* 5, no. 10 (1982): 13.

45. Oath from American Drug Free Powerlifting Association, ADFPA membership

card, ADFPA powerlifting file, Judy Gedney papers, H. J. Lutcher Stark Center; J. Gedney, telephone interview with J. Todd, 1983.

46. R. Klein, "Using the Polygraph for Drug Testing," *Powerlifting USA* 6, no. 5 (1982): 13–14.

47. J. Gedney, e-mail to J. Todd, June 26, 2004.

48. Brother Bennet, "Message from the ADFPA President," *Powerlifting USA* 7, no. 4 (1983): 25.

49. C. Cotter, "Message from the USPF President," *Powerlifting USA* 6, no. 1 (1982): 24; Brother Bennet to P. Rader, personal letter, September 11, 1982, Rader Powerlifting files, H. J. Lutcher Stark Center.

50. C. Cotter, "Message from the USPF President," *Powerlifting USA* 6, no. 6 (1982): 17; C. Cotter, "Rules Passed and Other Decisions Made by the USPF Executive Committee since Dayton," *Powerlifting USA* 7, no. 1 (1983): 36.

51. Cotter, "Message from the USPF President," *Powerlifting USA* 6, no. 6 (1982): 17.

52. APF advertisement, *Powerlifting USA* 6, no. 7 (1983): 58.

53. Advertising Flyer for APF/AMPF, Todd Powerlifting file, H. J. Lutcher Stark Center; E. Frantz, conversation with J. Todd, January 1983.

54. A. Bostrom, "Letter to Mike Lambert," *Power Hotline* 3, no. 14 (1984): 1; C. Cotter, "Message from the President," *Powerlifting USA* 8, no. 2 (1984): 30–31.

55. M. Lambert, "USPF Women's National Championships," *Powerlifting USA* 7, no. 9 (1984): 10; C. Cotter, "Message from the President," *Powerlifting USA* 8, no. 11 (1984): 21.

56. C. Cotter, "Message from the President," *Powerlifting USA* 7, no. 11 (1984): 25.

57. Cotter, "Message from the President," *Powerlifting USA* 8, no. 11 (1984): 21.

58. M. Lambert, "Women's Worlds," *Powerlifting USA* 7, no. 12 (1984): 7; J. Gedney, "From Judy Gedney," *Powerlifting USA* 8, no. 2 (1984): 52.

59. R. Shafer, "Women's Corner," *Powerlifting USA* 8, no. 2 (1984): 27.

60. E. Douglas, "APF Worlds," *Powerlifting USA* 10, no. 6 (1987): 11–14; Biasotto and Ferrando, "Brother Bennet."

61. M. Lambert, "Ernie Frantz Talks about His Meet," *Powerlifting USA* 8, no. 2 (1984): 31.

62. A. Bostrom, "Letter to Mike Lambert," *Power Hotline* 3, no. 14 (1984): 1; Cotter, "Message from the President," *Powerlifting USA* 8, no. 2 (1984): 30–31.

63. M. Sternberg, on-line interview with Eric Stone, April 9, 2004, www.apf-illinois .com/MarisInterview.html.

64. *Frantz, E. et al. v. United States Powerlifting Federation, Conrad Cotter and International Powerlifting Federation*, 85 C 06132, U.S. District Court, Northern Illinois, Eastern Division, Frantz Lawsuit files, H. J. Lutcher Stark Center.

65. M. Lambert, "Mike Lambert Looks at Powerlifting 1986: The New Season Begins," *Powerlifting USA* 9, no. 5 (1986): 8.

66. C. Cotter, "Message from the President," *Powerlifting USA* 9, no. 8 (1986): 24.

67. C. Cotter, "Message from the President," *Powerlifting USA* 9, no. 11 (1986): 2.

68. Ibid.

69. T. Kurlowicz, "APF Nationals," *Powerlifting USA* 9, no. 12 (1986): 13.

70. Top Ranked Lifter (A), "Response," *Powerlifting USA* 9, no. 10 (1986): 32.

71. C. Cotter, "Message from the President," *Powerlifting USA* 10, no. 2 (1986): 32–33; "Minutes of the USPF National Committee Meeting, 4 July 1986," *Powerlifting USA* 10, no. 2 (1986): 32–33.

72. R. Peters, advertisement, *Powerlifting USA* 10, no. 2 (1986): 72.

73. K. Beckwith, interview with J. Todd, Austin, TX, January 5, 2008.

74. J. Ladnier, interview with J. Todd and T. Todd, Atlanta, GA, October 4, 2004.

75. K. Beckwith, interview with J. Todd, Austin, TX, March 5, 2005; Natural Athlete Strength Association, www.nasa-sports.com.

76. Natural Athlete Strength Association, www.nasa-sports.com.

77. L. B. Baker, telephone interview with J. Todd, September 20, 2003; J. Rogers, telephone interview with J. Todd, October 9, 2003; D. Latch, e-mail to J. Todd, November 17, 2004; S. Runyon, telephone interview with J. Todd, September 21, 2003.

78. Latch to Todd, November 17, 2004.

79. Franz quoted in E. Douglas, "APF Worlds," *Powerlifting USA* 10, no. 6 (1987): 11–14.

80. K. Kidder, "Letter to Prospective Members," 2003, www.worldpowerlifting.org, copy on file at H. J. Lutcher Stark Center.

81. K. Kidder, telephone interview with J. Todd, September 30, 2003.

82. M. Lambert, "What's Going on with USA Powerlifting," *Powerlifting USA* 20, no. 7 (1997): 6–7, 90–91.

83. R. K. Merton, "The Unanticipated Consequences of Purposive Social Action," *American Sociological Review* 1, no. 6 (1936): 901.

84. A. Guttmann, *From Ritual to Record: The Nature of Modern Sport* (New York: Columbia University Press, 1987), 16.

85. Centre for Strategy and Policy, "Millennium Project POST-MODERNISM," www.open .ac.uk/oubs-future/Millennium/657.htm.

86. L. Pacifico, interview on *American Strength Legends*, June 17, 1999, www.mcshane -enterprises.com/ASL/pacificointerview.html.

87. J. J. MacAloon, "Doping and Moral Authority: Sport Organizations Today," in *Doping in Elite Sport: The Politics of Drugs in the Olympic Movement*, ed. W. Wilson and E. Derse (Champaign, IL: Human Kinetics, 2001), 205, 209, 210.

88. Ibid., 210.

# CHAPTER FOUR

# The Role of Physicians, Scientists, Trainers, Coaches, and Other Nonathletes in Athletes' Drug Use

GARY A. GREEN, M.D.

The traditional focus of antidoping efforts has centered on athletes and on those responsible for enforcing regulations (i.e., sports governing bodies and antidoping agencies). This ignores a host of personnel who are integrally involved with, influence, and may ultimately benefit from an athlete's use of performance-enhancing drugs. The athlete's decision to use these drugs is typically the end result of a process involving many other people. These ancillary personnel often have their own vulnerabilities that lead them to encourage, condone, or enable athletes' use of performance-enhancing drugs. To effect change, we must understand their roles in this system. Although the focus is almost always on the athlete who tests positive for performance-enhancing drugs, the circle of people who participate is much larger. The 1998 Tour de France doping scandal and the U.S. Bay Area Laboratory Cooperative (BALCO) affair demonstrate the number of people required for illicit ergogenic drug use. The same forces that tempt athletes to use such substances may also influence these ancillary personnel.

Another contributing factor is the lack of responsibility that envelops the athlete who is raised in the athletic milieu. From a young age, many athletes knowingly or unknowingly cede responsibility for some of life's basic decisions that are assumed by a variety of willing personnel. In many U.S. universities, elite athletes lead structured lives in which they are awakened by athletic personnel, eat at training tables, take prearranged classes, and attend practices. Much of their own responsibility for orchestrating their daily lives has been eliminated, and this can result in poor decision-making habits. The lack of responsibility may also contribute to an athlete's drug use: he or she may not question prescribed drugs or may unknowingly accept drugs from people who work in the athletic environment, such as physicians, athletic trainers, exercise scientists, or coaches. Unfortunately, the void in personal responsibility is often filled by unscrupulous individuals who are seeking economic or status gain at the expense of the athlete.

Involvement of personnel such as physicians, coaches, and athletic trainers in providing ergogenic drugs to athletes is not merely speculative. The National Collegiate Athletic Association (NCAA) performs a quadrennial survey of the drug use and abuse habits of NCAA athletes. The 2005 survey received responses from 19,676 male and female intercollegiate athletes across all NCAA divisions and revealed patterns of use for ergogenic, therapeutic, and recreational drugs.[1] One of the more interesting questions asked users of anabolic steroids to state their main source for the drugs; the responses are listed in table 4.1. Clearly, athletes receive anabolic steroids from a wide array of sources. Many of these sources are discussed in this chapter.

Before entering into a discussion of the types of personnel involved with drug use by athletes, we need to understand sports pharmacology. Sports pharmacology differs from traditional pharmacology by classifying substances according to reasons for their use, rather than pharmacological actions. For example, traditional pharmacology would categorize clenbuterol and albuterol together because they are both beta-2 agonists. Sports pharmacology, however, classifies drugs according to their usage—recreational, therapeutic, or ergogenic. Recreational drugs are often performance-decreasing (ergolytic); examples include alcohol, cocaine, marijuana, and heroin. Although sports organizations often test for these drugs and cite reasons for deterring their use, that topic is beyond the scope of this chapter.

The more important distinction is between therapeutic and ergogenic drugs. Therapeutic drugs are used to treat a particular medical condition, whereas ergogenic substances are taken with the sole intention of increasing performance. To help clarify this distinction, the World Anti-Doping Agency (WADA) has published an International Standard for Therapeutic Use Exemptions (TUEs) (see table 4.2).[2] The line between therapeutic and ergogenic can be blurred, however, and this may lead to erroneous or inappropriate use of ergogenic drugs. For example, returning to the drugs mentioned above, clenbuterol is banned by most sports organizations as a performance-enhancing anabolic agent, whereas albuterol is allowed for the treatment of asthma. One might argue that albuterol allows an athlete with asthma to improve his or her performance and should thus be considered an ergogenic drug. However, according to criterion III in

TABLE 4.1
*Where Do You Usually Get Your Anabolic Steroids? Responses to National Collegiate Athletic Association Survey, 2005*

| Source | Responses (% of total) |
| --- | --- |
| Friend or family | 17.4 |
| Other (nonteam) physician | 8.3 |
| Team physician | 4.9 |
| Retail store | 12.1 |
| Coach | 7.3 |
| Strength coach | 2.2 |
| Teammate or other athlete | 10.5 |
| Website / mail order | 13.9 |
| Athletic trainer | 5.6 |
| Pro scout or agent | 3.4 |
| Other source | 23.3 |

*Source:* Data from National Collegiate Athletic Association, 2005 *Study of Substance Use Habits of College Student-Athletes* (Indianapolis, IN: National Collegiate Athletic Association, 2006).

*Note:* N = 413 anabolic steroid users from a survey of 19,676 NCAA student-athletes.

table 4.2, the performance increases only to the point that the athlete would achieve if he or she did not have asthma.

## Physicians

The role of the physician in sport is traditionally limited to that of the team physician who performs preparticipation physical exams, provides medical coverage during events, and treats athletes for injuries sustained during athletic competition. However, the role has lately expanded to include providing information and education on drugs, functioning as the medical director of drug testing programs, and providing justification for TUEs.

The traditional responsibility of sports physicians is to provide medical care to athletes. While the established image of "sports medicine" in the United States is that of an orthopedic surgeon performing surgery on the injured athlete, there are legions of primary care physicians who practice sports medicine. Primary care sports medicine practitioners are generally physicians trained in the specialties of internal medicine, family medicine, or pediatrics. The distinction is important in that the primary care sports physician prescribes a much greater variety of medications than does the orthopedist. The primary care sports physician and orthopedist work in concert, and their working relationship can be com-

TABLE 4.2
*World Anti-Doping Agency International Standard for Therapeutic Use Exemption (TUE) Criteria*

I. The athlete should submit an application for a TUE no less than 21 days before participating in an event.

II. The athlete would experience a significant impairment to health if the prohibited substance or prohibited method were to be withheld in the course of treating an acute or chronic medical condition.

III. The therapeutic use of the prohibited substance or prohibited method would produce no additional enhancement of performance other than that which might be anticipated by a return of normal health following the treatment of a legitimate medical condition. The use of any prohibited substance or prohibited method to increase "low-normal" levels of any endogenous hormone is not considered an acceptable therapeutic intervention.

IV. There is no reasonable therapeutic alternative to the use of the otherwise prohibited substance or prohibited method.

V. The necessity for the use of the otherwise prohibited substance or prohibited method cannot be a consequence, wholly or in part, of prior nontherapeutic use of any substance from the prohibited list.

*Source:* Adapted from WADA, "International Standard for Therapeutic Use Exemptions," www.wada-ama.org/rtecontent/document/international_standard.pdf (accessed March 8, 2009).

pared to that between a cardiologist and cardiothoracic surgeon, or a neurologist and a neurosurgeon.

Physicians enter into a variety of arrangements with athletes, including the traditional doctor-patient relationship, and these can influence the use and abuse of ergogenic drugs. In the typical doctor-patient arrangement, the physician is obligated to first do no harm and to strive to improve a patient's health. This also includes a somewhat paternalistic attitude on the part of the physician, whereby the patient has implicit trust in the ability of the physician to act in the patient's best interest. A fiduciary responsibility is assumed by the physician toward the patient. For the athlete-patient, the physician may be conflicted as to what constitutes therapeutic and ergogenic use of drugs. For example, a 36-year-old professional male athlete has a physiological decline in testosterone level, but is that a medical condition requiring testosterone treatment? According to criterion III in table 4.2, this would not be considered therapeutic use.

A physician may be placed in difficult circumstances in which he or she is asked to balance competing interests. For example, the wishes of an athlete seeking top performance must be weighed against the doping-control regulations of the sport. An additional circumstance is treating the injured athlete. If anabolic steroids or human growth hormone would improve surgical recovery, can that use be justified in the interest of a favorable surgical outcome? Yet another scenario is a patient's request for prescription drugs so as to avoid safety issues associated with "black market" sources. Athletes frequently "doctor shop" until they find a physician who will acquiesce to their requests, and physicians must at times weigh the loss of income against ethical demands.

The physician-patient dynamic is further complicated when the physician has a relationship to a sports organization. Being a team physician for a high-profile sports team often has significant benefits for the physician in terms of prestige, income, and community visibility. The position of team physician can be so desirable that some U.S. professional teams have entered into "medical sponsorship" arrangements in which the role of team physician goes to the highest bidder (i.e., the physician compensates the team). The status that accrues to the physician and the desire to maintain that status create the potential for conflict. A physician may be pressured by the athlete or the employing organization to unethically prescribe ergogenic drugs. And because the athlete is not paying the physician, this often confuses the traditional doctor-patient relationship.

These three issues—the physician's desire to heal, the altered doctor-patient relationship, and team physician status—can make the physician vulnerable to unethically prescribing ergogenic drugs. Given the tight control of drugs such as anabolic steroids, it can also be lucrative for a physician to prescribe these medications for nonmedical reasons. Perhaps the most glaring examples of physician abuse are contained in the records of the former East Germany, where physicians played an integral role in the state-sponsored doping program.[3] It is also clear that physicians participated in the 1998 Tour de France doping scandal by monitoring the drug use of cyclists.[4]

On the positive side, physicians are involved with the antidoping efforts in many international federations. Physician involvement is required for all U.S. Anti-Doping Agency review panels of doping offenses. In addition, physicians may play a role in the treatment of the athlete addicted to ergogenic drugs. This addiction can often happen unintentionally. Mandell described the "Sunday Syndrome" in National Football League players who chronically used amphetamines to prepare for games and then required depressants to counteract the effects.[5] Some physicians also believe that a true addiction to anabolic steroids can develop, and treatment programs have been created to address such addictions. In my opinion, this is not a true physical addiction but rather a psychological dependence on a particular body type and performance level.[6]

Sports medicine has become an established specialty for both orthopedic and primary care physicians, and they play a great many roles in the care of athletes. Some of these roles may tempt a physician to violate antidoping efforts. A team physician may be tempted to hasten a return to play from surgery or injury by providing banned substances, such as anabolic steroids, in the belief that this

combination with many other drugs. The two-month history of anabolic steroid use shown in table 4.3 is fairly typical for a bodybuilder.[10] It would be difficult to convince a university's institutional review board to approve a placebo-controlled study at these dosages.

Also ethically complicated is the use of research subjects who are potentially eligible for drug testing. This is a quandary because, for research results to be applicable, the studies must necessarily use a cohort similar to Olympic athletes. As an example, I was part of a project to validate testing to detect recombinant erythropoietin (rHuEPO) before the 2002 Winter Olympics.[11] To develop the test, small amounts of rHuEPO were given to the volunteer research subjects. One of the criteria for inclusion in the study was that volunteers could not be subject to drug testing or actively competing. According to WADA's World Anti-Doping Code, "Research efforts should avoid the administration of prohibited substances or prohibited methods to athletes."[12] The risk, however, was that Olympic athletes who tested positive might challenge the testing on the basis that the test was not developed with a representative cohort and that, somehow, Olympic athletes metabolized rHuEPO differently from untrained individuals.

A more difficult issue arises for scientists working directly with athletes outside a university system. Their position is dependent on the athletes' or team's performance. Pressure may come from the team or from the individual scientist whose success or failure is directly related to the accomplishments of the athlete. The temptation to augment training with performance-enhancing drugs is often significant. When there is a banned substances list governing the sport, the obligations of the scientist are clear. Any use of a drug on the banned list with the sole intention of increasing performance is clearly a violation of the sport's policies. The difficulty comes either with substances that are new or when it is unclear whether particular substances are banned. An example is insulin. Until 1998, insulin was not banned in the Olympics, and it was added to the list following an inquiry from a Russian medical officer about the use of insulin in nondiabetic athletes.[13] In the nondiabetic athlete, insulin can theoretically be an anabolic hormone, and there have been anecdotal reports of bodybuilders using it for several years in combination with anabolic steroids and growth hormone.

Exercise scientists need to adhere to solid scientific and ethical principles with respect to legitimate research and traditional risk-benefit analyses. In the circle of athletics, the benefits of individual accomplishment can overwhelm the potential risks, not only to a particular athlete but also to the integrity of sport. Questions have been raised by Karen Maschke (see chapter 5) and others regarding the societal benefits of research into the use of performance-enhancing drugs in

TABLE 4.3

*Anabolic-Androgenic Steroid Use by a 23-Year-Old Bodybuilder over a Two-Month Period (with comparable physiological replacement dose)*

| Generic Drug (Trade Name) | Dosage | Physiological Replacement Dose |
|---|---|---|
| Methandrostenolone (Dianabol) | 75 mg subcutaneously every other day | 5 mg/day |
| Methenolone (Primobolin) | 150 mg subcutaneously every other day | 2.5–10 mg/day |
| Oxandrolone (Anavar) | 20 mg/day orally | 5–10 mg/day |
| Oxymetholone (Anadrol) | 100 mg/day | |

*Source:* Data from F. Tennant, D. L. Black, and R. O. Voy, "Anabolic Steroid Dependence with Opioid-Type Features," *New England Journal of Medicine* 319, no. 9 (1988): 578.

sport. Humankind clearly values sport, as demonstrated by the near obsession with sports in many societies throughout history. Research into deterring unethical drug use in sport clearly protects individuals who do not want to use drugs to compete and maintains the integrity of sport.

Research on finding safe and effective means to improve performance is more complex. With respect to recruitment and payment of subjects, researchers should follow proper guidelines so as not to offer improper inducements for research.[14] Whether exercise scientists function in a university or independently, they need to be guided by the same principles of scientific integrity that govern investigation in other fields: the risks and the benefits should be fully evaluated and balanced.

## Athletic Trainers

As a group, athletic trainers are vulnerable to a wide range of forces that affect their relationship with athletes. Although athletic trainers are usually employed by teams, their job performance ultimately depends on their ability to interact with individual athletes in a variety of situations. An athletic trainer spends a great deal of time with the athlete and serves many roles—confidante, motivator, nurse, doctor, and therapist, to name a few. The trainer is in a position to see both the strengths and weaknesses of the athlete, and there are often competing loyalties.

Until recently, the term *trainer* could refer to persons with a range of skill sets and educational backgrounds. The National Athletic Trainers' Association (NATA) has now taken steps in the United States to professionalize the occupation. A rigorous certification program ratifies someone as a "certified athletic trainer" (ATC) who is licensed and has completed a full program designed to meet the needs of athletes. When referring to this position, the NATA recommends the use of the term *athletic trainer* or *ATC*.

Although the NATA has made a great effort to improve the image of the profession, athletic trainers still have a great many responsibilities that fall outside traditional athlete care. Some examples include team transportation scheduling, keeping game statistics, and equipment management. All of these create distractions for ATCs and interfere with their ability to perform their core functions. In addition, the ATC has to work closely with the team physician, and a lack of communication from the physician often leaves the ATC in the position of having to interpret medical care for the athlete. This can further strain the athlete-ATC relationship and lead to increased stress for the ATC.

Athletic trainers work in a variety of situations, and each presents its own unique set of circumstances. One of the most common roles is serving as an ATC for a high school, intercollegiate, or professional team. Athletic trainers may also work with individual athletes, usually at the elite level, to assist in their training and/or recovery from injury. In this latter setting, ATCs should be differentiated from "personal trainers" who often have little formal training and no licensure requirements. One of the major conspirators accused in the BALCO case was a professional athlete's personal trainer who allegedly distributed anabolic steroids to professional athletes.

Athletic trainers often report to many different individuals, few of whom directly employ them. In a college or university setting, an ATC is paid by the institution and reports to the athletic director, but the coach can make demands on the ATC and influence his or her job security. The team physician can also make demands on the ATC, such as treatment for an injured player and return-to-play guidelines. All of these competing responsibilities can tug at the ATC.

Ensuring an athlete's compliance with therapeutic medications is one example of how these competing influences affect the ATC. In most medical situations, the physician prescribes therapeutic drugs directly to the patient. However, in yet another example of how athletes cede responsibility, in the sports environment medications are often prescribed in the presence of the ATC, who becomes responsible for ensuring the athlete's compliance. The ATC must be aware of an athlete's use of outside prescription drugs, over-the-counter medications, and dietary supplements, in addition to permissible therapeutic drugs. This creates a great deal of responsibility for the overburdened ATC, who may be cited for failing to "control" an athlete who tests positive for a banned substance.

With respect to ergogenic drugs, athletic trainers in university settings are rarely the source. However, ATCs can be in a position of knowing about an athlete's drug use. The ATC can be placed in the uncomfortable position of reporting drug use by someone with whom he or she works every day. In addition, it is not uncommon for ATCs to participate in institutional drug testing programs. They often are responsible for administering the program or doing various tasks such as collecting urine samples or delivering test notifications. This creates a role conflict: having to act in the neutral position of a drug-testing administrator on the one hand, and yet knowing about individual athletes' drug use on the other. In the case of a positive drug test, this creates the appearance of bias and can compromise the integrity of drug testing programs. Direct involvement of an ATC with an institution's drug testing program can also lower an athlete's trust and compromise the athletic trainer's ability to perform his or her primary functions.

Athletic trainers who work in the collegiate environment often consider themselves "neutral" on the topic of ergogenic drug use. However, this attitude can contribute to an atmosphere in which substance use is tolerated or tacitly encouraged. Athletes often interpret the lack of a strong message to signify approval for any illicit or unethical behavior they are considering. As a front-line player, the ATC must provide a clear signal to athletes about ergogenic drug use.

It is much more difficult to regulate athletic trainers who work individually with athletes. There is no institutional control, and these trainers are paid by the athletes to improve their performance. In addition, the athletic trainer's reputation is dependent on the athlete's performance, and there is a great incentive to augment training and recovery with ergogenic substances. As the provider of drugs, the trainer cements the relationship with the athlete and can exert a powerful influence over the athlete.

Taken as whole, athletic trainers form the backbone of sports medicine and contribute greatly to the overall health of the athlete. There are some tangible ways of improving their situation in order to deter athletes' ergogenic drug use. In my opinion, ATCs should not be directly involved with institutional drug testing programs. Although it may seem like an inexpensive and efficient way to do drug testing, putting athletic trainers in the middle of drug control compromises both the integrity of the program and the trainers' ability to perform their primary job. In an institutional setting, ATCs can have an integral role in the education of athletes about ergogenic drugs. The NATA has issued a position statement that it is working with its members to eliminate drug use from athletics and schools.[15] It is also essential that institutions play a role in empowering ATCs and allowing them to focus on their core mission (i.e., the care of athletes).

At the professional sports level, the role of an athletic trainer becomes even more complex. The potential financial rewards can tempt an athlete to take significant health risks. The ATC is often a willing participant in allowing the athlete to compete under these conditions. Drug use becomes just one more risk the athlete is willing to assume, and the risks of drug use are often dwarfed by the physical dangers of the sport. Under these circumstances, it is relatively easy to overlook ergogenic drug use. There may also be substantial financial rewards for the ATC who is associated with a successful professional team. Given these pressures, it is crucial to have an enforced league-wide antidoping policy at every level. As an example, Major League Baseball needed to address the issue of teams providing nutritional supplements that were often of questionable purity, with the attendant liability. In 2004, the league adopted a $10,000 fine for any personnel who provide a player with a nutritional supplement that results in a positive drug test. This sent a clear message to all personnel, but especially ATCs, who are often given the responsibility by the clubs to dispense dietary supplements. The athletic trainers are now in a much better position to refuse to dispense these products and to focus instead on the care of the athletes.

Athletic trainers maintain the front lines of sports medicine and are often the first ones to notice the signs and symptoms of drug use. Responsibility often falls to the ATC when an athlete fails to comply with a drug testing program. It is vital that ATCs are empowered to use this knowledge to provide education and support, and not condone use by turning a blind eye. Because ATCs often have limited control over their employment situation, it would be helpful if their environment were structured to maximize their ability to interact with athletes in a positive way with respect to ergogenic drug use.

Taking the ATC out of the loop of drug testing would be a concrete improvement. I recommend that teams use an independent third-party administrator to conduct their drug testing programs, rather than using the team's athletic trainer in this capacity. Although this adds to the cost of drug testing, it reduces the team's liability and certainly decreases the pressures on the ATC. This ATC can then serve more freely in the role of advocate and confidante in dealings with athletes. The cost for the third-party administrator should be calculated when a team considers a drug testing program.

Finally, the independent athletic trainer remains a problematic role. There will always be a large temptation to skirt the rules and a pool of athletes willing to assume the risk. Ranged against those forces are the penalties for violating the rules. In the case of ATCs, the NATA can revoke certification for ethical breaches. If the trainer is not NATA-certified, then it falls to the sport to enforce any penalties. The major consequence for an athletic trainer would be public identification in the case of a positive drug test or doping scandal and a ban on working with athletes from that sport. Prodded to some degree by the BALCO scandal, many professional sports leagues have banned all nonofficial personnel from their clubhouses and facilities. This allows at least some degree of institutional control over such people.

## Coaches

The most difficult position to confront is also the one that is most neglected and has the greatest potential to influence the athlete: the coach. Although coaches have total control over the athlete's playing career and influence everything from playing time to academics to leisure activities, coaches rarely address ergogenic substance abuse. One reason may be that coaches benefit most from improved performance. It is a fact of the profession that a coach's longevity and salary are usually determined by wins and losses. In the college ranks, a coach may graduate players, run a stellar program, and recruit excellent student-athletes, but this coach will still be fired if he or she posts a losing record. Yet, a great many peccadilloes will be tolerated if the coach is winning. The message that is sent to the coach is unmistakable: win or be gone. As coaches' salaries have risen, coaching tenure has decreased. In 2004, the coach of the Notre Dame football team was fired after fulfilling three years of a five-year contract, despite a winning record. Contrast that to the legendary University of California, Los Angeles, basketball coach John Wooden, who began coaching in 1948 and did not win a championship in his first 16 years. He then had 10 national championships in 12 years. One wonders whether a university would be that patient in the current environment.

Even more directly involved with the athletes are assistant coaches. They have little job security, work long hours at relatively low salaries, and, as a result, are fairly itinerant. According to the National Football League Coaches Association, roughly one-quarter of the 560 assistant coaches in the league either are fired or change teams each season.[16] They may often be called on to perform tasks that the head coach neglects or delegates, and they may also have confidential knowledge of an athlete's behavior. In large programs, the assistant coaches spend a great deal of time with the athletes, and it may be difficult for them to inform on their drug use. In addition, many such coaches are former players who may have used ergogenic drugs themselves and thus condone or encourage their use.

There is also an increasingly popular breed of coach that deserves special mention: the strength coach. Relatively unknown 20 years ago, strength coaches are now employed by most major universities and professional teams. Their popularity is reflected in the National Strength and Conditioning Association. Founded in 1978 with 76 members, it now boasts 25,000 worldwide members and offers educational programs and certifications for strength and conditioning coaches. Its mission statement concisely states: "As the worldwide authority on strength and conditioning, we support and disseminate research-based knowledge and its practical application, to improve athletic performance and fitness" (www.nsca-lift.org). Although the association has attempted to professionalize strength coaches, they are loosely regulated, and its mission statement does not mention limitations on performance-enhancing drugs. Because their own performance is directly measured by the strength gains of their charges, strength coaches are susceptible to condoning or encouraging illicit ergogenic drug use.

Scholastic and professional teams' educational programs should make a greater effort to educate coaches about ergogenic drugs and enlist their support in reducing their use. Coaches have a difficult line to tread. Their job is to extract the best performance from an athlete, but too much pressure in combination with reduced self-esteem leaves an athlete vulnerable to the seduction of illegal substances. Coaches wield tremendous influence over athletes and are a potentially untapped resource for education. Most educational programs on drug use are aimed at the athlete and neglect the coaches. It would obviously be efficient to take advantage of coaches' authority to deter ergogenic drug use. Coaches must be educated to recognize the signs of drug use and to understand the ways in which their demands encourage substance abuse. A coach's reaction to an athlete who experiences rapid weight and strength gains sends a strong message to the athlete and other members of the team. It is imperative that coaches become an integral part of the antidoping effort, as they often have the strongest influence over the athlete.

## Conclusion

In this chapter I have tried to raise awareness of the circles surrounding an athlete's decision to use performance-enhancing drugs. Just as an athlete can never accomplish great athletic feats without the support of many other personnel, drug use requires support from that same network, whether through denial, tacit approval, encouragement, or actively supplying the illicit substances. This is not to discount the athlete's own liability for using ergogenic substances, but to highlight that this is a multidimensional process. Indeed, one of the cornerstones of the WADA code is "strict liability" for an athlete's drug test. This is intended to restore some balance to the athletic milieu that reduces an athlete's personal responsibility. Physicians, scientists, trainers, and coaches can take steps to discourage athletes' use of illegal and unethical substances to gain a competitive advantage. Although these professions and occupations play different roles in the lives of athletes, they have in common the potential to be unduly influenced by the status and financial inducements that accompany sports.

It is obviously problematic to enforce compliance with drug-use regulations in the case of an autonomous physician, scientist, athletic trainer, or coach who works directly with an athlete outside the bounds of a university or institution. One part of the answer is to insist that identification should be made and penalties assessed not just for the athlete who tests positive but also for the people who aid and abet that athlete's drug use. Removing the status of being able to work with athletes and the financial rewards that accrue are two ways to penalize such people. WADA has attempted to ban coaches associated with athletes who test positive, and this may help deter the assistance that athletes require for their drug use. Given the huge inducements to violate antidoping rules, this seems a small step to offset such behavior.

The glory that athletes achieve is reflected in the people around them. However, just as a splash into a pond creates ripples, a positive drug test ruins more than just an athlete's career. Ancillary personnel need to be aware that significant consequences will also fall on those who assisted an athlete in the use of ergogenic drugs. Just as abusers of recreational drugs often damage the people around them, the negative publicity and disgrace of a positive drug test can also affect many others. Making certain that the coterie of personnel surrounding drug-using athletes also pay a price is one small but essential step in reducing ergogenic drug use.

### NOTES

1. National Collegiate Athletic Association, 2005 *Study of Substance Use Habits of College Student-Athletes* (Indianapolis, IN: National Collegiate Athletic Association, 2006), www.ncaa.org/library/research/substance_use_habits/2006/2006_substance_use_report.pdf.

2. World Anti-Doping Agency, "International Standard for Therapeutic Use Exemptions," www.wada-ama.org/rtecontent/document/international_standard.pdf.

3. W. W. Franke and B. Berendonk, "Hormonal Doping and Androgenization of Athletes: A Secret Program of the German Democratic Republic Government," *Clinical Chemistry* 43, no. 7 (1997): 1262–79; S. Ungerleider, *Faust's Gold: Inside the East German Doping Machine* (New York: St. Martin's Press, 2001).

4. W. Voet, *Breaking the Chain: Drugs and Cycling—The True Story* (London: Random House, 2002).

5. A. J. Mandell, "The Sunday Syndrome: A Unique Pattern of Amphetamine Abuse Indigenous to American Professional Football," *Clinical Toxicology* 15, no. 2 (1979): 225–32.

6. K. J. Browe, "Anabolic Steroid Abuse and Dependence," *Current Psychiatry Reports* 4, no. 5 (2002): 377–87.

7. World Anti-Doping Agency, "World Anti-Doping Code," www.wada-ama.org/rtecontent/document/code_v3.pdf.

8. S. Bhasin, T. W. Storer, N. Berman, C. Callegari, B. Clevenger, J. Phillips, T. J. Bunnell, R. Tricker, A. Shirazi, and R. Casburi, "The Effects of Supraphysiologic Doses of Testosterone on Muscle Size and Strength in Normal Men," *New England Journal of Medicine* 335, no. 1 (1996): 1–7.

9. S. W. Casner, R. G. Early, and B. R. Carlson, "Anabolic Steroid Effects on Body Composition in Normal Young Men," *Journal of Sports Medicine and Physical Fitness* 11 (1971): 98–103.

10. F. Tennant, D. L. Black, and R. O. Voy, "Anabolic Steroid Dependence with Opioid-Type Features," *New England Journal of Medicine* 319, no. 9 (1988): 578.

11. A. Breidbach, D. H. Catlin, G. A. Green, I. Tregub, H. Truong, and J. Gorzek, "Detection of Recombinant Human Erythropoietin in Urine by Isoelectric Focusing," *Clinical Chemistry* 49, no. 6 (2003): 901–7.

12. WADA, "World Anti-Doping Code."

13. G. A. Green, "Insulin as a Drug of Abuse in Sport?" *Diabetes Technology and Therapeutics* 6, no. 3 (2004): 387–88.

14. N. Dickert and C. Grady, "What's the Price of a Research Subject? Approaches to Payment for Research Participation," *New England Journal of Medicine* 341, no. 3 (1999): 198–203.

15. National Athletic Trainers' Association, "Official Statement on Steroids and Performance Enhancing Substances," March 7, 2005, www.nata.org/statements/official/steroidstatement.pdf.

16. *Los Angeles Times*, January 31, 2004.

# CHAPTER FIVE

# Performance-Enhancing Technologies and the Ethics of Human Subjects Research

KAREN J. MASCHKE, PH.D.

Since 1928, various international sports organizations have banned the use of certain substances and technologies—referred to here as sports enhancement, or performance-enhancing, technologies—by athletes who participate in their events. The International Olympic Committee (IOC) established its first list of banned substances in 1967, and in 1999 it convened the World Conference on Doping in Sport. This event led to the creation of the World Anti-Doping Agency (WADA), which in March 2003 released a World Anti-Doping Code. Backed by all major sports federations and nearly 80 governments, the WADA code harmonizes antidoping regulations "across all sports and all countries of the world" and is a core document that provides "a framework for anti-doping policies, rules and regulation within sport organisations and among public authorities."[1] In addition to the IOC list of banned substances and the WADA code, numerous amateur and collegiate sports organizations in the United States have adopted antidoping codes for their athletes.

One reason for prohibiting athletes' use of some enhancement technologies is the harm these substances or technologies might pose to human health. Another reason stems from the belief that the meaning of sport is debased when athletes use enhancement technologies. With reference to the Olympic games, Catlin and Murray point out that by banning performance-enhancing technologies, the IOC and other organizations are attempting to ensure "that all athletes compete on a level playing field." The meaning of sport, they assert, is about victory going "to the athlete with the best combination of natural ability, stamina, courage, willingness to undergo intense and difficult training, and strategic cunning," not victory going to the athlete who uses sports enhancement technologies to enhance his or her performance.[2]

Although Catlin, Murray, and others might be right about the meaning of sport,[3] humans have attempted to enhance athletic performance at least since the Greek era. Sports enhancement technologies used centuries ago were probably not subjected to rigorous experimental methods. Nonetheless, over the years, athletes and coaches obviously shared information about technologies they believed had enhanced athletic performance. With the advent of formal human clinical trials in the twentieth century, some information about technologies that might enhance athletic performance has been obtained from studies conducted for therapeutic purposes. For example, the U.S. Food and Drug Administration (FDA) has approved several drugs to treat disease-related anemia. The drugs include genetically engineered recombinant erythropoietin (rHuEPO), which mimics natural erythropoietin (EPO), the hormone that increases the production of red blood cells (erythrocytes). Recent reports of rHuEPO use include admissions by several cyclists in the Tour de France that they had used the drug.[4] The "dual-use" problem (i.e., technologies developed for therapeutic purposes and then used to enhance athletic performance) will probably increase. Indeed, there is concern that some athletes will use gene-transfer technologies (and may already have done so), now being tested in humans and animals, that are designed to increase muscle bulk and strength for patients with muscular dystrophy and other degenerative disorders.[5]

The dual-use problem is an unintended consequence of therapeutic research. Yet, therapeutic research has social and scientific value because it might identify safe and effective treatments for human diseases and disorders. But what about research whose purpose is to identify technologies that might enhance athletic performance? Human research with sports enhancement technologies raises ethical and policy challenges that have yet to be fully explored. This chapter provides a brief sketch of some of the published accounts of sports enhancement research, describes the ethical framework for research with humans, considers whether this research meets established ethical criteria for research with humans, and poses policy questions for the sports and research ethics communities.

## Research with Performance-Enhancing Technologies

It is difficult to quantify how many human studies have been conducted involving technologies that might enhance athletic performance. A search on PubMed and the search engine Google using the terms *drugs and sports, sports enhancement, sports enhancement research, amphetamines, steroids, creatine,* and other terms related to sports enhancement (e.g., *blood doping, altitude training,* and *EPO*), turned up dozens of articles, abstracts, and media accounts of technologies tested in humans that might enhance sports performance. Research participants included healthy nonathletes, as well as healthy athletes. Some of the healthy athletes had competed in elite national and international amateur and professional sporting events.

In 1959, *JAMA* published the findings of two studies that examined the effect of amphetamine on athletic performance. In the Smith and Beecher study, six different experiments were conducted with small samples of highly trained college weight throwers, swimmers, and runners. The study participants were given amphetamine two to three hours before they performed in experimental athletic sessions. The American Medical Association, the Medical Research and Development Board of the U.S. Army, and the U.S. Public Health Service helped finance the study. Smith and Beecher reported that a majority of the athletes improved their performance after amphetamine use, with the magnitude of improvement highest for weight throwers. By contrast, Karpovich reported in the same volume of *JAMA* that his study of amphetamine use in a small sample of swimmers and runners produced conflicting results regarding improvement in athletic performance.[6]

Twenty-one years after the *JAMA* articles appeared, Chandler and Blair of the University of South Carolina reported the effect of amphetamine sulfate use on selected physiological components related to athletic success in six healthy male college students. At the time the study was conducted, nonprescription amphetamines were illegal under the U.S. Controlled Substances Act. Chandler and Blair reported that the Human Subjects Committee of the College of Health and Physical Education at the University of South Carolina approved the study and that "all requirements and legal documentation dictated by the Food [and] Drug Administration and the South Carolina Division of Narcotics and Drug Control were met."[7] The study revealed various improvements after amphetamine use in performance measurements for strength, muscular power, sprinting speed, acceleration, aerobic power, and anaerobic capacity. However, the study also suggested that amphetamine use masked fatigue.

Researchers have also conducted studies to determine whether anabolic-androgenic steroids increase muscle mass and strength. By the end of the 1960s, authorities in East Germany were requiring coaches and sports officials to systematically investigate the performance effectiveness of androgenic steroid use by

East German athletes, particularly girls and young women. In 1974, the Central Committee of the Socialist Party initiated a bill to create a formal, government-mandated sports enhancement research program. The bill provided, among other things, that androgenic steroids and other doping substances should "be further developed and optimized by research on doping in high-performance sports, with special emphasis on the development of new substances and the most efficient patterns of administration, considering both the requirements of the specific sporting event, the time of drug administration and withdrawal, and other methods to avoid detection at international meetings."[8]

East Germany's hormonal doping research program was a secret, state-sponsored program designed to produce medal-winning athletes in elite international sports events. Hundreds of physicians and scientists carried out the enhancement and detection research, administered drugs to athletes, and/or participated as "unofficial collaborators" with the Stasi, the government's secret police, in surveying and reporting problems with the state doping system and evidence of possible defection of athletes and others from East Germany.[9]

Other steroid research has been conducted openly, including a study sponsored by the U.S. National Institutes of Health (NIH) that published its findings in 1996 in the *New England Journal of Medicine*. When the article was published, steroids had been on the IOC's banned substance list for 20 years. The authors noted that the results of previous research on anabolic-androgenic steroids were inconclusive: "Some of the studies were not randomized; most did not control for intake of energy and protein; the exercise stimulus was often not standardized; and some studies included competitive athletes whose motivation to win may have kept them from complying with a standard regimen of diet and exercise." The authors discovered from their study that, especially when combined with strength training, supraphysiological doses of testosterone increased fat-free mass and muscle size and strength in normal male subjects.[10]

In 1999, *JAMA* published the findings of a study that examined whether androstenedione, a testosterone precursor that acts like a steroid, increased strength. The study was conducted by researchers in the Department of Health and Human Performance at Iowa State University. Experimental and Applied Sciences Inc. of Golden, Colorado, a company that manufactured oral androstenedione, financed the study. King and coauthors reported that oral administration of androstenedione to 30 healthy young men during an eight-week resistance training program did not "increase serum testosterone concentrations or enhance skeletal muscle adaptations to resistance training in normotestosterogenic young men" and that use of this drug may result in potentially serious adverse health consequences.[11]

A year later, Leder and colleagues reported in *JAMA* that androstenedione administered orally for seven days to young, healthy men increased serum testosterone and estrogen levels, particularly when administered at higher doses. They concluded that "these increases could lead to anabolic or untoward effects in susceptible populations" and that "long-term studies of androstenedione use are needed."[12] The study was funded by an unrestricted grant from Major League Baseball and the Major League Baseball Players Association and by grants from the NIH.

Both of the androstenedione studies were conducted amid the controversy over Mark McGwire's admission that he used the substance during the 1998 baseball season when he hit 70 home runs for the St. Louis Cardinals, breaking Roger Maris's single-season record of 61 home runs. Although, at the time, "andro" could be sold as a dietary supplement under the Dietary Supplement Health and Education Act of 1994, its use was outlawed by the IOC, the National Football League, and the National Collegiate Athletic Association. McGwire and others argued that because andro was a legal, over-the-counter supplement and Major League Baseball did not ban its use by players, there was nothing wrong with his using it.

Although both of the *JAMA* studies indicated that andro might have adverse health effects, the findings of King and colleagues' study showing no strength increase were significant in the light of the politics surrounding federal regulation of the substance. If the King study had found that andro was muscle building, the substance would have met all four of the criteria for being listed as a prohibited schedule III drug under the Anabolic Steroid Control Act of 1990. Because the study used small doses of andro and a small sample of non-elite athletes, the finding that andro did not increase muscle strength was almost guaranteed. This was good news for the study's sponsor, which would have had to cease manufacturing and selling a substance that met the definition of a schedule III drug had the findings about strength been different.

Despite the safety concerns that both studies raised, Major League Baseball did not ban the use of andro until the summer of 2004. The ban was announced after the FDA, using a provision of the Food, Drug, and Cosmetic Act, warned 23 companies in March that they could face enforcement actions if they did not stop distributing products sold as dietary supplements that contained andro.[13] Later that year, Congress passed and President George W. Bush signed the Anabolic Steroid Act of 2004, which eliminated the "muscle building" criterion as a requirement for a substance to be listed as a schedule III controlled substance, which means that it can be sold only with a prescription.[14]

Creatine, another substance sold as a dietary supplement, has also been tested in humans to determine whether it has performance-enhancing potential. According to one news account, creatine is the most widely used sports supplement and "has been subjected to the most clinical research."[15] In response to studies by Soviet scientists during the 1970s and 1980s indicating that runners using creatine enhanced their performance, the Central Institute of Physical Culture officially recommended its use, and supplements of the substance were given routinely to USSR national athletes.[16]

In 1999, Graham and Hatton conducted a meta-analysis of creatine research and found that the studies they examined produced inconsistent findings due to poor study designs, small sample sizes, and differing dosage regimens. Although the studies included in the meta-analysis did not report any serious adverse effects from creatine use, Grahan and Hatton noted that most of the studies did not formally assess safety issues.[17] Thus, there is scant evidence that creatine enhances performance and virtually no evidence regarding its safety profile. The IOC does not include creatine on its banned substances list, and researchers continue to test its enhancement effect on athletic performance. For example, in 2003, Belgian researchers reported in the *International Journal of Sports Medicine* that a one-week regimen of creatine-pyruvate supplementation in well-trained cyclists does not have a beneficial impact on endurance capacity or intermittent sprint performance.[18] Yet, despite research findings suggesting that creatine has limited enhancement value, professional athletes in the United States reportedly use the supplement regularly. Moreover, creatine use is on the rise among high school athletes.[19] Because it is designated as a dietary supplement under the Dietary Supplement Health and Education Act of 1994, the FDA does not regulate creatine as a drug. It is sold over the counter, and estimates of U.S. sales revenues are as high as $100 million per year.[20]

Researchers have also conducted blood doping experiments to determine the effects of this intervention on athletic performance. Blood doping involves the use of autologous, homologous, or heterologous blood or red blood cell products to enhance the uptake, transport, or delivery of oxygen.[21] Research has shown that increasing the concentration of red blood cells can increase oxygen capacity, which increases physical endurance. During the 1970s and 1980s, Soviet researchers were conducting blood doping research and Soviet athletes were regularly using blood doping to prepare for competition. All the while, Soviet authorities denied that their athletes were using the procedure, and the research activities were state secrets.[22]

While the Soviets conducted clandestine blood doping research, scientists from other countries openly conducted and published the results of their blood doping studies.[23] The 1972 article by Ekblom and coauthors is often cited as the pioneering study that provided evidence of the performance-enhancing effects of blood doping. Ekblom and colleagues removed a quart of blood from four individuals, separated the red blood cells, refrigerated them for four weeks, and then transfused them back into the subjects, who were able to run up to 25 percent longer than before the procedure was conducted.[24]

In 1987, *JAMA* published the report of a study by Brien and Simon that was designed to determine the effects of the infusion of red blood cells in six highly trained male distance runners. The research—which was sponsored by the NIH, its National Heart, Lung, and Blood Institute, and the Blood Systems Research Foundation—revealed that autologous infusion of red blood cells (400 mL) increased athletic performance in a 10-kilometer race. The authors concluded that enhanced athletic performance was "probably due to an increase in oxygen delivery to the working muscles" and that "done with autologous reinfusion under careful medical supervision, as in this case, the procedure is safe." They also noted that the "procedure of 'blood doping' . . . is controversial." "Autologous transfusion has raised ethical questions," they noted. "It is regarded by the International Olympic Committee as dishonest. Our purpose here was not to encourage dishonesty in sports but rather to explore the effects of increase in RBC [red blood cell] mass on runners' performance."[25]

Elite athletes reportedly switched from autologous blood doping to the use of rHuEPO when the FDA approved use of this substance in 1989 to treat anemia in patients with chronic renal failure. rHuEPO is a synthetic hormone that increases red blood cell count and thus the capacity to carry oxygen. The IOC placed rHuEPO on its banned substances list in 1990. In 1991, Ekblom and Berglund published an article in the *Scandinavian Journal of Medicine and Science in Sports* in which they described the effects of subcutaneous injections of rHuEPO on submaximal and maximal exercise in healthy male subjects.[26] Other researchers conducted studies to determine whether a valid and reliable test could be developed to detect EPO doping in humans.[27] The Australian Federal Government and the IOC funded research known as the EPO 2000 Project. The research team included individuals from the Australian Institute of Sport, the Australian Sports Drug Testing Laboratory, Australian Government Analytical Laboratories, and the Children's Hospital of Harvard Medical School. The researchers noted that the ethics committee of the Australian Institute of Sport approved the study in accordance with the Declaration of Helsinki, a research ethics code that the World Medical Association first adopted in 1964.[28]

Researchers have also studied the effects of altitude on physical endurance. Baker and Hopkins examined 17 published studies, conducted with athletes, that were designed to determine whether living and training at high altitude enhanced athletic performance, and 8 published studies with athletes that examined the effect of "living high, training low."[29] Since publication of the Baker and Hopkins review, additional studies have been undertaken involving simulated altitude exposure. In 2001, Australian researchers reported that houses with simulated altitude levels do not mimic the effects of rHuEPO doping. Based on the results of a study conducted with well-trained athletes and healthy nonathletes, the researchers concluded that "simulated altitude facilities should not be considered unethical based solely on the tenet that they provide an alternative means of obtaining the benefits sought by illegal r-HuEpo doping."[30]

In 2001, the Nike Corporation initiated an altitude training study known as the Oregon Project. Directed by former Olympic runner Alberto Salazar, the project was designed to determine whether a "living high, training low" regimen could improve the performance of elite American distance runners. Several elite runners agreed to live in a five-bedroom house in Portland, Oregon, in which nitrogen was pumped into the house to simulate living at high altitude. Levine and Stray-Gunderson, researchers who have conducted many altitude studies with elite athletes, are among those who claim that the "living high, training low" method is an effective way of improving athletic performance.[31] In the fall of 2006, WADA announced that it would not add hypoxic tents to its 2007 prohibited list.[32]

## Ethical Dilemmas of Research on Sports Enhancement

During the twentieth century, various professional codes, guidelines, laws, and regulations were crafted to establish an ethical framework for conducting research with humans. Although opinion remains divided over how certain ethical principles should be interpreted and applied, there is consensus that for research with humans to be ethical, certain criteria must be met. Human research should be conducted in accordance with a written protocol that describes (1) the purpose of the study; (2) the drug, device, agent, biological substance, practice, or other intervention that is being tested; (3) the risks and benefits of the interventions being tested and the procedures being used; (4) the criteria for subject inclusion and exclusion; (5) the methods of experimentation; (6) the duration of the study; and (7) the procedures for collecting and analyzing the data. Individuals recruited to participate in studies must give their voluntary informed consent to be research subjects, and researchers must be qualified to conduct the research. Federal regulations in the United States require institutional review boards to review and approve all federally funded research with humans.[33] The United States is one of only a handful of countries that legally require an ethics board to review research protocols. However, the Declaration of Helsinki as well as several national policies and professional codes state that human research protocols should be approved when appropriate by an independent ethics review committee.[34]

Although informed consent issues have dominated the public and professional discussion about research with humans, the social value and scientific value of a study are also important elements of what makes human research ethical.[35] The two major international ethics codes, the Nuremberg Code and the Declaration of Helsinki, express the principle that research with humans should have social and scientific value. The Nuremberg Code says that "the experiment should be such as to yield fruitful results for the good of society, unprocurable by any other methods or means of study, and not random or unnecessary in nature" and that "the experiment should be so designed and based on the results of animal experimentation and a knowledge of the natural history of the disease or other problem under study that the anticipated results will justify the performance of the experiment." Likewise, the Declaration of Helsinki says that "medical research involving human subjects should be conducted only if the importance of the objective outweighs the inherent risks and burdens to the subject. This is especially important when the human subjects are healthy volunteers."[36]

Assessing the social and scientific value of research that may enhance athletic performance and the risks and benefits of such research illuminates the tension between the desire to acquire scientific knowledge about human performance and legitimating or encouraging the use of such knowledge to enhance athletic performance. Yet, the potential value of such studies includes (1) determining a technology's safety profile, (2) developing methods to detect the use of banned technologies, and (3) determining whether technologies enhance athletic performance.

Well-designed safety studies might provide knowledge that could be used to dissuade athletes from using harmful technologies and to encourage sports organizations to add these technologies to their banned substances list. However, to obtain meaningful results, some technologies might have to be tested at dosage levels that could harm research participants. For instance, because athletes have reportedly used anabolic steroids in amounts far in excess of therapeutic levels, research to determine the safety profile of these substances would need to use high dosage levels. Ethics review boards might be wary, though, of approving studies in healthy individuals that had a high risk, low benefit ratio.

There may also be social and scientific value in conducting studies designed to develop methods for detecting the use of banned technologies. Athletes who participate in events governed by codes of conduct are expected to comply with explicit norms of behavior and may be required to undergo drug testing as a condition of participation. Thus, valid and reliable tests are needed to identify athletes who use banned substances and to reduce the number of false positive results, so that athletes complying with relevant codes are not penalized on the basis of inaccurate test results. However, like safety studies, detection research can also carry a high-risk, low-benefit profile. Detection research may require use of doses that could endanger a participant's health, and studies with banned substances may put participants at risk of being disqualified from competition. In chapter 4, Gary Green notes that one of the exclusion criteria for a study designed to develop a test to detect rHuEPO use was that research participants could not be actively competing while in the study or be subjected to drug testing. Detection research runs the risk of violating the provision in the WADA code that says research "should avoid the administration of prohibited substances or prohibited methods to athletes." However, unless valid and reliable methods of detection are developed, athletes who test positive are likely to challenge the scientific validity and reliability of their results.

When research is designed solely to determine whether technologies enhance athletic performance, the ethical dilemmas are more pronounced, especially if the research involves banned technologies. However, there may be value in learning that a technology—even a banned one—does not enhance athletic performance. Coaches and professional organizations might be able to use this information to persuade athletes to stop wasting their time and money on technologies that are not beneficial and that might harm them in some way. Moreover, as Green points out, "by the very nature of their work, exercise scientists seek performance enhancement through improvements in such areas as biomechanics, human physiology, equipment, nutrition, and ergogenic substances" (see chapter 4). The tension lies in wanting to learn whether and how humans can enhance athletic performance and upholding the values of "ethics, fair play, and honesty" in sport.[37]

## Conclusion

The social and scientific value gained from research with technologies that might enhance athletic performance includes developing methods for detecting the use of banned technologies, determining the nature and extent of potential health harms of performance-enhancing technologies, and identifying which technologies enhance athletic performance and how. Yet, research designed solely to identify performance-enhancing technologies raises dilemmas for sports organizations that ban certain technologies, for exercise and other sports scientists, for research funders, and for the ethics boards that review such research. For technologies that are on banned lists, it seems likely that relevant stakeholders would support research to identify methods for detecting use and to learn about safety issues, despite the unintended consequence that the research might provide evidence that the banned technology enhances athletic performance.

But should research be conducted with banned technologies solely to learn more about their enhancement potential? What about research with technologies that are not banned, such as "nitrogen houses," creatine, oral bovine colostrum supplementation, and others? Sports research also includes studies designed to help athletes train better and more safely. The dilemma is whether the kinds of study described above undermine the international movement to transform sport into an enhancement-free enterprise. From a policy perspective, that dilemma raises questions about what "sports enhancement" means, whether sports should be enhancement-free, and if so, whether research designed solely to improve enhancement should be permitted to go forward. These are questions ripe for a thorough and sustained national and international discussion among sports researchers, funders, sporting organizations, and ethics review boards.

ACKNOWLEDGMENTS

I would like to thank Tom Murray, Gary Green, and two anonymous reviewers for their helpful comments on earlier drafts of the chapter.

NOTES

1. World Anti-Doping Agency, "The World Anti-Doping Code," 2003, www.wada-ama .org/rtecontent/document/code_v3.pdf. Quotation from the 2007 revisions to the World

Anti-Doping Code. WADA, The World Anti-Doping Code: The 2007 Prohibited List, International Standard," effective January 1, 2007, www.wada-ama.org/rtecontent/docu ment/2007_List_En.pdf.

2. D. H. Catlin and T. H. Murray, "Performance-Enhancing Drugs, Fair Competition, and Olympic Sport," *JAMA* 276, no. 3 (1996): 237.

3. Ibid.; R. Butcher and A. Schneider, "Fair Play as Respect for the Game," *Journal of Philosophy of Sport* 25, no. 1 (1998): 1–22.

4. In September 2006, two of Lance Armstrong's teammates from the 1999 Tour de France admitted they had used rHuEPO while training for the race. J. Macur, "Two Ex-Teammates of Cycling Star Admit Drug Use," *New York Times*, September 12, 2006.

5. T. Friedman, "Potential for Genetic Enhancements in Sports," testimony before the President's Commission on Bioethics, July 11, 2002, www.bioethics.gov/transcripts/ jul02/index.html.

6. G. M. Smith and H. K. Beecher, "Amphetamine Sulfate and Athletic Performance," *JAMA* 170, no. 5 (1959): 542–57; P. V. Karpovich, "Effect of Amphetamine Sulfate on Athletic Performance," *JAMA* 170, no. 5 (1959): 558–61; see also J. C. Wagner, "Stimulants and Performance," www.sportsci.org/encyc/drafts/Stimulants.doc.

7. J. Chandler and S. Blair, "The Effect of Amphetamines on Selected Physiological Components Related to Athletic Success," *Medicine and Science in Sports and Exercise* 12 (1980): 66.

8. W. W. Franke and B. Berendonk, "Hormonal Doping and Androgenization of Athletes: A Secret Program of the German Democratic Republic Government," *Clinical Chemistry* 43, no. 7 (1997): 1268.

9. Ibid., 1263.

10. S. Bhasin, T. W. Storer, N. Berman, C. Callegari, B. Clevenger, J. Phillips, T. J. Bunnell, R. Tricker, A. Shirazi, and R. Casburi, "The Effects of Supraphysiologic Doses of Testosterone on Muscle Size and Strength in Normal Men," *New England Journal of Medicine* 335, no. 1 (1996): 1–7.

11. D. S. King, R. L. Sharp, M. D. Vukovich, G. A. Brown, T. A. Reifenrath, N. L. Uhl, and K. A. Parsons, "Effect of Oral Androstenedione on Serum Testosterone and Adaptations to Resistance Training in Young Men: A Randomized Controlled Trial," *JAMA* 281, no. 21 (1999): 2020.

12. B. Z. Leder, C. Loncope, D. H. Catlin, B. Ahrens, D. A. Schoenfeld, and J. S. Finkelsetin, "Stenedione Administration and Serum Concentrations in Young Men," *JAMA* 283, no. 6 (2000): 779–82.

13. U.S. Department of Health and Human Services, "HHS Launches Crackdown on Products Containing Andro and FDA Warns Manufacturers to Stop Distributing Such Products," press release, March 11, 2004, www.fda.gov/bbs/topics/news/2004/ hhs_031104.html.

14. The White House, "Statement by the Press Secretary," press release, October 22, 2004, www.whitehouse.gov/news/releases/2004/10/20041022-13.html.

15. J. Briley, "For Young Athletes, Limited Gains—At High Risk," *Washington Post*, April 9, 2002.

16. M. I. Kalinski, "State-Sponsored Research on Creatine Supplements and Blood

Doping in Elite Soviet Sport," *Perspectives in Biology and Medicine* 46, no. 3 (2003): 445–51.

17. A. S. Graham and R. C. Hatton, "Creatine: A Review of Efficacy and Safety," *JAMA* 39, no. 6 (1999): 803–10.

18. R. Van Schuylenbergh, M. Van Leemputte, and P. Hespel, "Effects of Oral Creatine-Pyruvate Supplementation in Cycling Performance," *International Journal of Sports Medicine* 24, no. 2 (2003): 144–50.

19. Briley, "For Young Athletes."

20. M. H. Williams, R. B. Kreider, and J. D. Branch, *Creatine: The Power Supplement* (Champaign, IL: Human Kinetics, 1999).

21. WADA, "World Anti-Doping Code: The 2007 Prohibited List."

22. Kalinski, "State-Sponsored Research on Creatine."

23. Ibid.; B. Berglund and P. Hemmingsson, "Effect of Reinfusion of Autologous Blood on Exercise Performance in Cross-Country Skiers," *International Journal of Sports Medicine* 8 (1987): 231–33; A. J. Brien and T. L. Simon, "The Effects of Red Blood Cell Infusion on 10-km Race Time," *JAMA* 257 (1987): 2761–65; A. J. Brien, R. J. Harris, and T. L. Simon, "The Effects of Autologous Infusion of 400 mL Red Blood Cells on Selected Hematological Parameters and 1,500 m Race Time in Highly Trained Runners," *Bahrain Medical Bulletin* 11 (1989): 6–16; B. Ekblom, A. N. Goldberg, and B. Gullbring, "Response to Exercise after Blood Loss and Reinfusion," *Journal of Applied Physiology* 33 (1972): 175–80; M. H. Williams, M. Lindhjem, and R. Schuster, "The Effect of Blood Infusion upon Endurance Capacity and Ratings of Perceived Exertion," *Medicine and Science in Sports* 10, no. 2 (1978): 113–18.

24. Ekblom, Goldberg, and Gullbring, "Response to Exercise after Blood Loss."

25. Brien and Simon, "Effects of Red Blood Cell Infusion," 2761, 2765.

26. B. Ekblom and B. Berglund, "Effect of Erythropoietin Administration on Maximal Aerobic Power," *Scandinavian Journal of Medicine and Science in Sports* 1, no. 2 (1991): 88–93.

27. M. Audrane, R. Gareau, S. Matecki, F. Durand, C. Chenard, M. T. Sicart, B. Marion, and F. Bressolle, "Effects of Erythropoietin Administration in Training Athletes and Possible Indirect Detection in Doping Control," *Medicine and Science in Sports and Exercise* 31, no. 5 (1999): 630–45; R. Parisotto, M. Wu, M. J. Ashenden, K. R. Emslie, C. J. Gore, C. Howe, R. Kazlauskas, K. Sharpe, G. J. Trout, and M. Xie, "A Novel Method Utilizing Markers of Altered Erythropoiesis for the Detection of Recombinant Human Erythropoietin Abuse in Athletes," *Haematologica* 85 (2000): 546–72.

28. Parisotto et al., "Novel Method."

29. A. Baker and W. G. Hopkins, "Altitude Training for Sea-Level Competition," in *Sportscience Training and Technology* (Internet Society for Sport Science, July 20, 1998), www.sportsci.org/traintech/altitude/wgh.html.

30. M. J. Ashenden, A. G. Hahn, D. T. Martin, P. Logan, R. Parisotto, and C. J. Gore, "A Comparison of the Physiological Response to Simulated Altitude Exposure and r-HuEpo Administration," *Journal of Sports Sciences* 19, no. 11 (2001): 831–37.

31. B. D. Levine and J. Stray-Gunderson, "A Practical Approach to Altitude Training: Where to Live and Train for Optimal Performance Enhancement," *International Journal of*

*Sports Medicine* 13 (1992): S209–12; B. D. Levine and J. Stray-Gunderson, " 'Living High—Training Low': Effect of Moderate-Altitude Acclimatization with Low-Altitude Training on Performance," *Journal of Applied Physiology* 83 (1997): 102–12.

32. The WADA Ethics Panel was asked for its opinion and, after considerable deliberation, rendered its judgment that using hypoxic tents or chambers to simulate "live high, train low" was inconsistent with the spirit of sport as described in the WADA code. The panel made no recommendation with respect to any ban, as this judgment involves additional factors such as the performance-enhancing properties of the technology, the risk of harm, and the views of the relevant sports communities. The WADA List Committee, with input from the Ethics Panel, decided not to ban the use of this technology at this time. Personal correspondence with Thomas Murray, chair, WADA Ethics Panel.

33. U.S. Department of Health and Human Services, Protection of Human Subjects, 45 CFR 46 (2001).

34. World Medical Association, Declaration of Helsinki, "Ethical Principles for Medical Research," September 10, 2004, www.wma.net/e/policy/b3.htm; Canadian Institutes of Health Research, "Tri-Council Policy Statement, Ethical Conduct for Research Involving Humans," October 20, 2005, http://pre.ethics.gc.ca/english/pdf/TCPS%20October%20 2005_E.pdf.

35. B. Freedman, "Scientific Value and Validity as Ethical Requirements for Research: A Proposed Explication," *IRB: A Review of Human Subjects Research*, November–December 1987, 7–10; E. J. Emanuel, D. Wendler, and C. Grady, "What Makes Clinical Research Ethical?" *JAMA* 283, no. 20 (2000): 2701–11; D. J. Casarett, J. H. T. Karlawish, and J. D. Moreno, "A Taxonomy of Value in Clinical Research," *IRB: Ethics & Human Research* 24, no. 6 (2002): 1–6; C. Grady, "Thinking Further about Value: Commentary on 'A Taxonomy of Value in Clinical Research,' " *IRB: Ethics & Human Research* 24, no. 6 (2002): 7–8.

36. Nuremberg Code, 1949, http://ohsr.od.nih.gov/guidelines/nuremberg.html; World Medical Association, Declaration of Helsinki, "Ethical Principles for Medical Research."

37. WADA, "World Anti-Doping Code," 2003, 3.

# CHAPTER SIX

# Toward an Understanding of Factors Influencing Athletes' Attitudes about Performance-Enhancing Technologies

## Implications for Ethics Education

ROBERT J. DONOVAN, PH.D.

There is a considerable literature on ethical issues concerning the use of performance-enhancing drugs and nutritional supplements, particularly with respect to substances banned by the International Olympic Committee (IOC) and the World Anti-Doping Agency (WADA). Although Dingelstad and coauthors suggest that technological advantages in wealthier countries should be taken into account in ethical discussions on performance enhancement in sport, there has been little debate on the ethics involved in the use of existing and emerging performance-enhancing technologies.[1] The U.S. Anti-Doping Agency reportedly established a group in February 2002 to look at the ethics of performance-enhancing technologies,[2] but as of early 2009, this group had not published any findings.

A report by Loland includes a discussion of doping, highly specialized nutritional supplements, high-altitude chambers, and genetic technology as performance-enhancing technologies.[3] However, in this chapter I distinguish performance-enhancing *substances* ingested by the athlete from noningested performance-enhancing *technologies*. Performance-enhancing technologies include advances in equipment and clothing, technologies of oxygenation enhancement, and, with far greater implications for society at large, gene doping and gene modification. The technology that appears to be of most current interest is that of creating an atmospheric environment so that the athlete can "live high, train low," as Nike has done in its Oregon Project. The "Nike house" is constructed so that athletes eat, sleep, and spend their leisure time in a high-altitude, reduced-oxygen atmosphere, and train at sea level.[4]

Consistent with Loland's discussion of his "thick" theory of sport,[5] I agree that the performance-enhancing technologies of most ethical interest are those that enhance performance with no additional effort by the athlete and are administered by experts. Hence, in this discussion I exclude technologies that enable performance enhancement by providing feedback (such as heart monitors) but do not themselves enhance performance. Also, because performance-enhancing *drugs* are banned but potentially performance-enhancing nutritional supplements (such as creatine and Tribex) are not, I refer where relevant to *banned* performance-enhancing substances.

This chapter aims to contribute to discussions on the role of educational interventions in enhancing positive moral reasoning about the use of performance-enhancing technologies by reviewing the factors thought to influence athletes' use of performance-enhancing substances and technologies in general, and their use of banned drugs in particular. The chapter first establishes an ethical base for considering performance-enhancing technologies, then summarizes Donovan and colleagues' model of factors affecting athletes' attitudes and intentions toward banned performance-enhancing substances and extends this to include acceptance or otherwise of performance-enhancing technologies.[6] I then describe the influence of broad sociocultural forces and sport-specific social and economic forces in predisposing athletes to the use of performance-enhancing substances and technologies. The chapter then considers the stages of development in children and the factors affecting moral development. Finally, I attempt to bring these aspects together to delineate what is required to minimize the various forces that make athletes vulnerable to temptations to use banned substances and performance-enhancing technologies and what is required to enhance the forces that make athletes resilient to such temptations.

## Establishing an "Ethical" Base by Declaring Performance-Enhancing Technologies against the Rules

Several arguments have been proposed for banning performance-enhancing substances, the main ones being that such substances (1) provide athletes with an unfair advantage and hence are a breach of "fair play," (2) are potentially harmful to health, and (3) are against the rules of the sport and therefore constitute cheating.[7] The "cheating" argument is that the use of banned substances involves deception, destroys trust between participants, and hence undermines the social practice of sport. Other arguments are that the use of banned substances harms the image of sport and forces other athletes to use potentially harmful substances to remain competitive.[8]

A common counterargument is that the playing field is not level anyway, given differences in athletes' financial and social circumstances and hence differential access to equipment, clothing, coaching expertise, nutritional advice, and medical management. The "harm" argument is also open to question in that many sports are inherently risky, extreme training regimens are not necessarily healthy, and not all banned substances are harmful, particularly if administered under medical supervision. Similarly, although public opinion appears to be overwhelmingly against the use of banned performance-enhancing substances, the argument that the use of banned drugs harms the image of sport does not seem to be supported by at least some events and surveys.[9] For example, in spite of numerous drug "scandals," cycling remains as popular as ever, and baseball star Mark McGwire's admission to using androstenedione (banned by WADA but not, at that time, by baseball's governing body) had no discernible effect on the record breaker's popularity, although his later, unforthcoming appearance at a congressional hearing may have damaged his public image.[10]

Given the drive for competitive advantage inherent in sport itself, in current circumstances, any performance-enhancing substance or technology that is not excluded by the rules is open for public consideration by athletes and their entourages. It is questionable, therefore, whether an ethical base could be established against the use of specific performance-enhancing technologies or substances if these were permitted under existing rules. Hence, establishing a moral or ethical base for banning substances or technologies may first require that they be declared "against the rules." Houlihan also came to this conclusion as a basis for countering doping.[11]

Athletes willingly and, in the main, unquestioningly accept the rules relating to how their game is played or how their event is organized and run. While some individuals push the rules to limits more than others, even when officials are not present (as in "social games"), the social contract generally ensures compliance with the rules. Being "against the rules," therefore, is not easily counterargued and can apply equally to performance-enhancing substances and performance-enhancing technologies.

Rules that fit the following criteria are far more likely to be obeyed than rules that do not:

1. The rules are imposed by organizations perceived to have legitimate authority in the area.
2. The rules are seen to be justified.
3. The rules are seen to be applied equally across all athletes.
4. The rules are seen to be implemented without denigration of transgressors.
5. Penalties for transgression are applied fairly and equally across athletes.[12]

Criteria 1 and 2 are the most important in terms of achieving athletes' compliance. The perceived justification for a rule returns us to the current arguments for and against the banning of performance-enhancing drugs. One overriding principle might be that although a level playing field does not, and is unlikely to ever, exist without a rethinking of what we want sport to be, the extent of inequality can be controlled by restricting the use of substances and technologies that enhance performance without effort by the athlete and would increase the already existing relative inequalities.[13] That is, for technological enhancements in any area, it is likely that those athletes already enjoying superior access to finance, equipment, training methods, dietary management, and so on, would be the athletes to benefit most from unfettered access to any performance-enhancing substance or technology.[14] When ill-health effects are used as further justification for bans, scientific evidence is essential to convince athletes, coaches, and others of the credibility of the justification.

I suggest that the primary focus should be on adherence to the rules, supported by moral reasoning as to how a deliberate breaching of rules to gain an unfair advantage over one's competitors undermines the very basis of sport. This would be facilitated by providing athletes and their entourages with an understanding of sport as a social institution with a moral base. One advantage of an emphasis on rules is that, provided athletes have a strongly developed conventional commitment to playing by the rules, then additional moral justifications may not be essential for all athletes.

## Factors Influencing Attitudes toward Banned Performance-Enhancing Drugs

Donovan and coauthors proposed an overall model of factors assumed to predict an athlete's attitude toward using a banned performance-enhancing drug.[15] Although developed with banned substances in mind, the model components can be used to predict athletes' attitudes to permitted performance-enhancing substances and technologies, simply by excluding those components relating to compulsory testing and sanctions for transgressions. The model can be used to assess any individual's (coach's, doctor's, parent's, etc.) attitudes toward performance-enhancing technologies and substances, not just athletes' attitudes.

Based on a review of public health interventions in general and on the drugs discussed in the sports literature, Donovan and colleagues' model proposed six major inputs to an athlete's attitudes and intentions with respect to the use of performance-enhancing drugs: (1) individual *personality factors*: optimism, inner-outer directedness, risk-taking propensity; (2) *threat appraisal*: a cognitive and emotional appraisal of the likely negative outcomes of using a banned performance-enhancing substance or technology—including the likelihood of being caught, the severity of the penalties, and ill-health effects; (3) *benefit appraisal*: a cognitive and emotional appraisal of the likely positive outcomes of using a banned performance-enhancing substance or technology, including social and financial rewards; (4) *reference group appraisal*: perceptions about relevant others' attitudes to using a banned performance-enhancing substance or technology; (5) *personal morality*: moral standing with respect to using a banned performance-enhancing substance or technology and whether this use is consistent with one's perceived sporting values; and (6) *legitimacy*: beliefs about whether laws governing performance-enhancing substance or technology use are justified and applied fairly and equally across all athletes (see figure 6.1).

Of particular interest is reference group appraisal. Reference groups may not be passive referents. Many members of the athlete's entourage have their own motives for wanting the athlete to win, including parental pride, a coach's or trainer's professional status, and financial support for the sporting organization. Hence athletes are often under pressure from these referents to excel and, in some cases, to use banned substances and new technologies.[16]

Two market factors facilitate or inhibit the translation of attitudes and intentions into behavior: the *affordability* of drugs and their *availability*. The cheaper and more easily available the drugs, the more likely are those with even tentative positive attitudes toward drug use to succumb to trial and regular use. Young athletes are unlikely to be able to afford drugs, but their coaches and team doctors may have the means. There is substantial evidence that members of the athlete's entourage are sources of drug supply and drug management.[17] Pharmaceutical companies clearly have much to gain from developing new drugs that provide performance-enhancing benefits for athletes, as well as from improving the efficacy and convenience of administering existing drugs. For example, pharmaceutical companies are reportedly attempting to develop a long-acting

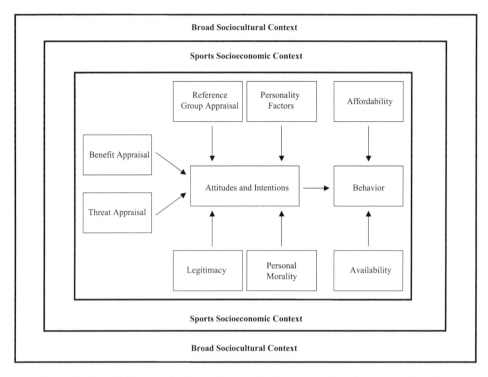

*Figure 6.1.* Overall framework for predictors of athletes' use of performance-enhancing drugs and performance-enhancing technologies

*Source:* Adapted from R. J. Donovan, G. Egger, V. Kapernick, and J. Mendoza, "A Conceptual Framework for Achieving Drug Compliance in Sport," *Sports Medicine* 32, no. 4 (2002): 269–84.

erythropoietin (EPO) requiring a once-weekly injection only.[18] The recent case of tetrahydrogestrinone (THG) manufacture by BALCO (the Bay Area Laboratory Cooperative) seems to be a case in which a company directly targeted the athlete market for performance-enhancing substances.

In this chapter, the components in figure 6.1 are considered as embedded in two overlapping contexts: the *socioeconomic context* of sport per se, which itself is embedded in the broader *sociocultural context.* The model suggests that in the absence of a strong individual ethical base, and in an environment supportive of drug taking, deterrents are necessary to dissuade athletes from using banned performance-enhancing substances or technologies. When a strong ethical base exists in an environmental context that is antidoping, however, athletes are unlikely to use banned performance-enhancing substances or technologies. The broad sociocultural context and the sports subcontext influence all of these factors to a greater or lesser degree.

## Sociocultural Context

Numerous elements of the broad sociocultural context can influence social norms that facilitate individuals' and groups' use of performance-enhancing technologies and substances. Perhaps the most relevant are the ready acceptance of new technologies that save time and effort, the search for miracle drugs and technologies to prolong life and prevent suffering, the widespread use of licit and illicit drugs in the general population, and a general demand for enhancement technologies (e.g., with respect to body image and cognitive functioning). I suggest that all these factors, along with a public health shift in emphasis from disease cure to disease prevention, provide a predisposing context for athletes—and others involved in sport—to accept performance-enhancing drugs and technologies. As the authors of one report put it: "Isn't doping use just a sign of the times, like we take vitamin pills and Viagra?"[19]

### *Labor-Saving Devices and "Miracle Cures"*

Since the industrial revolution, the emphasis in developed countries has been on scientific and technological advancement, including a drive to make the performance of household and occupational tasks quicker and easier (e.g., the washing machine; assembly-line robots) and an almost obsessive desire for medical advances to prolong life. While cultural values still include reward for hard work, athletes, like the rest of us, have a sociocultural predisposition to see the use of technology to increase productivity (and with less time and effort) as not only acceptable but also a worthy and admirable goal. Athletes who see themselves as "workers" could be even more susceptible than others to the use of performance-enhancing technologies. French cyclist Erwan Mentheour, when he admitted to using EPO and other banned substances, reportedly said: "That was part of the job."[20]

Advances in food technology and nutrition abound. Many food products (even our milk and cereals) are "vitamin enriched," and the market for so-called functional foods is expected to expand substantially in the coming years. Functional foods are natural foods that provide physiological benefits (or reduce the risk of chronic disease) beyond their basic nutritional functions; examples are carotenoids in vegetables, flavonoids in fruit, fiber in oats, omega-3 fatty acids in fish and seafood.[21] "Nutraceuticals," these components isolated from the food and sold in pills or capsules, are already well established in the health-conscious wider population and in athletic circles. In short, the young athlete grows up in a food culture accepting of technology to enhance the physiological benefits of foods. Similarly, our "pill" culture that seeks to avoid pain and suffering provides a disposition toward the use of performance-enhancing substances that assist in recuperation after injury, reinforced by a culture that seeks and promotes aids for "speedy recovery," all within an overall value placed on instant rather than deferred gratification.

There have been dramatic innovations in medical technology in the past 50 years, including organ transplants and cardiac bypass surgery.[22] Efforts are now focused on artificial devices to replace human organs, with perhaps the two most successful to date being the already established cochlear implants that allow the profoundly deaf to hear and the emerging use of artificial hearts. As transplants and artificial organs become more commonplace, the view of the human body as cyborg would find ready acceptance in a sporting culture characterized by a high value placed on technological advances. It is likely that such a view would be accepting of performance-enhancing substances and technologies.[23]

Overall, the factors noted above provide a favorable sociocultural disposition toward scientific and technological efforts that make life easier, prolong life, and enhance the quality of life, and do so with minimal effort on the part of the beneficiary. Such a disposition is easily generalized to performance-enhancing technologies in sport.

## A Culture Accepting of Recreational Mood-Altering Substances

While it is true that virtually all cultures have, over the centuries, cultivated mind-altering substances, only in the past century have sophisticated manufacturing and marketing technologies led to the supply of these substances becoming one of the largest businesses in the world. Breweries, distilleries, vignerons, tobacco manufacturers, pharmaceutical companies, and marijuana, heroin, and cocaine distributors now constitute multi-billion-dollar businesses. The illicit drug trade in North America (United States, Canada, Mexico) was estimated to be worth $142 billion in retail sales in 2003, with annual sales for the U.S. alcohol industry of $115 billion in the same year.[24] While tobacco use is declining in developed countries, substantial proportions of these populations still smoke, and tobacco consumption is increasing in developing countries. Consumption of coffee, tea, and caffeine-based sodas continues, with "extra" caffeine and other energy-based drinks targeted to young people in particular. In short, athletes are part of a wider culture accepting of the use of legal substances to achieve mood and "energy" effects.

It is commonly noted that the increase in doping in sport coincided with the increasing use of illegal recreational drugs in the general population in the 1960s, with the implication that both phenomena represented an increased liberalism and acceptance of experimentation with drugs.[25] While society in general "officially" frowns on illegal drug use, the fact is that substantial proportions of the population (including at least one recent U.S. president and the young relatives of another) have at some time tried an illicit drug. Hence there is no clear moral proscription on even illegal drug use for many young athletes, and European sports officials report that promoting antidoping messages is difficult in a broader social context that accepts recreational drug use.[26]

## A Culture Accepting of Clinical Drug Use

Among legal pharmaceuticals, the number of annual antidepressant prescriptions in the United States has trebled since 1988, the year that Prozac (fluoxetine), the first of the new antidepressants, was released.[27] Similarly, in Australia in 2001, antidepressants were the most used prescription drug in the central nervous system category. While to some extent these data indicate the growing pandemic of clinical depression throughout the world, they also represent a cultural acceptability of legal drugs for mood control and enhancement.[28]

Licit drug use is also increasing among the young, as more and more doctors seem willing to prescribe these drugs, and more and more parents are seeking a "magic pill" to solve their children's behavioral and mood problems. For example, the number of young people in the United States prescribed antidepressants, though small, appears to have trebled since 1988—perhaps, in many cases, to control attention-deficit hyperactivity disorder rather than depression.[29] While the absolute numbers are small, occasional media publicity gives an impression that the use of these substances is far more widespread than in reality and hence increases cultural acceptability of drug use.

## A Culture Accepting of Enhancement in General

Three areas of note in the social acceptance of enhancement procedures are the use of body image–enhancing drugs, the use of cognitive-enhancing drugs, and cosmetic surgery.

Several studies support the finding of increased social pressure on young people to use drugs to attain an "ideal" body image.[30] Some have noted, for example, that when the GI Joe doll arrived in stores in 1964, he had a body shape most boys could aspire to and achieve, but today's GI Joe dolls have muscular bodies that would be difficult to emulate without steroids.[31] One U.S. survey reportedly found that half of the boys aged 11 to 17 years chose an ideal body image that was possible to attain only by steroid use, and another found that 45 percent of college men were dissatisfied with their muscle tone.[32] These are fertile fields for steroid marketers.

Cognitive performance enhancement includes the use of drugs to aid memory, think faster, and focus attention by individuals who have no clinical need for such aids. For example, university students worldwide are reported to use Ritalin (methylphenidate) to enhance their ability to study by focusing attention and perhaps enhancing memory.[33] Such use is not surprising in societies that place great value (and great rewards) on competitiveness and achievement. As with performance-enhancing technologies (as distinct from performance-enhancing *drugs*) in sport, there seems to have been little discussion on the ethics of cognitive-enhancing drug use among the "intellectually intact."[34] However, as Whitehouse and coauthors note, in a competitive culture of high rewards to the winners, if people believe that cognitive enhancers will provide a competitive edge, then not only will consumers seek out these products, but the pharmaceutical industry will be more than happy to oblige them. Butcher claims that research is already progressing in this direction.[35]

Cosmetic surgery can be viewed as enhancement to achieve a physical appearance rewarded by the broader society. Cosmetic surgery has undergone substantial growth since the 1980s, and the American Society of Plastic Surgeons reported that Americans had 9.2 million cosmetic surgical procedures in 2004, up 24 percent since 2000.[36] Nonsurgical cosmetic procedures accounted for nearly 7.5 million procedures performed in 2004, with Botox injections being the most common (3 million procedures performed). The top five surgical procedures (in order) were liposuction, nose reshaping, breast augmentation, eyelid surgery, and facelift. Such surgery also raises the issue of what might be termed "performance-enhancing surgery," such as the Lasik vision-corrective procedure, reportedly used by some golf and motor-racing sportspersons.[37]

*Disease Prevention versus Disease Treatment:*
*The Health Promotion Era*

The shift in public health to a health promotion / disease prevention focus in the past 30 years or so also may have contributed to a sociocultural context accepting of performance-enhancing substances and technologies. As public health and medical science resulted in the control and eradication of infectious diseases and in safe food production and water supplies, attention turned to the emerging major causes of morbidity and mortality such as cardiovascular diseases and cancers. Epidemiologists declared that these were primarily "lifestyle diseases," resulting from what we eat, drink, and smoke, and how active we are. Hence the emphasis shifted to ensuring that healthy people remained healthy by reducing their risk factors for these lifestyle diseases. Medical scientists and epidemiologists also began to identify vitamins, minerals, and other substances that seem to protect against some diseases (e.g., folate, fiber, antioxidants), thus supporting the use of supplements and dietary management. This public health emphasis on increased healthiness occurred at the same time that medical and nutritional professionals increased their involvement in sport, thus providing a supportive environment for an emphasis on performance enhancement through dietary management, nutritional supplements, and other technologies.

Overall, the factors described above provide a context in which the use of performance-enhancing substances and technologies is consistent with much of what occurs and is condoned in society at large. We now turn to socioeconomic influences that impinge directly on the sports context.

## The Sporting Cultural Milieu

We live in an era in which sport has both international and domestic political ramifications. This was perhaps most evident in the former East Germany's systematic doping of athletes and the state-supported widespread use of blood doping in the Soviet Union in the 1970s and 1980s.[38] It is evident today in the vast sums of money supplied by governments to win gold at the Olympics.[39]

Several sports-related factors have been identified that are thought to facilitate athletes' acceptance of performance-enhancing substances and technologies, whether banned or permitted; these include the medicalization of sport, the commercialization of sport, and the intensification of sporting schedules.

These factors are themselves influenced by broader social trends and are interactive rather than mutually exclusive.

## The Medicalization of Sport

Waddington sees the medicalization of sport as part of what sociologists have described as the medicalization of life in general.[40] The 1950s and 1960s saw rapid and significant changes in the discovery, manufacture, and marketing of pharmaceutical drugs that were more effective and had fewer adverse side effects than previous drugs.[41] This general pharmaceutical revolution resulted in athletes having a greater array of drugs to choose from. This era also coincided with an increasing involvement of doctors in the medical management of athletes, leading to a rapid growth in sports medicine since the 1960s.[42] Coupled with the broader public health change from disease treatment to health promotion, sports medicine shifted from not only treating injuries but also advising on enhancing performance, including the use of legal drugs and nutritional supplements. The increased use of legal substances can be seen as facilitating, or the drugs even acting as gateway substances to, the use of banned performance-enhancing substances and technologies.

Doctors have substantial authoritative influence over their patients, and this includes athlete-patients. This influence can be positive or negative, and sports doctors frequently face dilemmas when treating athletes for injuries and responding to athletes' requests.[43] Unfortunately, studies indicate that doctors are one of the major sources of banned drugs for athletes.[44]

## The Commercialization of Sport

Achievements in sport have been rewarded from the time of the ancient Olympics. In fact, it is claimed that these rewards ultimately led to corruption, with bribery, cheating, and drug taking being commonplace. However, not until after the industrial revolution did commercialism and professionalism begin to flourish in sport, including links to the media.[45] Sport became a social institution as well as big business, with substantial rewards for all involved, not just the athletes, and the alleged increase in doping since the 1960s was concurrent with the massive increases in money invested in sport. Furthermore, this "de-amateurization" of sport has contributed to a sporting culture in which the focus is on external goals rather than on participation for intrinsic rewards.[46]

The 1960s also coincided with the rapid expansion of TV networks and international communication links, bringing sporting events to audiences worldwide. For business corporations, sport is entertainment, and the media have played an ownership role as well as a broadcast role. For example, News Corporation's Fox Entertainment Group until recently owned the Los Angeles Dodgers and still retains a minority holding in the baseball team. Media exist to deliver audiences to advertisers, and sport is a primary way of accomplishing precisely that. Sponsorship has concurrently become a major promotional tool, quadrupling in the 1990s, with corporations around the globe estimated to spend more than $24.6 billion in sponsoring sports, arts, entertainment, causes, and events in 2001.[47] Sporting multimillionaires are now commonplace, with many athletes earning far more money from commercial sponsors than from their sport.

By any measure, it is clear that the financial rewards in professional sport are far greater now than in the 1950s. The large amounts of money available to winners are an obvious inducement to use performance-enhancing substances and technologies, whether legal or not. For elite athletes who consider sport their job, the temptation to use banned substances and technologies is exacerbated by the possibility that other athletes competing for the same prizes may be using performance-enhancing substances or technologies. Injury downtime also becomes economically important, putting pressure on athletes to use whatever means are available to reduce injury time.

## The Intensification of Sporting Schedules

Concurrent with the increased commercialization of sport has been an increase in the number and frequency of competitive events, particularly in recent years.[48] In sports for which world rankings determine entrance to high-prize events, the pressure is on athletes to participate frequently just to stay in the top rankings. In other cases, media organizations create events, and the financial pressure is then on federations and clubs to participate.

The physical demands placed on athletes by an increased frequency of participation are therefore getting greater and greater. This physical (and mental) stress is further exacerbated by the ever-increasing performance level in sports, with physical strength gaining in importance relative to training and technical skills.[49] This is due partly to improved training, better diets, and better management, but also to increased competitiveness. Pressure to remain at peak performance comes from the simple fact that there are dozens of other, often younger, athletes ready to take one's place, and in some sports, the age of entry at the elite level is getting younger and younger. One implication of this is that athletes are becoming professional at a younger age and, because of commercialization pressures, are leading a life apart from mainstream youth, in which training schedules, diets, supplements, and medications dominate and the individual's most intensive interactions—other than with parents and family—are with trainers, coaches, sports physicians, dieticians, and sports officials.[50] In short, as athletes become increasingly focused on performance and on "gold goals" and as all aspects of their life and lifestyle are increasingly geared toward that narrow focus, decision making can become distorted as such narrow parameters are used as relevant criteria.

The problem of tempting economic rewards is made worse by the unequal distribution of wealth in many sports, where winners dominate the share of funds and losers (sometimes differing little in talent from the winners) earn only a small fraction of the winner's take.[51] Similarly, some sports clubs and individuals are more attractive to audiences than others and hence attract greater sponsorship and other funds. It is likely that the greater the (perceived) inequality of wealth distribution, the greater is the temptation to use a performance-enhancing technology or substance.

## The "Dark" Side of Sport

Although sport, at least in its amateur context and in terms of Olympic ideals, is associated with teaching positive civic values, there seems to be increasing concern that this is not always so and that, in fact, sport may be teaching negative values and behaviors.[52] This has even led to a questioning of the efficacy of using sport in social interventions aimed at reducing illegal drug use and criminal behavior among young people.[53]

This "dark" side of sport has no doubt always been around among some players and their entourages.[54] However, it is likely that the increased commercialization of sport, with its promises of fame and fortune, combined with the unrealistic expectations of fans, family, friends, coaches, and countries, generates an environment in which a "win at all costs" mentality is not just accepted but actively encouraged. In Eitzen's view, the imbalance of financial rewards noted above contributes to a "winning is the only thing" attitude.[55] This attitude is seen to facilitate the use of banned performance-enhancing substances and technologies and to encourage other unethical practices, such as normative cheating (e.g., pretending to be fouled) and normative violence (accepting on-field violence as part of the game and endorsing intimidation of opposing players).[56] Eitzen notes several characteristics of such a subculture: the aggressive behavior of spectators;

parental pressure on children to perform; coaches engaging in inappropriate tactics; organizations being reluctant to take action against high-profile transgressors; and team doctors assisting players by dispensing banned performance-enhancing drugs, dispensing painkillers inappropriately, and assisting athletes to pass a drug test.[57] In a rather grotesque example, Eitzen cites the case of a high school football coach who painted a chicken gold and had his players stomp it to death in the locker room before a game against a team called the "Golden Eagles."[58]

The work of Stoll and Beller indicates that while sport may reinforce values of loyalty, sacrifice, and teamwork, it often does not reinforce or teach values of honesty, responsibility, and justice.[59] Rather, sport may teach selfishness, envy, hostility, and bad temper. In short, without appropriate intervention, sport may not teach good moral reasoning, but rather teach bad moral reasoning. Given evidence that children's involvement in sport can be related to *less* mature moral reasoning and *higher* aggression and that the beginning athlete's moral reasoning will be influenced by the sporting culture within which his or her career develops, it is crucial that the basis for moral arguments against the use of performance-enhancing substances and technologies should be established from an early age.[60] This is particularly important given the influence of parents on a child's moral reasoning. The behavior of some parents is such that some junior sporting organizations require parents to sign a code of conduct—an agreement that they will not belittle or berate their own child, will not intimidate or show aggression to opposing players and spectators, and will not loudly criticize the referee's decisions—before their child can join the club.

## Moral Development in the Context of Socioemotional Development

Recent years have seen a markedly increased focus on the period from conception and birth to the early years of life as crucial for an individual's later health and well-being.[61] Researchers and practitioners around the globe are realizing that the earlier the intervention in areas such as behavioral problems in children, the greater is the likelihood of both short-term and long-term success. Programs such as Head Start in the United States and the Building Blocks and Positive Parenting Program ("triple P") in Australia are based on research into early childhood development.

Research such as that of Sroufe and colleagues, Williams and colleagues, and many others has identified "pathways" to prosocial behaviors and better health and, conversely, to antisocial behaviors and ill-health.[62] Of particular interest here is the child's socioemotional development. Sroufe and colleagues delineated six stages of socioemotional development from conception to 17 years of age (see figure 6.2).[63] Within each of these six stages, four related and interdependent developmental themes (*a* through *d* in figure 6.2) underpin healthy prosocial development: attachment and connectedness, emotional regulation, autonomy and identity, and moral development (which begins in stage 2; all others begin in stage 1). All of these are based on satisfactory social interactions with parents and caregivers, siblings, peers, and others in an ever-widening social domain. From the perspective of our discussion here, the concept of attachment is of prime importance in influencing moral development.

*Attachment* refers to an enduring positive emotional link between an individual and a caregiver (e.g., infant and parent; pupil and teacher) established through repeated positive interaction over time. *Connectedness* refers to an individual's sense of belonging to a particular group or entity. Connectedness is established by repeated positive interactions over time and particularly through opportunities to contribute to the group, opportunities for skill learning within the group, and social recognition by the group of one's achievements (i.e., a feeling that the group values the individual's contribution).[64] When attachment to an institution is strong and fulfilling, the individual is likely to adopt the institution's values and norms. That is, participation, learning, and recognition within the family lead to strong family bonds and internalization of the parents' values; participation, learning, and recognition in the classroom lead to strong attachment to the school and internalization of educational and civic values; and participation, learning, and recognition within a sporting club lead to strong bonds to the club and internalization of the sporting values held by that organization. Individuals who fail to form attachments to core institutions in society are vulnerable to forming attachments to outlaw, antisocial, or fringe groups whose members do not share the same set of values as mainstream society. Participation, learning, and recognition within deviant groups will lead to strong bonds with those groups and internalization of those groups' values. Such groups have emerged in the form of "doping communities" of athletes in which doping is seen as normal and those opposed to doping are viewed as outsiders.[65] This underlines the importance of the sporting culture that the young athlete enters. When coaches foster a winning or performance culture rather than a culture of mastery or intrinsic reward, athletes will most likely adopt weaker moral reasoning around concepts of fair play.[66] If the athlete is already under pressure from parents who condone a "whatever it takes" attitude, then the likelihood of accepting

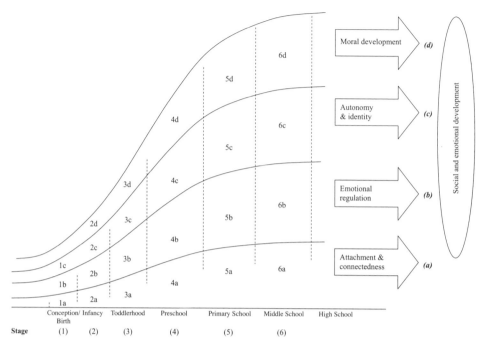

*Figure 6.2.* Overall framework for predictors of athletes' use of performance-enhancing drugs and performance-enhancing technologies

*Source*: Adapted from R. J. Donovan, G. Egger, V. Kapernick, and J. Mendoza, "A Conceptual Framework for Achieving Drug Compliance in Sport," *Sports Medicine* 32, no. 4 (2002): 269–84.

banned performance-enhancing substances and unacceptable technologies will be high.

Like young people in general, young athletes interact with a widening array of organizations and groups (or domains) as they make their way in the world. Some of these groups will have different if not conflicting values, leading to strains between values taught by parents and values expressed by peers or by some sections of the media. In a pluralistic society, there are countless opportunities for one's values and ethics to be modified as one interacts in different situations. The more consistent the values between the individual's intersecting worlds, the more likely it is that the individual's values not only will be reinforced but also will remain unchallenged. Conversely, the more contradictory the values of these intersecting groups, the more likely it is that the individual's values will be challenged.

The scheme in figure 6.2 suggests that attachment and connectedness underpin these other developments and that moral development is enabled by optimal development in all underlying themes. It also suggests that moral development accelerates in the primary school stage (5–12 years of age) and is almost complete by 15 years. When these developmental stages are mapped against a young athlete's career path, we can see that moral development is already well under way by the time many potentially elite athletes begin intensive training and is often complete by the time they reach their peak. This highlights how crucial it is to commence moral reasoning in sport at a very early age, and how such early training could have substantial payoffs in prevention down the track.

## Toward a Comprehensive Approach to Ethics in Sport

Based on the above discussion, figure 6.3 illustrates the three levels of intervention required for a comprehensive approach to teaching moral reasoning in sport as a means of preventing doping and other illegal activities: *individual-level* interventions targeting the beliefs, attitudes, and behaviors of individuals per se; interventions targeting the *sporting subculture*—that is, the beliefs, attitudes, and behaviors of those who represent the organizations and institutions involved in the sports "industry" and who have the power to influence the values of others, either by example or through their power to make and change policies and regulations in the various sporting domains; and *sociocultural* interventions targeting the beliefs, attitudes, and behaviors of those who have the power to make and change policies and regulations in areas influencing broader social forces.

### Individual-Level Interventions

Much education at the individual level has been targeted at athletes, but the evidence suggests that intensive educational interventions also should target those who may encourage or even supply banned substances or may foster values not conducive to good moral reasoning: that is, parents, teachers, coaches, trainers, and sports physicians. Given the primary role of parents in moral development, particularly in the early years, parents are a primary target group for interventions.[67] Parents (and teachers) have a major impact in establishing a positive moral identity when children are young, and such modeling effects can be lasting even though children, as they grow older, adopt other models such as sports heroes and entertainment stars.[68] Survey research shows that the primary role models for young people are their family and close relatives and confirms the

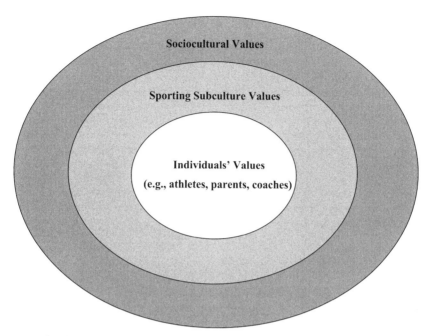

*Figure 6.3.* Three intervention levels for moral reasoning in sport

importance of educational interventions targeting the parents of young athletes and the necessity for early intervention.[69]

Some sporting organizations require parents and athletes to accept a code of conduct as a condition of membership for the child. While this is a good start, requiring parents to attend one or more workshops on sporting values and moral reasoning would be far better. Similarly, while some institutions include values and moral reasoning in their courses for coaches, trainers, sports physicians, and sports psychologists, others do not. Including these in the relevant curricula could be made a condition of accreditation. Sports physicians require specific assistance in dealing with the ethical dilemmas they face in the doctor–athlete-patient relationship that are very different from those of the usual doctor-patient relationship.[70] The use of performance-enhancing substances and techniques is only one of several ethical issues facing sports physicians and should not be treated in isolation from these other issues. Various materials produced by Stoll, Beller, and colleagues at the University of Idaho Center for Ethics provide examples for targeting teachers, athletes, parents, coaches, and fans.[71]

Given the evidence that children's involvement in sport can be related to *less* mature moral reasoning, it is crucial that the basis for moral arguments against the use of performance-enhancing substances and technologies be established from an early age.[72] The evidence indicates that children as young as five years of age are capable of distinguishing between morals and conventions and of understanding the universality, generalizability, and nonarbitrariness of morality.[73] Furthermore, the literature on socioemotional and moral development suggests that it may well be too late to teach moral reasoning if we wait until the athlete is 16 to 17 years old. It would be more beneficial to teach moral reasoning to all children from their first year of school, and this "curriculum" should include games and sports examples from everyday experiences. (Some specific suggestions for these educational activities are discussed below.) As children grow older and enter a sporting career trajectory, specific moral reasoning in sports components could be included in their coaching or related school subjects.

## Sporting Subculture Interventions

Individual-targeted interventions, particularly when included in curriculum materials, would have a cumulative impact at the sporting subculture level. However, it is necessary also to target groups and institutions that influence sporting values, such as sports journalists, sports physicians, commercial sponsors, pharmaceutical companies, event marketers, and sporting equipment and clothing manufacturers. Educational efforts here could begin with encouraging the adoption of appropriate codes of conduct by these groups. For example, pharmaceutical companies should have strict procedures for restricted distribution and handling of drugs that have performance-enhancing benefits, and event marketers could implement broader distributions of prize money among competitors so as to lessen the earnings disparities between "winners" and "losers." It is beyond the scope of this chapter to discuss these interventions beyond stating that they are essential to supporting individual-level interventions.

Officials and members of national and international sports federations and Olympic committees also require targeted educational interventions. While some might consider this presumptuous, there have been sufficient scandals in the Olympic movement and sports federations to suggest that periodic workshops on moral reasoning could be of value. Because officials and members might be approached by laypersons for their opinions on ethical dilemmas, these workshops could also be valuable for disseminating better informed and more accurate messages to such inquirers.

## Broad Sociocultural Interventions

Dubin, in his investigation of doping in Canada after the Ben Johnson affair, concluded that cheating in sport is simply a symptom of the unprincipled pursuit of wealth and fame that exists in society at large. This view seems to be shared by others familiar with elite sport. For example, Yesalis is quoted as saying that "unless we deal with the social environment that rewards winning at all costs and an unrealistic physical appearance, we won't even begin to address the problem."[74]

While the capacity of antidoping organizations and centers for ethics to mount educational campaigns to influence the broader social domain is clearly limited, one avenue might be to advocate for values-based learning from a very early age in schools. This would involve incorporation of values in the curricula for all subjects, in the school administration, and, in fact, in the life of the school, rather than the teaching of values as separate entities. To date, there are few published systematic and comprehensive interventions that teach children general values and moral reasoning. However, the values policy instituted at the West Kidlington primary school in Oxfordshire in the United Kingdom is one such example.[75] In this "whole-of-school" approach, each month's designated value (there are 22 values in total) is discussed and illustrated in all school activities and courses within the school curriculum. By means of example, discussion, and encouragement, students are taught to consider their behavior and to observe which actions have the best results for themselves and their community. The methods vary with the age of the children, in accordance with their increasing cognitive capacity to understand and discuss more abstract concepts—which, however, are always grounded in experiences or examples. Furthermore, through parental engagement, the values taught at school are projected into children's lives at home and hence into society at large. Modeling by teachers also plays a major role.

## Some Strategies for Educational Interventions

Education can be described as development of the ability to analyze, elaborate, and interpret information to aid in decision making. It involves a core set of information and a core set of analytic skills, including the ability to seek further relevant information to aid in further analysis. Moral education (and reasoning) involves similar cognitive processes and can therefore be learned through formal educational interventions.[76] Thus far, it is suggested that antidoping education has tended to emphasize the provision of information rather than the development of analytic skills in moral reasoning. Educational programs constructed to deal with ethics in sport should involve substantial interactive processes and active involvement in the analysis of ethical dilemmas, both in general and in a sporting context. Binder's *Fair Play for Kids*, a successful intervention that teaches "fair play" values (which received the Award of Merit from the International Commission for Fair Play for fair play education in schools), is based on two learning processes identified in the literature as important for helping children aged 8 to 11 years develop their ability to make moral judgments: (1) the identification and resolution of moral conflicts and changing roles and perspectives; and, because children at this age tend to see their world from an egocentric point of view, (2) the use of games, simulations, and role-plays to provide them with opportunities to put themselves in someone else's shoes.[77] Talk, or cognitive aspects, are an important component of the process of conflict resolution and moral decision making, and most of the activities in the program are accompanied by a "Let's Talk" section.[78]

More recent curriculum theory related to moral and ethical education complements and extends Binder's Kohlberg-based framework. For example, Nussbaum's work suggests a focus on the lived experiences and moral conflicts of real people in real situations, as opposed to intellectual discussions of abstract moral dilemmas, and an emphasis on narrative—drama, poetry, and story—as an important tool for ethical education.[79] Current thinking suggests that teachers should be encouraged to develop positive learning environments in which young people have opportunities to question and talk about moral stories and dilemmas and to practice different ways of acting and behaving. Hence interventions should feature poems, stories, and excerpts from plays that feature human conflicts and human emotions of moral dilemmas in life in general, as well as in sports situations.

Regardless of specific learning strategies, there is substantial evidence that educational interventions in moral reasoning can be successful in advancing moral growth, including in the area of fair play.[80] We can therefore be optimistic that appropriate interventions would yield positive results in developing athletes with good moral reasoning.

## Conclusion

Educational interventions to teach moral reasoning in sport should be embedded, as far as is possible, in more comprehensive values-based and moral reasoning interventions. Interventions should be targeted at as young an age as possible, given the evidence that children as young as five years old are capable of understanding the basic tenets of morality and distinguishing the domains of morals and conventions. Clearly, the methods and examples would vary by age, but the level of sophistication should always be challenging rather than too easily grasped. Moral reasoning in sport should be taught through experiential methods of narrative and drama, as well as through logical reasoning and discussions. Providing "reasons why" is particularly important to support acceptance of desired moral stances at all ages.

The influence of the social domains within which the young athlete moves must also be targeted. While there is little we can do to directly influence broader social forces such as materialism and other values that influence the use of banned substances and technologies, if values-based education were to be accepted universally from the first year in schools, this could yield young athletes more resistant to negative social influences and could even affect social forces in the longer term. However, substantial efforts can also be made to influence the sporting subculture so that desirable values are reinforced and undesirable broader social forces neutralized where possible.

Given the various counterarguments against banning certain substances and technologies, interventions to foster moral reasoning in sport could demarcate the social conventional domain from the moral domain, but equally emphasize both as important for the functioning of sport and the creation and reinforcement of positive sporting values. The primary focus should be on adherence to the rules, with clear moral reasoning as to how deliberate breaching of the rules to gain an unfair advantage over one's competitors undermines the very basis of sport.

Finally, sporting norms and rules are more likely to be complied with if athletes have some input into these norms and rules, particularly as athletes develop along their career trajectory. At the very least this means that in educational interventions, athletes must be given more than a list of banned substances and technologies—they must be given good arguments for the bans and the opportunity to debate these arguments.

NOTES

1. D. Dingelstad, R. Fosden, B. Martin, and N. Vakas, "The Social Construction of Drug Debates," *Social Science and Medicine* 43, no. 12 (1996): 1829–38.

2. A. Tilin, "The Ultimate Running Machine," *Wired*, October 8, 2002, www.wired .com/wired/archive/10.08/nike_pr.html.

3. S. Loland, "Sport Technologies: A Moral View," *Sport Technology: History, Philosophy and Policy* 21 (2002): 157–71.

4. Tilin, "Ultimate Running Machine."

5. Loland, "Sport Technologies."

6. R. J. Donovan, G. Egger, V. Kapernick, and J. Mendoza, "A Conceptual Framework for Achieving Drug Compliance in Sport," *Sports Medicine* 32, no. 4 (2002): 269–84.

7. P. J. Arnold, *Sport, Ethics and Education* (London: Cassell Education, 1997); M. Barnard, "Drugs and Darwin Fuel Athletes," *North Statesman* 11 (1998): 523; D. H. Catlin and T. H. Murray, "Performance-Enhancing Drugs, Fair Competition and Olympic Sport," *JAMA* 276, no. 3 (1996): 231–37; J. Parry, "Ethics and Doping," paper presented at IEC Scientific Conference: Doping in Sport, 2004, www.blues.uab.es/olympic.studies/doping/parry.htm; I. Waddington, *Sport, Health and Drugs: A Critical Sociological Perspective* (London: E. & F. N. Spon, 2000).

8. PMP Consultancy, *Studies to Combat Doping in Sport*, Lot 2 Final Report to the European Commission, Education and Culture Directorate-General, London, November 1, 2001.

9. Harris Interactive, "Despite Scandals and Allegations of Performance Enhancing Drug Use, Olympic Reputation Remains Untarnished," September 26, 2000, www.harrisinteractive.com/news/printerfriend/index.asp?NewsID=153; H. Stamm, M. Lamprecht, M. Kamber, B. Marti, and N. Mahler, "Public Perceptions on Doping in Sport," *International Journal of Pharmacy and Practice* 10 (2002): R28.

10. Barnard, "Drugs and Darwin Fuel Athletes."

11. B. Houlihan, *Dying to Win: Doping in Sport and the Development of the Anti-Doping Policy* (Strasbourg: Council of Europe Publishing, 1999), www.sponsorship.com.

12. T. R. Tyler, *Why People Obey the Law* (New Haven: Yale University Press, 1990).

13. Restricting the use of substances and technologies that enhance performance without effort by the athlete is recommended by Parry ("Ethics and Doping") and discussed by Loland ("Sport Technologies").

14. E. Parens, "Is Better Always Good? The Enhancement Project," *Hastings Center Report* 28, no. 1 (1998): S1–15.

15. Donovan et al., "Conceptual Framework."

16. KPMG, *Aren't We All Positive? A Social and Economic Analysis of Doping in Elite Sport* (Hoofddarp, Netherlands: Bureau voor Economische Argumentatie, 2001).

17. PMP Consultancy, *Studies to Combat Doping*, 37–40.

18. K. Birchard, "Past, Present and Future Drug Abuse at the Olympics," *Lancet* 356, no. 9234 (2000): 1008.

19. KPMG, *Aren't We All Positive?* 4.

20. Quoted in E. Davy, "Drugs and Sport," *Current Science* 86, no. 2 (2000): 8.

21. Agriculture and Agri-Food Canada, "Functional Foods and Nutraceuticals," March 20, 2008, www4.agr.gc.ca/AAFC-AAC/display-afficher.do?id=1170856376710.

22. J. Le Fanu, *The Rise and Fall of Modern Medicine* (New York: Carroll & Graf, 1999).

23. Parry, "Ethics and Doping."

24. United Nations Office on Drugs and Crime, *World Drug Report* (Vienna: Vienna International Centre, June 2005); "Economics of Alcohol and Tobacco—U.S. Alcohol Sales

and Consumption," www.libraryindex.com/pages/2127/Economics-Alcohol-Tobacco-U-S -ALCOHOL-SALES-CONSUMPTION.html.

25. M. Verroken, "Drug Use and Abuse in Sport," in *Drugs in Sport*, 3rd ed., ed. D. R. Mottram, 29–62 (London: Routledge, 2003).

26. PMP Consultancy, *Studies to Combat Doping*, 34.

27. J. M. Zito, D. J. Safer, S. dosReis, J. F. Gardner, K. Soeken, M. Boles, and F. Lynch, "Rising Prevalence of Antidepressants among U.S. Youths," *Pediatrics* 109, no. 5 (2002): 721–27.

28. C. Murray and A. Lopez, eds., *The Global Burden of Disease* (Cambridge, MA: Harvard University Press, 1996).

29. J. M. Zito, D. J. Safer, S. dosReis, J. F. Gardner, L. Magder, K. Soeken, M. Boles, F. Lynch, and M. A. Riddle, "Psychotropic Practice Patterns for Youth: A 10-year Perspective," *Archives of Pediatric Adolescent Medicine* 157, no. 1 (2003): 17–25.

30. "Sports Medicine: Muscular Body Images Pressure Girls, Boys into Misuse of Anabolic Steroids," *Health and Medicine Week* 26, no. 5 (2001): 4–5; G. Kanayama, H. G. Pope, and J. L. Hudson, "'Body Image' Drugs: A Growing Psychosomatic Problem," *Psychotherapy and Psychosomatics* 70, no. 2 (2001): 61–65.

31. Mediascope, "Muscle Madness: The Ugly Connection between Body Image and Anabolic Steroid Use," Mediascope Press Issue Briefs (Studio City, CA: Mediascope, 2000).

32. Ibid.

33. J. Butcher, "Cognitive Enhancement Raises Ethical Concerns," *Lancet* 362, no. 9378 (2003): 132–33.

34. P. J. Whitehouse, E. Juengst, M. Mehlman, and T. H. Murray, "Enhancing Cognition in the Intellectually Intact," *Hastings Center Report* 27, no. 3 (1997): 14–22.

35. Ibid.; Butcher, "Cognitive Enhancement."

36. "9.2 Million Cosmetic Plastic Surgery Procedures in 2004 in USA, up 5% on Previous Year," *Medical News Today*, March 18, 2005, www.medicalnewstoday.com/articles/ 21454.php.

37. Yesalis, cited in PMP Consultancy, *Studies to Combat Doping*, 34.

38. M. I. Kalinski, "State-Sponsored Research on Creatine Supplements and Blood Doping in Elite Soviet Sport," *Perspectives in Biology and Medicine* 46, no. 3 (2003): 445–51; Verroken, "Drug Use and Abuse."

39. KPMG, *Aren't We All Positive?* 10.

40. Waddington, *Sport, Health and Drugs*, 120–21.

41. Le Fanu, *Rise and Fall*, 206–17.

42. PMP Consultancy, *Studies to Combat Doping*, 33.

43. B. Saloman, "Ethics in the Locker Room: The Challenges for Team Physicians," *Occupational Medicine* 17, no. 4 (2002): 693–700.

44. P. Laure, "Doping in Sport: Doctors Are Providing Drugs," *British Journal of Sports Medicine* 31, no. 3 (1997): 258–59.

45. KPMG, *Aren't We All Positive?* 10–13.

46. Waddington, *Sport, Health and Drugs*, 123–24.

47. KPMG, *Aren't We All Positive?* 9; International Events Group, www.sponsorship .com.

48. KPMG, *Aren't We All Positive?* 21–22.

49. Ibid., 24.

50. Ibid., 26.

51. Ibid., 13–17.

52. J. M. Beller and S. K. Stoll, "Moral Reasoning of High School Student Athletes and General Students: Empirical Study versus Personal Testimony," *Pediatric Exercise Science* 7, no. 4 (1995): 352–63; J. A. Crone, "Toward a Theory of Sport," *Journal of Sport Behaviour* 22, no. 3 (1999): 321–40; D. A. Kreager, "Unnecessary Roughness? School Sports, Peer Networks, and Male Adolescent Violence," *American Sociological Review* 72 (2007): 705–24; A. Nattiv, J. C. Puffer, and G. G. Green, "Lifestyles and Health Risks of Collegiate Athletes: A Multi-Center Study," *Clinical Journal of Sports Medicine* 7, no. 4 (1997): 262–72; T. Wandzilak, T. Carroll, and C. J. Ansorge, "Values Development through Physical Activity: Promoting Sportsmanlike Behaviors, Perceptions, and Moral Reasoning," *Journal of Teaching in Physical Education* 8 (1988): 13–22.

53. T. Crabbe, "A Sporting Chance? Using Sport to Tackle Drug Use and Crime," *Drugs: Education, Prevention and Policy* 7, no. 4 (2000): 381–91.

54. D. S. Eitzen, "Ethical Dilemmas in American Sport," *Vital Speeches Day* 62 (1996): 6.

55. Ibid.

56. Crone, "Toward a Theory of Sport."

57. D. S. Eitzen, "Ethical Dilemmas in American Sport: The Dark Side of Competition," in *Sport in Contemporary Society*, 5th ed., ed. D. S. Eitzen (New York: St. Martin's Press, 1996); D. S. Eitzen, *Fair and Foul: Beyond the Myths and Paradoxes of Sport* (Lanham, MD: Rowman & Littlefield, 1999).

58. Eitzen, "Ethical Dilemmas in American Sport: The Dark Side of Competition."

59. S. K. Stoll, *Who Says This Is Cheating? Anybody's Sport Ethics* (Dubuque, IA: Kendall/Hunt, 1993); J. M. Beller and S. K. Stoll, "Declining Role of Moral Values Found among Athletes," *Chronicle of Higher Education*, March 31, 1993; Beller and Stoll, "Moral Reasoning of High School Student Athletes."

60. B. J. Bredemeier, M. Weiss, D. Shields, and B. Cooper, "The Relationship of Sport Involvement with Children's Moral Reasoning and Aggression Tendencies," *Journal of Sport Psychology* 8 (1986): 304–18.

61. A. A. Williams, S. R. Zubrick, and S. R. Silburn, *Foundations of Social and Emotional Development: A Continuum* (Perth: Institute for Child Health Research, 2001).

62. L. A. Sroufe, R. G. Cooper, and G. DeHart, *Child Development: Its Nature and Course*, 3rd ed. (New York: McGraw Hill, 1996); Williams, Zubrick, and Silburn, *Foundations of Social and Emotional Development*, 88–111.

63. L. A. Sroufe, *Emotional Development: The Organization of Emotional Life in the Early Years* (New York: Cambridge University Press, 1996).

64. R. F. Catalano and J. D. Hawkins, "The Social Development Model: A Theory of Antisocial Behaviour," paper presented at the Safeco Lectureship on Crime and Delinquency, Seattle, WA, 1986.

65. PMP Consultancy, *Studies to Combat Doping*, 31, 34–35; A. J. Schneider, "Cultural Nuances: Doping, Cycling and the Tour de France," *Sport in Society* 9, no. 2 (2006): 212–26.

66. Y. Ommundsen, G. C. Roberts, P. N. Lemyre, and D. Treasure, "Perceived Motivational Climate in Male Youth Soccer: Relations to Social-Moral Functioning, Sportspersonship and Team Norm Perceptions," *Psychology of Sport and Exercise* 4 (2003): 397–413.

67. A. A. Bucher, "The Influence of Models in Forming Moral Identity," *International Journal of Educational Research* 27 (1998): 619–27; J. G. Smetana, "The Role of Parents in Moral Development: A Social Domain Analysis," *Journal of Moral Education* 28, no. 3 (1999): 311–21.

68. T. Lickona, *Raising Good Children: Helping Your Child through the Stages of Moral Development* (New York: Bantam Books, 1989); Bucher, "Influence of Models."

69. Bucher, "Influence of Models"; RoperASW, *2003 Roper Youth Report* (New York: NOP World, 2003).

70. Saloman, "Ethics in the Locker Room."

71. University of Idaho, "Curriculum and Materials Offered by the Center for Ethics," 2004, www.educ.uidaho.edu/center_for_ethics.

72. Bredemeier et al., "Relationship of Sport Involvement."

73. O. Lourenco, "Making Sense of Turiel's Dispute with Kohlberg: The Case of the Child's Moral Competence," *New Ideas in Psychology* 21 (2003): 43–68.

74. C. L. Dubin, *Commission of Inquiry into the Use of Drugs and Banned Practices Intended to Increase Athletic Performance* (Ottawa: Canadian Government Publishing Centre, 1990); C. E. Yesalis quoted in "Sports Medicine," *Health and Medicine Week* 26, no. 5 (2001): 2.

75. F. Farrer, *A Quiet Revolution: Encouraging Positive Values in Our Children* (London: Rider, 2000).

76. Beller and Stoll, "Moral Reasoning of High School Student Athletes."

77. D. Binder, *Fair Play for Kids: A Handbook of Activities for Teaching Fair Play*, 2nd ed. (Ottawa: Fair Play Canada, 1995).

78. Smetana, "Role of Parents in Moral Development."

79. M. C. Nussbaum, *The Fragility of Goodness: Luck and Ethics in Greek Tragedy and Philosophy* (New York: Cambridge University Press, 1986).

80. Beller and Stoll, "Moral Reasoning of High School Student Athletes"; S. L. Gibbons and V. Ebbeck, "The Effect of Different Teaching Strategies on the Moral Development of Physical Education Students," *Journal of Teaching in Physical Education* 17 (1997): 85–98; S. L Gibbons, V. Ebbeck, and M. R. Weiss, "Fair Play for Kids: Effects on the Moral Development of Children in Physical Education," *Research Quarterly for Exercise and Sport* 66 (1995): 247–55; Crone, "Toward a Theory of Sport"; A. Nattiv, J. C. Puffer, and G. G. Green, "Lifestyles and Health Risks of Collegiate Athletes: A Multi-Center Study," *Clinical Journal of Sport Medicine* 7, no. 4 (1997): 262–72; T. Wandzilak, T. Carroll, and C. J. Ansorge, "Values Development through Physical Activity: Promoting Sportsmanlike Behaviors, Perceptions, and Moral Reasoning," *Journal of Teaching in Physical Education* 8 (1988): 13–22.

# PART II

# CONCEPTUAL MAPS AND ETHICAL IMPLICATIONS

# CHAPTER SEVEN

# Ethics and Endurance-Enhancing Technologies in Sport

THOMAS H. MURRAY, PH.D.

Some sports reward explosive acceleration—for example, the 100-meter sprint. Some, such as the shot put and weightlifting, require enormous strength. Other sports tax human physiology for extended periods. These include some of the most celebrated Olympic events: distance swimming, Nordic skiing, the pentathlon, and the signature event of the Games, the marathon. The Tour de France, arguably the most famous annual competition in the world, sends men on bicycles up long, steep mountain roads; most of the Tour's daily stages last for hours and cover more than a hundred miles.

Sporting competitions such as these push people to the limits of their endurance. Small wonder that athletes search vigilantly for anything that might enhance their ability to press on. The search for endurance-enhancing technologies is a part of this quest to maximize one's performance and to gain, or at least not cede, a competitive edge.

Historically, the most common way to increase endurance was to train—hard and long. As athletes, coaches, and trainers have learned more about exercise physiology, they have learned how to train smarter, building up the particular systems in the body that affect endurance. Lungs can increase their capacity to transfer oxygen into the bloodstream; muscles can burn stored fat more efficiently; brief intervals of great intensity can, surprisingly, build stamina, not just strength.

In time, people became interested in the effect of altitude on performance. Athletes who trained near sea level found that their performance fell off sharply when they competed in thin mountain air. The availability of oxygen to tissues straining at their maximum is a limiting factor for human endurance. With less oxygen available at higher altitudes, athletes learned to spend time at altitude, acclimatizing their bodies to work with diminished oxygen. One notable change in the body is an increase in number of red blood cells (erythrocytes) that carry oxygen from the lungs to oxygen-craving tissues. Why not, then, move permanently to the mountains?

Within limits, and on the whole, one's capacity to excel in endurance sports increases with an increase in the concentration of erythrocytes in the blood. Regular exposure to the thin air of mountain climes results in an increased concentration of erythrocytes. The problem for an elite athlete is that the thinner air limits the exertion one can sustain, so one cannot train as hard in the mountains as at sea level. The solution? Train near sea level, rest at high altitude—a strategy known as "live high, train low."[1] As I write this chapter, sitting here in the Hudson Valley of eastern New York State, the "train low" half of the strategy is readily available, but "living high" would be tough. The geologically ancient mountains of this part of the world are not nearly tall enough to make that much of a difference. Eons of erosion have worn them down to beautiful but not towering nubs, at least compared with the Rockies, Andes, Alps, Apennines, or Himalayas.

Human ingenuity has responded by, in effect, bringing the mountain air down to whoever has a few thousand dollars to buy a hypoxic chamber or has a wealthy sponsor who can create an entire suite of hypoxic rooms. The basic idea is to simulate high altitude by reducing the partial pressure of oxygen, which can be accomplished through pumping in extra nitrogen. An athlete can train to exhaustion at sea level, and then go off to sleep in a tent or room that simulates altitudes of 2000, 3000, even 4000 meters or higher. Train low, live (at mechanically simulated) high.

There is a much more direct way to increase your erythrocytes. Erythropoietin (EPO) is a hormone, produced by the human body, that signals the blood-producing hematopoietic stem cells in bone marrow to make more erythrocytes. Researchers isolated the gene template for EPO and genetically engineered it into cell culture production systems so that it could be made by the vat full. This biosynthetic EPO (recombinant EPO, or rHuEPO) is a godsend to people with chronic anemia, patients undergoing cancer treatment whose bone marrow has been battered into submission, and people who must undergo regular hemodialysis because their kidneys are failing. When EPO was approved for sale, it took about a nanosecond for cyclists and other athletes to figure out that it might be a quick and easy way to bolster their endurance, to get their hands on it, and—if the oft-repeated reports are true—to overdose and kill themselves.[2] EPO may well be the most important performance-enhancing drug in sport; before tests were developed to detect it, athletes could use it with little fear of sanction; and EPO is widely believed to be highly effective at boosting performance in endurance events.[3]

Other drugs are in development that might affect endurance, though none have emerged as a serious challenger to biosynthetic EPO and its descendents. Recent research on muscle growth and function in rodents that uses gene transfer has raised fears—and hopes?—that gene "doping" will soon be used to create genetically engineered superathletes.[4] The imminence of genetic enhancement appears to be greatly exaggerated. Still, the prospect that gene transfer could eventually, at some future time, be used to manipulate athletes' anatomy and physiology is a challenge to the meaning of sport. But, I will leave that discussion to the future and focus here on the endurance-enhancing technologies and strategies that athletes are using today.

## Is Worrying about the Ethics of Enhancement Mistaken or Fruitless?

More than a few commentators have argued that we shouldn't waste our moral fervor on agitating against the use of performance-enhancing drugs in sport. Some accuse those who do have ethical concerns of being conceptually confused, morally mistaken, or simply wasting their breath. Of the many arguments offered, five are worth considering in some detail. We can call them: the claim of incoherency, the line-drawing problem, antipaternalism and the presumption in favor of liberty, the "resistance is futile" mantra, and the heroic/Romantic/Promethean vision.

### The Claim of Incoherency

What's the difference between a special swimsuit that allows one to slip through the water with less resistance and a drug that boosts endurance? Both technologies permit swimmers to go faster and farther. Some skeptics claim that there are no conceptually or ethically coherent differences among the multitude of means that athletes can use to improve their performance.[5]

Many years ago I suggested a hypothetical case to test this claim.[6] Imagine that someone presented herself at the start line for the Boston marathon. She had the proper registration papers, a number pinned to her jersey, and clever footwear—with wheels on the bottom. Our imaginary marathoner was wearing rollerblades. Imagine further that the organizers of the event had not contemplated the outrageous possibility that someone would want to compete in the Boston marathon on rollerblades and therefore had not expressly banned them. The laws of physics and the limits of human physiology favor the rollerblading marathoner. Suppose she covers the 26-plus miles faster than anyone else. Should we say that she has legitimately won the competition? Or would we be convinced that she has undermined the meaning of the marathon, which is meant, after all, to be run not skated? She no more deserves to be considered the winner of the Boston marathon than a man who clears the highest bar in the high jump with the aid of a trampoline deserves a medal in his event. The rollerblading marathoner and the trampoline-aided high-jumper have both violated the underlying meaning of their respective sports. If they can be said to have won, it was by trickery, a gimmick. Yes, there could be a marathon on rollerblades and a high jump on trampolines. But they would be different events—not the marathon as foot race; not the high jump as unaided leap and acrobatic transit over the bar.

The argument from incoherency cannot explain what every competitor or admirer of the marathon or high jump knows: that there most certainly is a difference between running shoes and rollerblades, trampolines and unaided leaps. We grasp these conceptual distinctions with no difficulty; with equal ease, we understand that they matter morally. So, the skeptic may say, I admit that people can make coherent distinctions among various methods of enhancing performance—but where do you draw the line?

## The Line-Drawing Problem

Once it is acknowledged that we can see the difference between, say, "live high, train low" and administering a drug such as EPO, we still have the problem of deciding where on the continuum of means for enhancing endurance we should draw the line between acceptable and unacceptable. The challenge grows with the availability of intermediate technologies such as hypoxic chambers. The skeptic's accusation is a serious one: that any line we can draw will be unavoidably arbitrary.[7] If the skeptic is correct, we have a serious problem.

The skeptic's complaint confuses two senses of the concept *arbitrary*. Most often, we use the word to criticize something for which no principled defense can be offered. When a despot orders one person to be killed and another to be given a fortune, for no reason other than it amuses him, this is a morally heinous and arbitrary act. More domestically, a parent who for no good reason rewards one child and punishes another is likewise acting arbitrarily. So, when critics claim that it is arbitrary to distinguish between "live high, train low" and use of EPO, they assume that no principled reason can be offered for that distinction. But, the critics are conflating the morally suspect type of arbitrariness with a related but distinct use of the same word.

Most of the rules of sport are arbitrary. Why is the distance between bases in baseball 90 feet? Why not 80 or 100 feet? Why is the distance from the rubber on the pitcher's mound to home plate 60 feet 6 inches? Imagine that baseball decided that this was indeed an arbitrary number and that every pitcher should be free to choose how far from the batter he stood. What would prevent pitchers from moving so close to home plate that no hitter could possibly swing a bat fast enough to catch up with the pitch? Batters would be reduced to bunting—holding the bat over the plate, hoping to make contact with the ball. There would be no outfielders, because no batter could hit the ball hard enough to get it out of the infield; no home runs, no extra base hits of any kind; just a lonely batter trying to react quickly enough to place a ball fair, a pitcher, catcher, and seven infielders. It would be a very different game than the baseball we know—less complex, less interesting.

So, baseball is well justified in drawing a line specifying a particular distance between the pitcher's rubber and home plate. But why 60 feet 6 inches? Why not 60 feet, or 61 feet, or 66 feet? The official distance is unquestionably arbitrary in the sense that some other distance could have been chosen. At 60 or 61 feet, the game would look pretty much as it does now. At 66 feet, batters would have milliseconds more to recognize a pitch and swing. The balance between pitcher and batter would shift ever so slightly in favor of the batter. But it would still be recognizable as baseball. (Like most sports, baseball has made small adjustments such as raising and lowering the pitcher's mound to fine-tune the balance between pitcher and hitter. A higher mound gives an advantage to pitchers; a lower mound, to batters. The current distance of 60 feet 6 inches became the rule in 1893.)[8]

When good reasons can be provided for drawing some line, and good reasons can be given for drawing it at this particular place—even if a case can be made that it would be equally sensible to draw it a little to one side or the other—then the particular line (60 feet 6 inches in the case of the pitcher's rubber and home plate) can be justified. It can still be described as "arbitrary"; after all, a distance of 60 or 61 feet would also be defensible. But this is a different sort of arbitrariness than random punishments and rewards, with their aura of moral indefensibility. To recapitulate, one can draw ethically defensible lines on a continuum when there are good reasons for drawing a line somewhere (or else pitchers would stand on top of batters) and good reasons for drawing the line at a particular place, even though other points along the continuum might be equally plausible.

The means that athletes can use to increase endurance don't form a continuous, unbroken, one-dimensional function like the distance from pitcher's rubber to home plate. Rather, they differ from one another in multiple ways. Sorting out which of those differences are significant and how much weight to give each dimension is not a simple task. But neither is it an impossible task. And, if it is done responsibly, it is not "arbitrary" in any ethically troubling way.

## Antipaternalism and the Presumption in Favor of Liberty

Even if meaningful distinctions can be drawn among the many ways of enhancing performance, shouldn't athletes' liberty to decide which means to use and which risks to accept be respected?[9] At a minimum, there should be a presumption in favor of individual liberty and against paternalism, at least for adult athletes. What reasons, then, can be offered to restrict athletes' liberty to choose whether to use endurance-enhancing drugs such as EPO?

A common assertion in the 1970s and 1980s was that performance-enhancing drugs were harmful and that they should be banned lest athletes hurt themselves. Athletes, in my experience, found this paternalistic concern unpersuasive. In a sport such as football—in which 300-pound behemoths hurl themselves at one another, painful injuries are an everyday event, and disabling, career-ending ones depressingly common—the prospect that a drug might cause some vague harm at some time in the indefinite future is not a powerful deterrent. Competitors in the Winter Olympic sports of luge and skeleton careen down twisting icy tracks at speeds in excess of 80 miles per hour with no more protection than a skinsuit and a helmet. Cyclists descending after a steep mountain climb can hit speeds of 60 miles per hour or more, wearing even less, their only points of contact with the road consisting of two skinny tires. To tell such athletes, "Don't use a performance-enhancing drug because you might hurt yourself," is to invite incredulity and scorn. Paternalism can be seen in such circumstances not as authentic concern for athletes' well-being but as rank hypocrisy.

In research done at The Hastings Center in the early 1980s, we learned from athletes that framing the decision whether to use performance-enhancing drugs as principally a question of individual liberty was a mistake.[10] Athlete after athlete described the enormous pressure they felt to use drugs when they believed their competitors were gaining a competitive edge. The metaphor used over and over was that of a level playing field. When the field is tilted in favor of those using performance-enhancing drugs, the pressure is on all competitors to level that field once again. One way to level the field is to assure that no one is gaining an edge through drugs by effectively prohibiting drug use. Another way—exemplified by athletes in certain sports at certain times—is to use the same drugs your competitors are using. The pressure to level the field, to not surrender a competitive advantage, is persistent and pervasive. When the margin between glory and anonymity is measured in fractions of a second or an inch, and when drugs can slice a second off a race or add a couple of inches to a leap or throw, that pressure can be terribly difficult to resist. Some athletes do resist; some even triumph despite competing against drug-assisted competitors. But others succumb—not because they see endurance- or other performance-enhancing drugs as glorious celebrations of personal liberty, but because, after many years of striving, they are reluctant to lose just because the field is tilted against them. In sport, the decision whether to use performance-enhancing drugs is not a purely self-regarding choice, and individual liberty is not the principal factor determining the ethics of that decision.

## *"Resistance Is Futile"*

Skeptics could concede that coherent distinctions can be made and defensible lines drawn, and that unbridled liberty does not trump concerns about fairness and integrity. But, they might add, none of that matters because you can't do anything to prevent the use of performance enhancers.[11]

The first thing to notice about this assertion is that it is not, in the first place, a moral argument. There is no claim here that using performance-enhancing drugs is ethically good; only that their use cannot be prevented. (I use the qualifying phrase "in the first place" because it could be argued that trying to prevent the unpreventable leads to ethically undesirable secondary consequences such as inconsistent and unfair enforcement, corruption, and disrespect for and loss of faith in legitimate authority. But it is important to remember that the "resistance is futile" objection does not in any way defend endurance-enhancing drug use in sport as ethically legitimate.)

In outline, the argument is a set of empirical predictions. People will do X despite efforts to prohibit X, and undesirable consequences Y and Z will follow. Sometimes the argument is buttressed by historical analogies: the prohibition of alcohol in the United States was in the end futile and led to many bad consequences, not least the rise of organized crime. A more sophisticated version of the argument describes the social forces and incentives driving people to do

X: coaches push their athletes to win; fans get excited when records are broken; star athletes can make a fortune in salary and endorsements. Sometimes the predictions are plausible. But not always. And the "resistance is futile" argument implies that only perfection is acceptable, which is contradicted by the entirety of human experience.

Societies prohibit all sorts of things: theft, murder, sexual assault, bribery, blackmail, and extortion, to name a few. I know of no society that doesn't experience all of these offenses despite the prohibition against them. Does anyone seriously want to argue that because people will steal anyway, we should not bother to prohibit theft? Or that because people will kill anyway, we should tolerate murder? Prohibitions that have the support of the community, even though they are occasionally, even frequently violated, can nevertheless be necessary and justifiable. The problem with Prohibition was not that it was a prohibition but that it was forced through by a censorious minority without persuading the millions of Americans who drank wine, beer, and liquor that they should give it up. It lacked moral and cultural legitimacy.

There is little doubt that many athletes—I venture to guess the vast majority—would be content to forego banned performance-enhancing drugs if they were confident that their competitors had done the same. (An exception may be for drugs that also prevent injury or speed healing; whether there are now such drugs, or will be in the future, they will pose an interesting challenge for the ethics of performance-enhancing drugs in sport.) The challenge for those who care about sport is to create an environment for competition in which honest athletes can trust that the playing field is—mostly—level. Resistance is futile only if most people don't believe in the prohibition in the first place, or if those who do believe in its legitimacy lose all faith in its equitable enforcement.

## Heroic/Romantic/Promethean Dreams

Human beings remake themselves. When old ideas about class and caste fade, people remake the social order and their place within it. When the technology to alter our bodies emerges, humans learn to effect change, to remanufacture themselves—to remake themselves by human hand according to their own will. Some such manufactures strike us as amusing, insignificant, or petty: aging movie stars whose Botox-smoothed faces lack all expressiveness; women and men whose bodies have been sucked or tucked to conform to culturally idealized aspirations for youthful shapes. Other manufactures are admired: athletes who achieve extraordinary levels of fitness, strength, and endurance by dint of hard work and self-discipline.

The heroic/Romantic/Promethean dream celebrates self-making.[12] It takes human nature, particularly the human body, as a canvas on which human will and technology can—and should—inscribe its own visions. This is a radical view of the place of endurance-enhancing drugs in sport, or for that matter the place of mechanical prostheses, surgical enhancements, or gene doping. The incoherency and line-drawing objections are on their face at least neutral about the ethical desirability of drugs in sport. The heroic/Romantic/Promethean critique isn't neutral at all. It takes the ability to remake ourselves according to our own wishes and designs to be the moral hallmark of our species, a thing to be prized. Human willfulness is elevated above all other human capacities. Pure will is in charge, exercising its power over our bodies, moods, memories, and mind.

This twenty-first-century vision of the triumph of the will carries its own moral ambiguities. Take anorexia. Noelle Caskey, a feminist film critic, describes a view of this disease: "Anorexia is the cultivation of a specific image as an image—it is a purely artificial creation and that is why it is so admired. Will alone produces it and maintains it against considerable odds."[13] The view that Caskey portrays, for people who see anorexia as a terrible and sometimes lethal disease, may seem unintelligible, profoundly mistaken, and perverse. Its very premise—that anorexia is a free, conscious, willful choice—is dubious to the point of bizarreness; the desirability of thinness, especially among young women, the principal victims of anorexia, is culturally shaped. But this view is a faithful expression of the heroic/Romantic/Promethean dream in which the act of willful manufacture is what matters, not the particular goals and goods pursued.

The unfettered emphasis on human will and power is dangerously unbalanced. Will and techne are important aspects of our humanity. But they can be applied foolishly or malevolently, as we are reminded every day. As moral agents we cannot escape the responsibility of self-reflection and self-criticism: Will this exercise of human will and power advance human good? Will it deepen injustice or restore a measure of justice? Will it respect what in us is worthy of value or undermine it?

In the end, the heroic/Romantic/Promethean dream applied to sport begs all the important moral questions. Its adoption as a guiding principle in sport would lead to the dominance of the performance principle.

# The Performance Principle

Maximum performance, by any and all means, is the ultimate goal under the performance principle. The performance itself is all that matters; the means have no value beyond their contribution to that performance (see Jan and Terry Todd's discussion of powerlifting in chapter 3). Doing away with all limitations on the use of performance-enhancing technologies in sport, whether rooted in skepticism about the enforceability of limitations, conceptual squabbles, or Promethean fantasies, leads to an embrace of the performance principle.

It is impossible to stare at the sun without being blinded; in a like manner, it may be difficult to imagine what an unhindered view of sport ruled by the performance principle would reveal. Will all of sport come to resemble the drug-fueled forms of powerlifting? By its nature, the performance principle is reluctant to accept any limits on manipulations of the athlete's body or equipment.

For a batter in baseball, visual discrimination is crucial. What would we say about a baseball player who undergoes surgery that improves his vision to 20/10? Who uses contact lenses that result in a comparable improvement? Suppose hitters discovered that, depending on the lighting conditions, lenses with a certain tint would allow them to pick up the ball's spin more rapidly so that they can discern whether the pitch is a fastball, curve, or slider. Would there be any objections to this technology? Baseball now prohibits corking bats, but what will it do about the bats of the future, which may be made from trees genetically engineered for lightness, density, resilience, and whatever other physical properties maximize the bat speed and power a hitter can generate? Finally, it's not hard to imagine an entire pharmacy for baseball: one drug to improve reaction time, a second for increased concentration, and the old standby, anabolic steroids, for strength.

The governing body for cycling imposes limits on equipment and on modifications of athletes' bodies. In road racing, bikes must not be lighter than a specified weight and must have traditional triangular frames; cyclists must not use EPO or otherwise raise their hematocrit above a certain level.

Why the limit on how light a bike may be? The most important reason is probably safety. The first thing to bear in mind is that the long steep climbs typical of a stage race like the Tour de France push cyclists to their physical limits. Every ounce carried on the athlete's body or on the bike extracts its price. Experts do precise calculations showing how many seconds are added to a climber's ride up a mountain for every additional gram he carries. Product designers are continually devising ways to make bike components lighter. Unfortunately, at the edges of technological innovation, these new products also tend to be weaker and more likely to fail. That may be a mere inconvenience if it's the tape wrapped around the handlebar. But if it's the handlebar itself that breaks, the cyclist will lose control and the consequences could be catastrophic. If the brakes, or wheels, or the frame disintegrate when the cyclist is descending at 50 or 60 miles per hour after a steep climb, death is a possibility—not only for that cyclist but for all those who follow him to the paving.

The inexorable pressure to get an advantage on the competition would drive cyclists to use lighter and lighter components with the completely predictable result that parts will fail, sometimes catastrophically. Better for all competitors to observe a minimum weight limit for their bikes: no one is tempted to further risk their life on an ultralight, extremely fragile, bike. What would the performance principle say about such limits on equipment?

Cycling has seen its share of performance-enhancing drugs, with EPO and stimulants the best known and, probably, most effective in that sport. How should cycling think about genetic modifications designed to enhance performance? Suppose that in the future there were effective ways to genetically supercharge muscles, increase lung volume and cardiac capacity, and tinker with bone marrow stem cells so that they made the optimum concentration of oxygen-carrying cells in the blood. What should be sport's response? Believers in the performance principle would have to embrace these modifications of human anatomy and physiology. Indeed, it is difficult to see how the performance principle could support any limits on even the most bizarre and risky genetic modifications. Like cyclists eager to shave every gram off their bike's weight, athletes guided by the performance principle would be driven to ever-greater risks to their health and life. The meaning of the sport itself would be distorted beyond recognition. Contests between people of different natural talents amplified by differences in self-discipline, perseverance, and fortitude would be replaced by contests between genetic manipulators in which indifference to the athlete's long-term health is a positive advantage, and moral scruples only get in the way.

Wherever the performance principle triumphs, sport may come to look like the drug-friendly forms of powerlifting. But sport cannot escape the ever-present desire to set limits; nor can it avoid coming to terms with the meaning of competition. Even the most extreme forms of powerlifting, as far as I know, prohibit athletes' use of jacks to lift the free weights. Limits and rules are unavoidable in sport. The proliferation of governing bodies in powerlifting testifies to a struggle over the meaning of the sport, as much as it may also reflect a fight over money and power. The question of the meaning of the competition never goes away, despite the performance principle's refusal to take the question seriously.

What, then, can serve as a guide to the meaning of sport and the ethics of enhancement? Ideas about human nature and the "natural" provide a possible path. Three of those paths have been prominent in discussions about biomedical enhancement technologies and sport.

## Three Conceptions of Human Nature in Relation to Sport

Can some notion of what is "natural" serve as a robust guide for the ethics of endurance-enhancing technologies in sport? The President's Council on Bioethics, in its report *Beyond Therapy*, tries to develop a case for the "natural" as a positive ethical guide, not merely in sport but in all realms of human performance. In the *Oxford Handbook of Bioethics*, I called this view "human nature as normative guide."[14]

A fundamental question is what an understanding of biotechnological enhancement in sport reveals about the ethics of enhancement in other realms of human life. The example of superior performance chosen in *Beyond Therapy*—excellence in sport—is misleading because it fits the authors' preferred framework too neatly, in two ways. First, it permits an excessively individualistic and physical account of the ethics of enhancement. Second, it mistakes the particular for the general. The particular, in the case of sport, is indeed the goal of specific forms of excellent performance within a strict context of rules that both constitute the practice and attempt to ensure fairness in the competition. But other equally if not more important human practices have other sorts of goals. For medicine, the ends include healing, health, comforting the afflicted, preventing premature death. We may hope that the healer flourishes in this role, and we should construct our social institutions and practices to encourage such flourishing. But there is not the same intimate and direct relationship between biotechnological enhancement and inauthenticity in the case of the healer and his practice as there is in the case of the athlete and hers.

We may regret that a dedicated physician feels compelled to resort to large quantities of caffeine to stay alert and look after patients on his watch, but such doctors are not, in the words of *Beyond Therapy*, compromising "our choosing and willing identity itself, since we are choosing to become less than normally the source or the shapers of our own identity." Nor, by drinking that vente full-caff, does our doctor "mock the very excellence of our own individual embodiment that superior performance is meant to display." And our physician would probably be dumbfounded were he to be confronted with this description of his actions: "by using these technological means to transcend the limits of our natures, we are deforming also the character of human desire and aspiration, settling for externally gauged achievements that are less and less the fruits of our own individual striving and cultivated finite gifts."[15]

The authors of *Beyond Therapy* recognize that they have a problem; that adhering faithfully to human nature as a normative guide leads to unintelligible descriptions and untenable conclusions. What about modafinil to help soldiers stay awake so that they can better defend their lives and their country? The example of the antitremor drug–aided surgeon that I introduced years ago also appears, and, again, *Beyond Therapy* blinks: an individual's nature can be defiled in the service of some greater good: "When we override our own boundaries, we do so or should do so for the sake of the whole, and only when the whole itself is at stake, when everything human and humanly dignified might be lost." It adds a qualification: "And we should do so only uneasily, overriding boundaries rather than abandoning them."[16] So, human nature as normative guide is not infallible. We are justified in "overriding" its counsel under certain circumstances. The lofty rhetoric in which *Beyond Therapy* couches its glum acknowledgment that the boundaries set by our natures can and should be violated under certain circumstances conceals even as it concedes. It conceals the difficult human judgments that must be made about the panoply of enhancement technologies in the many spheres of human endeavor. In this context, sport is easy; life is hard.

Human nature is not an unfailingly reliable guide to what is good. Alongside love, courage, loyalty, and fortitude—admirable human qualities—we are also capable of hatred, cowardice, treachery, and laziness. The last four are every bit as naturally human as the first four. Not all that is natural is good. And although there may be much in the unnatural, human-made world that is morally problematic, there is an abundance of things that are, on the whole, good. Vaccines, for instance, are artifacts constructed by humankind that alter our physiology. The most successful vaccines induce changes lasting a lifetime. Vaccines prime our immune system to respond rapidly and savagely to microbes that invade and attempt to colonize our body. Vaccines are created by human ingenuity; they manipulate our bodies by tricking our immune systems. They are decidedly unnatural. And they do an enormous amount of good. Smallpox has been vanquished; poliomyelitis persists in only a few places, its complete elimination stalled not so much because of flaws in the vaccine as by fear, ignorance, myth, and politics.

The claim that human nature is a guide to what is good and right is only one view about human nature. The second possibility is embodied in the fantasies of the heroic/Romantic/Promethean dreamers. Call this the "human nature as raw material" view. It emphasizes the plasticity of our natures.[17] We modify our bodies with exercise and drugs, but also with tattoos, piercings, liposuction, Botox, and cosmetic surgery. Genetic manipulation is still in its infancy, but eventually scientists are likely to learn how to use it with reliable and mostly predictable results. A few individuals have gone beyond the quotidian and done such things as having computer chips implanted; at least one person is trying to grow horns. For some, the body may be a canvas and the modifications they inscribe on the body are intended as an artistic expression of human limitations, human possibilities, or whatever theme animates their creative vision. Others want to escape the limits human nature imposes by imposing their will on the body through technology.

As long as humans are doing the manipulating, though, they will have to choose which human capacities they favor. Advocates of the heroic/Romantic/Promethean celebrate our ability to create technology along with our unfettered will that chooses how to employ those technologies. They view human nature as raw material to be manipulated to the limits of technology and human imagination. Aside from will and technology, all other human capacities are open to modification. We can tune our moods, attentiveness, and preferences along with our anatomy.[18]

There is a powerful though unspoken hierarchy of value at work here. Two aspects of human nature, our willfulness and our ability to create tools, are elevated above all other human capacities. Implicit in this view is that capacities such as the ability to love, to feel happy or sad, to form relationships, to feel empathy—the list goes on—are simply less important. Or more precisely, their place in the hierarchy of value is established by each person who imposes his or her will on human nature. But in the heroic/Romantic/Promethean view, plasticity is the rule, and tinkering with human nature is celebrated as an expression of human willfulness and cleverness.

There is a middle path. Human nature may not be an infallible guide to what is good and true, but it shapes our experience, gives form to our fears and longings, and sets the foundation on which we may flourish—or not. Human nature is not limitlessly malleable, as adherents to the heroic/Romantic/Promethean would have it. Elevating our capacity for willful manipulation above all other human capacities diminishes the significance of all other aspects of our nature. It also opens wide the door to narcissistic preoccupation, arrogance, and catastrophically bad judgments about which human capacities to tinker with, and to what end.

The middle path is to see human nature as establishing the contours of the given. We are creatures of a particular kind—even if one aspect of our kind is the ability to imagine, and occasionally to achieve, intentional, partial, redesign. But this is merely one aspect, not the most or only important one. Our natures are irreducibly complex and morally ambiguous. We are capable of great nobility, courage, love, and creativity; we are equally capable of baseness, cowardice, indifference, and pedantry. Our natures are also inescapably social. We rely crucially on the care of creatures like us to survive our many years of dependency. Our flourishing—our emotional growth and our happiness—depends on our relationships with others at least as much as it depends on what we can do with and to ourselves. This view of human nature, that it sets the contours within which we may flourish or fail to do so, gives fair weight to our embodied humanness without romanticizing either our given nature or fantasies of escape from that nature.

Sport is perhaps the paramount public expression of our embodied humanness. Achieving excellence in sport requires a base of natural physical talents and the honing and perfection of those talents through a wide array of other human capacities such as the ability to study and learn from coaches, as well as human virtues such as perseverance, dedication, and a willingness to suffer in pursuit of a valued goal. Basketball coaches say you can't teach height. But neither is height a moral virtue. Becoming a great basketball player is made easier by being very tall; speed, strength, quick reaction time, large hands, and gracefulness are also natural advantages, susceptible in varying degrees to willful alteration. (You can build on natural strength by assiduous training; there's not much you can do to make your hands larger.) But moral virtues are required to transform those talents into athletic success. Technique must be learned by repetition and practice; skeletal muscles, heart, and lungs must be brought to their peak capacity by hour after hour of dedicated effort. Athletes in team sports must learn to cooperate, to lead, to motivate themselves and others. Different sports rely on different sets of natural talents and virtues. But all sports require some mix of both talents and virtues. Sport affirms our physical nature and, at the same time, human will and virtue. Human flourishing, as expressed by the pursuit of excellence in sport, highlights the importance of viewing human nature as the contours of the given.

# Sources of Ethical Concern over Biotechnological Enhancement in Sport

The fear in *Beyond Therapy* that biotechnological enhancement will undermine human nature comes closest to the mark when it aims at sport; but its focus on human nature gets us only half way toward understanding the ethics of enhancement.[19] Sport is a social practice. The meaning of sport is not revealed by a reading of human nature per se, no matter how deep and perceptive that reading may be. Humans' fascination with sport—broad but by no means universal— may reflect widely shared inner yearnings about integrating our bodies and wills; that fascination may also derive from a drive to perfect and express human excellences; but those yearnings and drives are given shape by communities that celebrate particular sports and set the rules within which those sports take form. Though few individuals may take the trouble to articulate it, there is a point, a goal, of the social practice of sport that is widely shared, if implicitly understood. The point of sport, at the risk of repetition, is to pursue human excellence through the virtuous perfection of natural talents.

Why the point of the social practice is fundamental to understanding the ethics of enhancement is best revealed by looking outside sport, at medicine, for example. Imagine a drug that eliminates the slight tremors that all people experience. These perturbations are scarcely noticeable in ordinary life. But imagine further that in the most precise and delicate neurosurgeries, those tiny involuntary motions, amplified by the surgeon's scalpel, result in damage to nerve cells that are not a target of the surgeon's knife. Most of the time the damage is too small to be noticed; occasionally, however, it causes permanent and discernable harm. Suppose that a drug is discovered or developed that does away with that normal tremor. The surgeon's hand is now steadier, the scalpel's path more precise, the damage to surrounding tissue diminished. Studies confirm that patients of surgeons who take the drug do better; they have fewer complications and bad outcomes. The person you love most in the world needs neurosurgery. Which surgeon do you choose: the one who swears that she will never use performance-enhancing drugs because they undermine human nature, or the one who promises that she uses the tremor-stopping drug every time she operates?

I don't see this as a difficult choice. Of course I want the surgeon most likely to cure my beloved daughter or son, spouse, grandchild, parent, or dear friend. If I were philosophically inclined I might want to tell the first surgeon that she is making a mistake. By focusing on human nature as the standard, she is missing the point of the practice of neurosurgery, which is simply healing the patient. Her own flourishing is morally important of course. But it is not the most important matter at stake. Indeed, a wiser understanding of surgeons' flourishing would see it as deeply intertwined with their patients' successful recovery. If the drug caused serious and prolonged side effects that threatened the health of surgeons who used it, that would be a very different story. We should not compel surgeons to take significant risks with their own health. But if the drug is harmless to the surgeon and benefits enormously that surgeon's patients, then any surgeon who understands the point of his or her practice should want to take the drug.

Just as healing is the point or goal or end of surgery, so the virtuous perfection of natural talents is the point or goal or end of sport. We understand sport, we grasp its meaning, when we see that sport aims to highlight the relationship between talents, what athletes do to perfect those talents, and athletic success. From this understanding comes a standard for judging the ethical acceptability of any particular form of endurance enhancement. Does the endurance-enhancing technology undermine the meaning of the sport? Does it do so by corrupting what we regard as natural talents—a likely interpretation of the effect of gene doping? Does it overwhelm the impact of virtuous activities, just as EPO can substitute for perseverance in building endurance?

For any given endurance-enhancing technology, there are three possible outcomes in relation to the ethical standard.

*A technology may be ethically desirable.* It may, for example, reduce the impact of factors other than natural talents and their virtuous perfection by reducing unequal access to the legitimate means of enhancing performance. Some commentators argue that hypoxic chambers level the playing field for athletes who, because of geography or lack of money, cannot "live high, train low" as can some other athletes who have the good fortune or financial resources to be able to live on a plain convenient to a mountain.

*A technology may be ethically permissible.* Technologies in this category do not strengthen the tie between talent, virtue, and performance, but neither do they undermine it. A top-quality coach usually costs money. Not every athlete can afford such a coach, although elite athletes often find a way to do so through the support of their national organizing committee or some form of sponsorship. Nevertheless, some athletes have easier access than others to superb coaching. Inequalities of access are as pervasive as inequalities of talent and virtue. The question must always be asked: Is this a tolerable inequality? The answer will depend on the magnitude of the inequality, the power of the technology to enhance performance (small effects on performance are more easily tolerated), and the relationship of this technology to what matters in sport: converting talent and virtue to athletic success. Good coaches help maximize the athletes' natural gifts at the same time as they teach hard work, smart training, and other virtues. In that sense, competent coaching has a claim to fall under the category of ethically desirable. It would be best if every athlete at whatever level of competition had access to the same quality of coaching as every other athlete at that level. For Olympic and professional athletes, this is roughly the case. For amateur athletes, access to excellent coaching varies enormously. But the sources of the variation are many, and their ethical relevance mixed. Yes, wealthy persons can afford to hire first-rate coaches without affecting their standard of living. But some dedicated amateurs are willing to make significant economic sacrifices to retain the services of a superb coach. Even the wealthy amateur will gain little benefit from a great coach unless he or she has some natural talents and is willing to work hard and suffer to hone those talents. I am not aware of anyone who argues that differential access to excellent coaching for non-elite athletes is an intolerable inequality.

*A technology may be ethically prohibited.* Endurance-enhancing technologies, like other performance-enhancing technologies, should be prohibited when they undermine the meaning of sport by interfering significantly with the relationship between natural talents, their virtuous perfection, and athletic success. Blood doping and EPO boost endurance irrespective of talents or virtues. Either technology may permit a less talented, less dedicated athlete to triumph over a more talented and harder-working one. This directly undermines what we value about sport. It is also unfair to the honest athlete who is doing precisely what we value in the spirit of sport.

The ethics of endurance-enhancing technologies in sport begins with an understanding and celebration of the meaning of sport; acknowledges the power of performance-enhancing technologies to tilt the playing field against the most talented and hard-working athlete; resists the triumph of the performance principle; and evaluates each new enhancement technology according to its impact on what matters most: natural talents and virtuous athletes.

NOTES

1. E. Heinonen, "Altitude Stimulation Systems," *Runners World*, March 2005; M. Dobie, "Elevated Expectations: Altitude Tents Help Improve Endurance, But Are They Ethical?" *Newsday*, January 29, 2002, A62.

2. T. D. Noakes, "Tainted Glory: Doping and Athletic Performance," *New England Journal of Medicine* 351, no. 9 (2004): 847–49.

3. T. Murray, "Erythropoietin: Another Violation of Ethics," *Physician and Sports Medicine* 17, no. 8 (1989): 39–42.

4. A. Miah, *Genetically Modified Athletes* (New York: Routledge, 2004).

5. N. Fost, "Banning Drugs in Sports: A Skeptical View," *Hastings Center Report* 16, no. 4 (1986): 5–10.

6. Murray, "Erythropoietin."

7. D. B. Allen and N. C. Fost, "Growth Hormone Therapy for Short Stature: Panacea or Pandora's Box?" *Journal of Pediatrics* 117, no. 1 (1990): 16–21.

8. http://en.wikipedia.org/wiki/Baseball_field#Pitcher.27s_mound (accessed March 2009).

9. T. Murray, "The Coercive Power of Drugs in Sports," *Hastings Center Report* 13, no. 4 (1983): 24–30.

10. T. H. Murray, W. Gaylin, and R. Macklin, eds., *Feeling Good and Doing Better: Ethics and Nontherapeutic Drug Use* (Clifton, NJ: Humana Press, 1984).

11. S. M. Rothman and D. J. Rothman, *The Pursuit of Perfection* (New York: Pantheon Books, 2003).

12. Ibid.

13. N. Caskey, "Interpreting Anorexia Nervosa," *Poetics Today* 6 (1985): 259–273; quotation from p. 268.

14. T. Murray, "Enhancement," in *The Oxford Handbook of Bioethics*, ed. B. Steinbock (Oxford: Oxford University Press, 2008).

15. President's Council on Bioethics, *Beyond Therapy: Biotechnology and the Pursuit of Happiness* (New York: Harper Collins, 2003), 150.

16. Ibid., 154.

17. Rothman and Rothman, *Pursuit of Perfection*.

18. J. Savulescu, B. Foddy, and M. Clayton, "Why We Should Allow Performance Enhancing Drugs in Sport," *British Journal of Sports Medicine* 38 (2004): 666–70.

19. President's Council on Bioethics, *Beyond Therapy*.

# CHAPTER EIGHT

# *Fairness in Sport*

## An Ideal and Its Consequences

SIGMUND LOLAND, PH.D.

Ideas of fairness play an important role in sport. The classical challenge to fairness is intentional rule violations or cheating. Cheaters search for exclusive advantages not available to rule-abiding competitors, and most people consider the results of cheating invalid and unfair. But issues of fairness arise in many other circumstances as well. Outdoor competitions are exposed to changing external conditions. When, in ski jumping, an increase in wind makes conditions more difficult for the last 20 jumpers, people talk of an unfair competition. Sometimes individual differences between competitors also give rise to discussions of fairness. In 2003, eminent professional golfer Annika Sörenstam's debut among male players caused heated public debate. Among the arguments was the view that Sörenstam was placed at an unfair physical disadvantage. Moreover, fairness easily becomes an issue when there are great inequalities in resources in the support of competitors and teams. Technologically advanced sports, such as Formula One car racing or alpine skiing, are sometimes considered unfair due to inequalities among competitors in equipment and technical support.

In this chapter, I examine the fairness ideal in sport and its consequences for practice. I first suggest an interpretation of fairness in terms of two interconnected moral principles, then provide a critical and systematic discussion of actual and possible procedures for realizing these principles in sport. After spelling out an interpretation of fairness in sport, I examine its possible implications for the use of performance-enhancing technologies, including doping.

## Fairness

With etymological roots in the old English *fæger*, the term *fair* can mean, among other things, "attractive," "beautiful," "unblemished," "clean," "just and honest," and "according to the rules."[1] From a review of the philosophical literature, Carr lists a series of more or less overlapping moral accounts of *fairness*

—not disadvantaging others

—being unbiased, impartial, or neutral in our treatment of others

—sharing burdens and benefits equally, or maintaining a proper proportion between benefit and contribution

—treating equal or similar cases equally or similarly

—adhering to the rules

—treating others with the concern and respect they deserve[2]

As is evident from the examples in my introductory paragraph, most of these accounts are relevant in the discussion of fairness in sport. For the sake of precision and to narrow the discussions somewhat, I will try to be more specific.

In Rawls's influential *A Theory of Justice* (1971), *fairness* is understood in two ways.[3] First, it is seen as an individual obligation that arises as a result of voluntary engagement in rule-governed practices. Rawls's argument, drawn from the writings of C. D. Broad and H. L. A. Hart, among others, goes as follows: "when a number of persons engage in a mutually advantageous cooperative venture according to rules and thus restrict their liberty in ways necessary to yield advantages to all, those who have submitted to these restrictions have a right to a similar acquiescence on the part of those who have benefited from their submission." In short, the intuitive idea is that it is wrong to benefit from the cooperation of others without doing one's fair share. Rawls makes explicit mention of games in this respect. Voluntary engagement in games gives rise to an obligation of fairness prescribing the need "to play by the rules and to be a good sport."[4] Here, then, is a background for the common understanding of cheating as a classic case of unfairness. Cheaters search for an exclusive advantage that depends on others' adherence to the rules. Cheaters are "free riders" benefiting from the cooperation of others without doing their fair share.

The second interpretation is to see fairness as certain structural characteristics of a particular situation of choice between moral principles. As a methodological tool, Rawls proposes the thought experiment of the "original position."[5] Here, free and equal persons concerned to further their own interests are to choose the basic structure or principles of the just society. However, they do not have free access to all relevant information in this regard. To eliminate reasoning based on pure self-interest and to ensure impartial decisions, a "veil of ignorance" is lowered before the decision makers. Behind this veil, they are blind to particular information about themselves and their position in society, such as their sex, race, and intelligence, their psychological profile, and their special talents or handicaps. However, they are given knowledge of general, relevant facts about human societies, such as facts about political affairs, economic theory, organization, and human (moral) psychology and well-being. The "original position" is considered a paradigmatic example of an impartial and informed setting—it is fair. The principles of justice arrived at here are seen to gain authority by the fairness of the procedures by which they arise.[6]

Rawls indicates that the idea of the original position can be a methodological tool of relevance in the examination of more general issues of the morally right, including, I assume, the morally right in sport.[7] In what follows, behind an imagined veil of ignorance that screens out self-interest but with access to relevant facts, I will search for an understanding of fairness in sport.

## Fairness in Sport

In the many and diverse social practices and institutions of modern societies, a variety of schemes of local justice can be found, depending on the goals of the practice or institution under examination.[8] In a lottery, we cultivate chance and rely on pure procedural justice. Physical education in school includes evaluation of students on the basis of a combination of effort, motivation, and skill. Fair procedures for evaluation have to include all these elements in an impartial manner.

To a larger extent, competitive sport builds on a meritocratic scheme of distributive justice. Goods, such as competitive advantages and victories, are distributed based on distinction in performance. Burdens, such as competitive disadvantages, penalties, and losses, are distributed based on lack of performance or violation of performance standards. The characteristic, structural goal of sports competitions is to measure, compare, and rank competitors according to performance of relevant skills within the framework of the rules.[9] The critical question here is how this goal can be reached in fair ways.

As demonstrated by the chapter's introductory examples, challenges to fairness can come from rule violations and cheating and from inequalities in external conditions, in competitors' individual characteristics, and in the strength of their support systems. A key principle to reach fair and valid outcomes seems to be that of *equality of opportunity to perform.*

However, as a formal principle, this is of little help in resolving dilemmas arising from the various procedures for evaluating performance in practice. For instance, where are we to draw the line in outdoor sports for degree of climatic inequalities? What is a fair classification of competitors in golf? To what extent are inequalities in technology and equipment acceptable in sport? There is a need here for substantial criteria for what should count as relevant and nonrelevant equalities and inequalities.

In this regard, sports vary. Each sport has its distinctive rules that define a local interpretation of the requirement on equality of opportunity to perform. In soccer, catching and throwing the ball with the hands is strictly forbidden, whereas in U.S. football this is a critical skill. In boxing, knocks to the head are rewarded, whereas in wrestling the same kind of conduct leads to disqualification. However, on closer inspection, and above local accounts of relevant and nonrelevant equalities and inequalities, we can find some more general ideas.

The "equality of opportunity to perform" premise can be given a Kantian underpinning. As potentially autonomous and rational moral agents, persons ought to be treated never merely as means but always as ends in themselves. This by no means indicates equal or identical treatment in all settings. On the contrary, in most human practices, certain inequalities are considered relevant, acceptable, and even admirable, whereas others are considered nonrelevant and/or problematic and should be eliminated or compensated for. The point is to treat everyone as equals.[10]

Inequalities in natural talents or circumstances of birth are not just or unjust in themselves. However, social interpretations and regulations (or the lack thereof) of the consequences of such inequalities can be problematic indeed. A principle of relevance here is the so-called *fair opportunity principle* (FOP).[11] FOP has been formulated in various ways in various ethical theories, but the following version seems to encapsulate the key points: we should eliminate or compensate for essential inequalities between persons that cannot be controlled or influenced by individuals in any significant way and for which individuals cannot be deemed responsible.

In sport, FOP has particular relevance as an operationalization of the "equality of opportunity to perform" principle, where "essential inequalities" are to be understood as inequalities with a significant impact on sporting performance. In what follows, and from behind the imagined Rawlsian veil of ignorance, I test this assumption by discussing actual and possible procedures to ensure equal opportunity to perform in practice.[12]

## Inequalities in External Conditions

Let me start with the most obvious example of challenges to fairness: inequalities in external conditions, such as in arena and weather conditions during competitions. These are not within the sphere of control of individuals, and in line with FOP they ought to be eliminated and compensated for. In direct competitions in which participants compete simultaneously, there seem to be few problems. In track and field, all competitors run identical distances on identical surfaces. In ball games, the size of courts and pitches is more or less accurately given in the rules, and players and teams change positions regularly. Inequalities in climatic conditions that cannot be controlled, such as a sudden gust of wind on a tennis court or a sudden clearing of the sky and a low evening sun in the second half of a soccer match, are distributed by chance in a drawing of positions. In this way, possible inequalities linked to surface or weather conditions are eliminated or at least minimized.

These procedures are generally accepted and uncontroversial. However, some sports pose more difficult challenges and call for additional procedures. In outdoor indirect competitions in which participants compete partially or fully separated in time, uncontrollable climatic inequalities may have a strong impact on performance. In skiing, temperature changes can significantly affect the gliding of the skis; in speed skating, sun and wind can make conditions very different from one pair of skaters to another. In most of these sports, the solution is to have seeded groups in which competitors at similar levels of skill compete close in time and, within each group, to draw starting numbers in a lottery. Competitors of similar levels of performance are given as equal conditions as possible. Within each seeded group, uncontrollable inequalities are distributed by chance. Hence, the impact of these inequalities on the evaluation of performance is minimized.

To sum up, the primary procedure for ensuring equal external conditions is standardization of arenas. Additional procedures, used in cases of uncontrollable inequalities in climatic conditions, are chance (by a drawing of positions) combined with a seeding of competitors.

## Inequalities Linked to Persons

As the introductory example of the golfer Annika Sörenstam demonstrates, issues of fairness arise in discussions of individual differences, too. In line with FOP, the critical criterion will be that if there are inequalities in person-dependent factors that will have an impact on performance that individuals cannot control or influence in any significant way, then these inequalities should be eliminated or compensated for.

This ideal is followed in sport in many ways. Obvious inequalities here are linked to sex, age, and, to a certain extent, body size. Competitors are classified according to sex and age in most sports. Moreover, in sports in which body mass is important to performance, such as in the martial arts, boxing, and weightlifting, there are weight classes.

However, a critical look at a variety of sports demonstrates a lack of consistency in classification matters. In many sports, sex and age classifications are not relevant.[13] Think of a continuum here. At one end we find sports such as the 100-meter sprint in which biomotor abilities such as explosive strength and speed are crucial.[14] Statistically, men are genetically predisposed to develop these abilities to a significantly larger extent than women, and the development of such abilities is at its peak in young men. In other words, in these sports, most young men have a significant advantage over women. Sex classification seems justified. Other sports, such as archery, shooting, sailing, and curling, are at the other end of the continuum. Here, technical and tactical skills are far more important. Such skills are not dependent to the same extent on biomotor abilities but must be learned through years of training and social interaction.[15] Performances are less dependent on genetic predispositions and more dependent on factors over which the individual has influence and control. Moreover, performances are usually more complex and open to a variety of genetic predispositions, or a variety of talents. A moderately fast soccer player can compensate for a lack of speed by strong tactical skills. Similarly, a player with moderate endurance can make up for this with brilliant speed and technique. In principle, in many of these sports, women can compete on an equal level with men, and older people with younger people. Inequalities in sex and age do not have a significant effect on performance. Today's classification patterns are expressions of traditional gender and age roles and seem hard to justify from a systematic, normative point of view such as that of FOP.

In other instances, classification does not seem to be taken far enough. Unlike sex classes, which are based on statistical generalizations, classification according to body size is based on individual characteristics—that is, according to each individual competitor's body composition. In boxing, in the martial arts, and in weightlifting, weight classes are part of the tradition and are uncontroversial. In the shot put or the discus, however, body mass (or rather mass velocity) is crucial to performance, too, but there is no classification by weight. Moreover, in sports such as basketball and volleyball, height is significant to performance. In gymnastics, being small is of decisive importance to master the many technical challenges of the apparatus. On the basis of FOP, when inequalities in body height and/or mass have a significant effect on performance, these inequalities are nonrelevant and should be eliminated or compensated for by height and weight classes. This would make sports such as basketball, volleyball, and gymnastics fairer.[16]

An additional comment is needed here. Athletic performances are the result of a large number of factors and inequalities in both genetic predispositions and environmental stimuli. One person with a good genetic predisposition for swimming may grow up next to a public pool with a good coach, whereas another person with identical predisposition never gets the chance to develop swimming skills. Two persons with different genetic predispositions for swimming may grow up side by side in a fortunate environment and with the same environmental stimuli but end up with significant inequalities in performance. Should we not, then, eliminate or at least compensate for far more inequalities between persons than those in sex, body size, and age? What about inequalities in muscle fiber composition, or in the potential for developing strong cardiovascular capacity and endurance, or in environmental stimuli?

My response would be as follows: FOP does not prescribe the elimination of or compensation for *any* inequality with a significant impact on performance, only those "that cannot be controlled or influenced by individuals in any significant way." Inequalities in sex, body size, and age are biological and physical invariables, and these inequalities qualify for elimination or compensation. Inequalities in genetic predispositions for strength or endurance, or in mental capacities such as willpower and determination, or in environmental factors, are not outside the sphere of individual effort and control and can be compensated for by hard training and effort. Moreover, as I argue below, extensive inequalities in background variables can be compensated for by standardization procedures in the competitions themselves. Restrictions on the application of FOP seem justified.

The broader ethical question is whether this fairness ideal holds water in a larger scheme of socioethical values. What is the value of competitive sport in society? Is it possible to defend ethically a ranking of persons in absolute hierarchies that, at least in part, depend on fortunate genetic predispositions? Eric Juengst explores these questions in more depth in chapter 9. My brief response here is that as long as elite sport does not represent the norm for the distribution of basic goods and burdens in society (and I do not believe anyone seriously holds that this should be the case), and as long as athletes are voluntarily engaged and competitions meet the fairness requirements proposed in this chapter, sport can be an acceptable and also an admirable practice in society.

Sport expresses an absolute perfectionist ideal in which individuals are evaluated and compared in exact and objective ways. Who is the fastest 100-meter sprinter in the world? What is the best football team ever? Although absolute perfectionism does not seem to carry strong ethical value, it offers fascinating stories of human possibilities (and limitations!) and can play an acceptable role, among a variety of other practices with other ideals, in modern, complex societies. In addition, sport can be a carrier of what we might call relative perfectionist ideals. The field is full of examples and narratives of how individual and team success grows from doing one's best with one's own particular talents and predispositions. The ideal plays a substantive role in strong sporting cultures and in the coaching and psychology of performance. Moreover, and more important in this respect, the striving for one's "personal best" seems to have significant bearing and value outside the sporting context.[17] In this sense, sport can become, in Thomas Murray's phrase, a sphere for the "virtuous perfection of natural talents" (see chapter 7) and thus be a strong and concrete expression of a general moral ideal of perfectionism. Here, then, is a possible justification of competitive sport on moral grounds.

## Inequalities in System Strength

The fair opportunity principle has consequences for inequalities in support systems, that is, in the economic, technological, human, and scientific performance-enhancing support for an athlete or a team. Inequalities in system strength depend to a large extent on the cultural, national, and socioeconomic context in which one is born and raised and in which one lives. Such contexts cannot easily be controlled or influenced by the individual. According to FOP, if system inequalities exert a significant effect on performance, they ought to be eliminated or compensated for. How can this be done? What procedures can be of relevance here?

The idea of eliminating or compensating for inequalities in background and resources has a long and troubled history in sport, not least with the ruling on amateurism in the Olympic movement. The origins of the idea are found in the British aristocracy in the eighteenth century. By banning people as sports professionals who earned money by manual labor, the upper classes were able to keep sport an exclusive sphere. Moreover, with rules on amateurism it was possible to emphasize the ideology of an aristocratic, noninstrumental, noble attitude toward life. Although there might be philosophically interesting ideals in the amateur ethos, its practical-political consequences have been repressive for the majority of sports participants.[18] Instead of trying to control and regulate athletes' background, we should look at possibilities of reducing unfair inequalities in system strength with procedures linked to the competitions themselves.

First, based on FOP, equipment and technology should be identical for all competitors, or at least standardized as far as possible, and all competitors should be given equal access. Standardization procedures are found in sailing and in the throwing events in athletics, but they are more or less absent in other sports, such as skiing. There seems to be no acceptable justification for these inconsistencies. In tight skiing competitions, the quality and preparation of skis has a significant effect on the outcome. These inequalities are the responsibilities of ski manufacturers and support systems, not of athletes, and they should be eliminated or at least compensated for by standardization routines.[19]

Second, as seen, for example, in international soccer—in which a few wealthy clubs, such as Spain's Real Madrid, England's Manchester United, and Italy's Juventus, control the market of star players—inequalities in economic strength significantly affect performance. Again, according to FOP, these are inequalities for which teams and players have little or no responsibility. They are unfair. And again, there are alternative procedures. For instance, for every season within the same series, economic resources could be distributed equally among all participating teams. The challenge thus becomes sport-relevant and within the sphere of responsibility of the players and the coach. In a situation of scarce but equal resources, the coach must make sport-specific analyses of what kind of players he or she needs and prioritize among them. Moreover, together with the players, the coach's task becomes to realize the collective potential of the group of players—that is, to make a well-playing team out of them.

Third, the fairness ideal requires elimination of, or at least compensation for, inequalities in scientific know-how. These, too, are inequalities for which the individual cannot be held responsible. In line with a general norm of democratic science, procedures should be installed to secure open publication of all findings on performance enhancement. Knowledge is a public good, and all parties involved ought to be able to enjoy the fruits of it. This does not necessarily mean that those who invest and succeed in sports research give away advantages for free and that those who benefit from the openness of knowledge are free riders who enjoy the efforts of others without doing their fair share. Whether we are talking of new physiological insights in endurance training or new waxing techniques in alpine skiing, selection and practical implementation of knowledge would still require sport-specific knowledge, experience, and skills. The crucial point here is that the main effect of procedures to open up knowledge would be to reduce unfair inequalities between competitors.

## Fairness and the Use of Performance-Enhancing Technologies

This chapter is part of a larger project on ethical, conceptual, and scientific issues in the use of performance-enhancing technologies in sport. Two aims of the project are to attempt to conceptualize and distinguish between acceptable and unacceptable performance-enhancing technologies and to provide a thorough evaluation of the ethical arguments concerning the use of such technologies. I believe that FOP can contribute to this project.[20]

In general, technology can be understood as a human-made means to serve human interests and goals.[21] Sports technology can be defined as a human-made means to serve human interests and goals in or related to sport. The logic of competitive sport is the evaluation and comparison of performance. And indeed, the most powerful and radical kind includes those technologies designed to have performance-enhancing effects.

Performance-enhancing technologies can be categorized in many ways. A prime category is enhancement of body techniques, or the instrumental use of bodily movement patterns to execute sporting skills and perform. Sometimes, innovations in body techniques cause value conflicts. New technical moves and movement patterns, such as Dick Fosbury's flop in the high jump or the so-called V-style in ski jumping, gave the innovators a competitive advantage over their opponents at the time of their introduction. Critical arguments are often linked to contingent esthetic viewpoints ("the Fosbury flop is ugly" or "the V-style is ugly") or to essentialist views on the traditional "nature" of a sport. Such arguments tend to be short lived. The predominant view is to see technical innovations as the results of trial-and-error processes among talented athletes and coaches and as creative and valuable developments of a sport. In line with FOP, the advantage of an innovative technique is considered a fair advantage because it is within the sphere of individual influence and control.

A more common understanding of sports technology is to see it as the material means with which athletes perform—that is, sports equipment. The interaction between athlete and equipment is crucial to good performances in all sports. To the good skier, the skis and poles become prolongations of the body with which she feels and interacts with the environment. In bicycling, the master racer and his bike appear as one unified, balanced whole. However, and perhaps more often than with body techniques, innovations in sports equipment are controversial from a fairness point of view. If one athlete has exclusive access to superior technology, he or she has an advantage over others that, according to FOP, should be eliminated or compensated for. As noted above, the key procedure here is standardization of, or at least equal access to and free choice between, various kinds of equipment.

A third category of sports technology consists of all kinds of performance-enhancing means used outside competition, in training, that require athletes' effort to have effect. Examples are weights and strength-training regimens and machines, treadmills for running, and wind tunnels for finding aerodynamic positions in speed sports such as cycling and downhill skiing. Again, controversies may arise. The introduction of systematic, daily training in the early 1900s was met by criticism and skepticism by proponents of amateurism and was considered an expression of a simple, instrumental attitude and as "unnatural" and unhealthy. Similar reactions occurred with the introduction of weight training in the 1950s.[22] Today, such views are seen as historical anachronisms. To the modern sports community, most training technologies that require athletes' effort and control are considered valuable and/or acceptable, at least as long as they do not represent unreasonable risks of harm.

The most radical ethical challenges to sport today are often linked to what can be called *expert-administered technology*. Expert-administered technology differs from training technology, as the category includes means that do not require athletes' effort and control but depend for their efficacy on external experts. I am talking now of everything from rather uncontroversial nutritional regimens, to high-altitude chambers to enhance oxygen transport and endurance, to doping, and perhaps to, in the future, genetic technology. The most powerful forms of expert-administered technology, such as doping and genetic technology, may have radical consequences for the welfare and health of the individual athlete and, in fact, for ideas of what sports performance and sport are all about. How far can FOP take us in this respect?

The underlying premise of the fairness principles defended here is the Kantian idea of persons as potentially autonomous moral agents who are to be treated, never merely as means, but always as ends in themselves. A minimum requirement for fairness in sport is equality of opportunity to perform in competitions. All competitors ought to compete under equal conditions and to be given equal access to the same kind of technology. But this is not enough. According to FOP, athletes and teams should be able to influence and control key aspects of their performances: performances should be within their sphere of responsibility. Expert-administered performance-enhancing technology tends to reduce the significance of athletes' effort, control, and responsibility. From the perspective of FOP, this is problematic. Sport is easily turned into a moral risk zone in which the welfare of individuals becomes increasingly dependent on the moral standards of their support systems and in which athletes can be exploited and treated as means toward system survival. From the perspective of FOP, what are thought to be harmless expert-administered technological variants, such as the high-altitude chamber, should be met with skepticism. Potentially harmful technologies such as doping should be banned.

These arguments do not suggest that FOP provides clear-cut distinctions between the acceptable and unacceptable in this regard. First of all, in a situation with mature and rational athletes who can make free and informed choices of the use of technology, the argument about athletes' vulnerability and exploitation seems without merit. However, such a scenario is unlikely to arise. Athletic performances are the result of many years and even decades of hard training from a young age, and few athletes have the necessary knowledge to make their own choices along the way. Second, there are gray zones here, and there is a need for continuous ethical examination of the nature of performance-enhancing technologies and their consequences. Thus far I have mentioned only briefly one of the main technological challenges to current sport—the possible use of performance-enhancing genetic technology. Scenarios of manipulation of genetic predispositions for sports performances—or sporting talent—raise a series of new questions.[23] Popular images of the genetically modified superathlete simplify the matter. A sports performance is an extremely complex result of a high number of interactions between genetic potential and environmental influence and can probably never be fully controlled and manipulated. Still, the technological possibilities are radical enough. For instance, there is a possibility for genetic manipulation toward both better-performing and healthier athletes. In such a setting, traditional arguments in the doping debate on the potential harm to athletes do not hold. Moreover, use of genetic technologies may challenge radically the idea of athletes as autonomous moral agents and turn sport into a moral front zone in which general ethical questions on the status of agency, freedom, and responsibility are tested and rethought. I cannot pursue these questions further here, but I assume that principles such as FOP, with their Kantian underpinnings, may contribute in interesting ways to the development of sound ethical positions.

## Conclusion

I have proposed here an interpretation of fairness in sport in terms of the principle of equality of opportunity to perform and its operationalization: the fair opportunity principle that prescribes the elimination of or compensation for essential inequalities that individuals cannot control or influence in any significant way and for which they cannot be held responsible. Furthermore, and inspired by Rawls's thought experiment on the original position, I have discussed systematically and critically some actual and possible procedures for realizing FOP in sporting practice.

Another question that I have touched on but not discussed is whether my interpretation represents a realistic ideal. Is it reasonable to assume that the principle and procedures suggested in this chapter can be implemented in today's competitive sports?

The requirement of equality in external conditions is uncontroversial. Competitors and organizations usually have an open mind toward improving their procedures here. When it comes to the consequences of the fairness principles for individual differences and system inequalities, however, practices and attitudes seem more ambiguous. Reclassification strategies, such as fewer sex and age classes and more classifications by body size, challenge traditional gender roles and conceptions of equality and would no doubt meet resistance. In elite sport, the great potential for payoff in terms of profit and prestige intensifies the hard quest for exclusive advantages. Regulative regimes designed to decrease system inequalities, whether standardization of equipment in international skiing or an equal distribution of economic resources in professional soccer leagues, require grand cooperation in a social setting that is dominated by short-term self-interest. The possibilities for implementation of fairness ideals and procedures look rather grim.

This pessimistic scenario, though, is built on a traditional vision of competitive sport. But the development of sport can go in other, newer directions. In a series of new activities that are growing in popularity in the younger generations, a change in the nature of performance may make the ethical questions discussed here less pertinent. In the so-called board sports—skateboarding, surfing, windsurfing, and snowboarding—the focus is not so much on objective performance measurements under standardized conditions as on technical and tactical skills, expressiveness, and esthetic values. The significance of strict classification and inequalities in system strength decreases, and the significance of nonmanipulative factors such as complex skills and expressive qualities increases. Requirements on fairness are less rigid and more easily met. Perhaps we are witnessing the emergence of a new sports paradigm that is less vulnerable to the ethical challenges faced by more traditional sports today.

## NOTES

1. *Webster's New World Dictionary of the American Language* (New York: Warner Books, 1984).

2. C. L. Carr, *On Fairness* (Aldershot, UK: Ashgate, 2000), 2.

3. J. Rawls, *A Theory of Justice* (Cambridge, MA: Harvard University Press, 1971).

4. Ibid., 112, 113.

5. Ibid., 136–37.

6. The distinction between two interpretations of fairness in Rawls's work must not be understood as rigid. In Rawls's contractualist approach, the two interpretations are interconnected. Fair decision procedures are thought of as giving just outcomes. Agreements between rational decision makers under fair conditions are considered to have a morally obligating force. For further discussion, see C. Kukathas and P. Pettit, *Rawls: A Theory of Justice and Its Critics* (Cambridge, UK: Polity Press, 1990), 18ff.

7. Rawls, *Theory of Justice*, 17.

8. For a discussion of "local justice" or of the many and diverse schemes of justice found in various social practices and institutions, see J. Elster, *Local Justice: How Institutions Allocate Scarce Goods and Necessary Burdens* (Cambridge: Cambridge University Press, 1992).

9. S. Loland, "Technology in Sport: Three Ideal-Typical Views and Their Implications," *European Journal of Sport Sciences* 2, no. 1 (2002): 1–11.

10. For further discussion and justification of the concept of equality used here, see R. Dworkin, "What Is Equality?" *Philosophy and Public Affairs* 10 (1981): 185–246.

11. Rawls, *Theory of Justice*, 40, 100ff.; T. Beauchamp, *Philosophical Ethics* (New York: McGraw-Hill, 1991), 372ff.

12. The following discussion is based on S. Loland, *Fair Play in Sports: A Moral Norm System* (London: Routledge, 2002).

13. T. Tännsjö, "Against Sexual Discrimination in Sport," in *Values in Sport*, ed. T. Tännsjö and C. Tamburrini (London: E. & F. N. Spon, 2000).

14. T. O. Bompa, *Theory and Methodology of Training: The Key to Athletic Performance*, 3rd ed. (Dubuque, IA: Kendall/Hunt, 1994), 259ff.

15. R. A. Schmidt, *Motor Learning and Performance: From Principles to Practice* (Champaign, IL: Human Kinetics, 1991).

16. Elsewhere I have proposed a variety of procedures for eliminating inequalities of this type. Loland, *Fair Play in Sports*, 56. In volleyball, basketball, and gymnastics, there could be two leagues for men with the critical height of 180 centimeters, and similarly for women with the critical height of 170 centimeters. In addition, changes could be made in equipment and arenas to make sure that competitors meet the same relative challenges; basket and net height could be adjusted in relation to the critical height that defines the class. In the shot put there could be similar classes, with average body mass, for each sex, as the differentiating criterion. Indeed, the specific classification criteria could be discussed and, based on experience and statistical information, other solutions might be better. However, these are discussions about the appropriateness of the procedures, not about the principle of classification (FOP) itself.

17. W. M. Brown, "Personal Best," *Journal of the Philosophy of Sport* 22 (1995): 1–10.

18. L. Allison, *Amateurism in Sport: An Analysis and a Defence* (London: Frank Cass, 2001); E. A. Glader, *Amateurism and Athletics* (West Point, NY: Leisure Press, 1978).

19. An original procedure to ensure equality of equipment is found in the so-called folk races—motorcar rallies with participation open to all. Inequalities in car quality are regulated by a rule that the winning car must be open to purchase by any other competitor for a low sum of money, say, $2000. If a competitor races with a car worth much more, this is considered an expression of vanity and a possible win gives little or no prestige.

20. Much of the discussion here is based on Loland, *Fair Play in Sports*.

21. D. E. Cooper, "Technology: Liberation or Enslavement?" in *Philosophy and Technology*, ed. D. Fellows (Cambridge: Cambridge University Press, 1998).

22. J. M. Hoberman, *Mortal Engines: The Science of Performance and the Dehumanization of Sports* (New York: Free Press, 1992).

23. A. Miah, "Bioethics, Sport and the Genetically Enhanced Athlete," *Journal of Medical Ethics and Bioethics* 9, no. 3–4 (2002): 2–6.

# CHAPTER NINE

# Annotating the Moral Map of Enhancement

## Gene Doping, the Limits of Medicine, and the Spirit of Sport

ERIC T. JUENGST, PH.D.

In biomedical ethics, one frequently encounters the belief that there is an important moral distinction between using biomedical tools and products to combat human disease and attempting to use them to "enhance" human traits.[1] Thus, people argue that using biosynthetic human growth hormone to treat an inborn growth hormone deficiency is praiseworthy as bona fide medical treatment, but the use of the same product to increase the height of a hormonally normal short child is not.[2] Similarly, while the use of human gene-transfer techniques to combat disease enjoys widespread support from secular and religious moral authorities, a line is usually drawn at using the same protocols to improve on otherwise benign human traits.[3] From cosmetic surgery and pharmacology to attempts to control the aging process, medical practices often seem to become ethically problematic when they move "beyond therapy" to the "pursuit of perfection."[4]

In sports ethics, the concept of "enhancement" is also used to draw a moral line: in this case, between practices and interventions that are legitimate for athletes to use in pursuit of victory and those, such as "performance-enhancing drugs," that are not. Here, in addition to questions about the potential harms of enhancement interventions to athletes, the concern is about the implications of enhancement for the practice of sport itself. Thus, commentators argue that enhancement represents a form of cheating, either by conferring an unearned or unfair advantage[5] or by breaking established sports norms,[6] or that it represents a perversion of the ethos or goals of sport as a social practice,[7] or that it simply dehumanizes both sport and athletes by engineering athletic accomplishments through artificial means rather than allowing them to emerge from natural performance.[8]

These two discussions of "enhancement" in applied ethics come together dramatically in the debate over the potential use of gene-transfer technologies to improve athletic performance. Sports philosophers and policymaking bodies have used the widespread bioethical suspicion of biomedical enhancement interventions to reinforce their efforts to prevent the potential "gene doping" of athletes, and biomedical ethicists are drawn to the debate as a dramatic example of taking genetic technology "beyond therapy" for nonmedical purposes. Thus, when the World Anti-Doping Agency (WADA) announces that "the nontherapeutic use of cells, genes, genetic elements or the modulation of gene expression, having the capacity to enhance athletic performance, is prohibited,"[9] the blended language sounds plausible to both camps. But are the biomedical and athletic conversations about the ethics of enhancement talking about the same moral phenomenon? The two conversations are clearly overlapping: each draws extensively on the other for analogies and analyses. But the moral significance of "enhancement" is explicated in several different ways in both bioethics and the philosophy of sport, which have different moral lessons for the problem of "gene doping." For sports officials, sports physicians, and athletes to make sound ethical judgments about gene doping, it will be important to have a clear map of these different interpretations of "enhancement." That map is what this chapter attempts to provide.

I begin by reviewing a set of ideas about enhancement that I have discussed generically elsewhere,[10] to show how they apply to the gene-doping context. I then attempt to get higher resolution in one corner of that map that seems particularly relevant to the gene-doping debate: interpretations of "enhancement" that turn on a distinction between the "natural" and the "unnatural" in the context of sport. On these interpretations, the fundamental moral failing of gene doping is that the athletic achievements it makes possible are not, in one way or another, *natural* achievements. Paying attention to these interpretations is important because it does lead to a clearer sense of the intrinsic values of sport most endangered by the prospect of gene doping, which a discussion of the "spirit of sport" attempts to explicate. To look ahead, following our conceptual map suggests that the problem of gene doping boils down to a concern to preserve *the hierarchical ranking of inherited talents* as a key feature of sport's celebration of human excellence. This is an ironic conclusion, because the most plausible moral concern flagged by "enhancement" conversations outside the sports setting is also about the creation of human social hierarchies out of the facts of human biological variation. In the end, I think that getting clear about what we mean by enhancement in the context of gene doping reflects a hard question back into the ethics of sport: far from celebrating human diversity, does sport intrinsically glorify a genetic prejudice that the world is working hard to evolve beyond in other spheres of human life?

## Enhancement versus Treatment

In biomedical ethics, the term *enhancement* is usually used to characterize interventions designed to improve human form or functioning beyond what is necessary to achieve, sustain, or restore good health. As such, it functions as a "moral boundary" concept for medical practice. Just as the concept of futile treatment is used to indicate the limits of medicine's obligations to perform interventions that cannot achieve medical goals, "enhancement" is typically used to mark the limits of professional obligations to pursue biomedical interventions that can achieve goals beyond medicine's. Like futile treatments, enhancement interventions fall outside medicine's proper domain of practice: patients have no role-related right to demand them of the profession, and physicians who do provide them bear a burden of justification for doing so that does not apply to medically necessary interventions. By extension, the concept of an enhancement boundary can be called on to help define the social role of the medical profession, demarcate the proper sphere of biomedical research, and help set limits on health care payment plans. "Enhancement" helps us frame the proper domain for biomedicine in these contexts by providing a conceptual cap for the enterprise in an era when its technological capacities seem to have fewer and fewer upper limits.

Using the enhancement concept to demarcate the proper limits of medicine will not be sufficient, of course, to address the problem of athletic gene doping, because the issue is more than simply a problem of professional medical ethics: it is also about what athletes, coaches, and teams should be allowed to do for sport. Nevertheless, if it were clear that performance-enhancing gene-transfer interventions were beyond the pale of biomedicine, there would be no reason for biomedical scientists to pursue their development, and no obligation for health professionals to help athletes acquire them. For example, International Olympic Committee Chair Arne Ljungqvist frames the whole issue of performance enhancement in this way: "Virtually all doping substances are medicines, most of them obtained only on prescription. They are intended for the prevention or cure of disease or alleviation of disease-related symptoms. Their administration to healthy young people is against basic pharmacotherapeutical principles and represents, therefore, medical malpractice."[11]

To the extent that biomedical scientists and physicians will serve an even greater gatekeeping role for gene doping than for pharmaceutical doping, bio-medical interpretations of enhancement should provide a useful starting point for our map.

When it is used as a medical boundary concept, enhancement, like futility, plays both descriptive and normative roles. We need to be able to identify the boundary when we encounter it—to be able to identify our efforts as either futile or enhancing—and we need to know what the boundary implies for our professional obligations to continue. For enhancement interventions, the descriptive and normative implications of calling them "enhancements" seem to be at cross-purposes. While futile treatments literally do no good, enhancements are by definition and description *improvements*: changes for the good. Yet, the moral function of calling them "enhancements" is to place them beyond the pale of proper medicine. For a profession dedicated to pursuing the improvement of its patients, the fact that enhancements act, descriptively, just like all the other improvements the profession strives to achieve makes it difficult to discern when an intervention transgresses the normative boundary that the concept purports to mark. This has provoked three major ways of operationalizing the enhancement concept, tailored to different kinds of line-drawing problems. The boundary it flags can be interpreted in terms of medicine's professional domain, or the limits of "normal human functioning," or the line between health and disease. Each of these has interesting connections with the topic of gene doping.

## Medicine's Professional Domain

One common approach to defining the line between treatment and enhancement appeals to the conventional limits of professional medical practice. Ljungqvist is appealing to this view when he accuses physicians of "malpractice" in administering "prescription" medicines against the "pharmacotherapeutical principles" of the profession. Under this view, "treatments" are any interventions that the professional standard of care deems useful and proper, while "enhancements" are interventions that fall outside a physician's professional purview, either as malpractice or nonmedicine. Thus, physician-prescribed physical therapy to improve muscle strength would be considered legitimate medical treatment, while weightlifting under a coach's supervision to achieve a particular physique would be considered an enhancement. Attempts by (and appeals to) professional societies to police their own frontiers by discouraging particular practices as "enhancement" rather than "treatment" reflect this approach,[12] and for those committed to a particular theory of the goals or domain of medicine, it can offer firm guidance.[13]

Interpreting enhancement in terms of medicine's professional domain can also resonate well with several contemporary social-scientific critiques of biomedicine suggesting that medicine has no intrinsic domain of practice beyond that which it negotiates with patients and society.[14] For those influenced by this relativism, the normative lesson for professionals concerned about their obligations in specific cases can be simple. Given medicine's fundamentally patient-centered ethos, one takes one's cues from the patient's value system and thus negotiates toward interventions that can help achieve the patient's vision of human flourishing.[15] Unfortunately, both versions of this approach provide little help to those attempting to use the treatment/enhancement distinction to regulate sports physiology research or to police gene doping. From a theoretical point of view, while the goal of most medical practice is to reduce suffering and prolong healthy life, at least some sports physicians argue that "sports medicine presents a more complicated picture": "Patients who are athletes do not necessarily want to get well or to be free of pain. For many athletes, the simple goal is to get back on the playing field able to perform. In the relatively healthy population of athletes, supporting athletic achievement (and not reducing suffering or prolonging life) becomes the physician's reason for being."[16]

Others in sports medicine might not subordinate health maintenance to the "performance principle" so dramatically in describing their goals. But to the extent that sports medicine does embrace the value of athletic performance and includes its maintenance, preservation, and recovery within the specialty's domain, then the sports physician's range of legitimate problems and interventions expands accordingly. *Contra* Ljungqvist, some forms of performance enhancement, such as gene doping, may well obey the pharmacotherapeutic principles *of sports medicine*, especially if, as we shall see below, they improve performance and prevent suffering at the same time.

Medical historians, moreover, can point out that, whatever its philosophical goals, sports medicine seems to have been a medical specialty particularly susceptible to the cultural beliefs and social values of the institutions and athletes it serves.[17] Libertarians, in turn, can embrace that relativism as a sign of the shared negotiation of medical services between sports physicians and their autonomous clients. If their clients in sport were to decide that (safe) gene doping addressed real needs in a legitimate way, and if the requirements of informed consent could be met, on what grounds could sports medicine spurn its development and use?

Just as other medical specialties accommodate fertility assistance, cosmetic surgery, and "antiaging medicine,"[18] it seems likely that sports medicine could adjust its conventional domain of practice to include gene-doping interventions if that was all that stood in the way of significant performance enhancement.

## Normal Functional Range

Fortunately, there is another approach to interpreting the treatment/enhancement distinction that is framed explicitly as a policy tool for separating legitimate health care needs from luxury services. The most developed exposition of this view is James Sabin and Norman Daniels's endorsement of what they call the "normal function" standard for determining the limits of "medically necessary" (and therefore socially underwritten) health service. Following Daniels's earlier work, they construe health care as one of society's means for preserving equality of opportunity for its citizens, and they define "health care needs" as those services that allow individuals to enjoy the portion of the society's "normal opportunity range" to which their full array of skills and talents would give them access. This is done by restoring or improving the patient's abilities to the range of functional capacities typical for members of his or her reference class (e.g., age and gender) within the human species. Any interventions that would expand an individual's range of functional capacities beyond the range typical for his or her reference class would be deemed a medically unnecessary enhancement.[19] Others have used similar understandings of human malady to help explicate a distinction between "negative" (e.g., therapeutic) and "positive" (e.g., enhancing) human genetic engineering.[20] The advantage of the normal-function approach is that it provides one relatively unified goal for health care, toward which the burdens and benefits of various interventions can be relatively objectively measured against one another, balanced, and integrated. The normal-function approach comes close to accurately reconstructing the rationale behind many "line-drawing" judgments by health care coverage plans and professional societies.[21] Unfortunately, this approach also faces conceptual challenges, which are especially acute for sports medicine's role as the gatekeeper to gene doping.

Some critics of the normal-function approach take issue with its focus on the "species-typical range" as inadequately sensitive to the diversity of biological ways in which human beings can flourish in life.[22] Unlike other parts of medicine, however, sports medicine does seem relatively well protected against a "fatal attraction to normalizing,"[23] The normative value of athletic performance encourages sports medicine to press athletes to the top of the normal range for their reference class and to narrow that class to the athlete's competitors. As Ljungqvist and Bernstein and colleagues point out, the "patients" at issue in sports medicine are already "healthy young people" at the top of the species-typical range of functionality. If general health care needs are those required to maintain a level of species-typical functioning adequate to support an "open future" of opportunity, sports medicine addresses the needs of those who have already narrowed their futures to opportunities that require atypical levels of functioning.[24] Establishing the "species-typical norm" for a particular human function is a difficult enough task, even where descriptive statistics can help. But when the boundary is "optimal" not "normal" functioning, the evidentiary foundations of the approach begin to come apart because we have no empirical or theoretical bases for determining the upper limit of human functional capacity. Indeed, optimal athletic performance, like cognitive functioning,[25] will always be a moving target, shifting ever upward—in part, because it is the part of the purpose of sport to continually challenge both personal and global records of athletic achievement.

The second serious problem for the normal-function approach is the challenge of prevention. Like "health maintenance organizations," sports medicine usually frames its mission positively, in terms of "health promotion" for athletes rather than merely the treatment and rehabilitation of sports injuries. While some efforts at health promotion, such as exercise, straddle the border of medical responsibility, efforts to prevent the manifestation of specific maladies in individuals are widely accepted as legitimate parts of medicine's mission and are located squarely on the treatment side of the enhancement boundary. One of the ways one can prevent sports injuries is to strengthen the body's ability to resist pathological changes before any diagnosable problem appears. But to the extent that these forms of prevention attempt to elevate bodily functions above the normal range for the individual (and, in some cases, the species), they seem to slide into what the normal-function approach would call enhancement.[26] If the normal-function account is taken seriously as a biomedical boundary marker, how does one defend this kind of prevention? Conversely, if preventive interventions like these are acceptable in medicine, what can it mean to claim that researchers and clinicians should be "drawing the line" at enhancement?

Most of the conceivable examples of "gene-doping" interventions would be examples of this conundrum, because they would improve athletic performance precisely by increasing athletes' resistance to muscle damage, hypoxia, metabolic poisoning, or fatigue beyond their normal functional range.[27] When optimal performance is achieved by functional range–extending prevention, has sports medicine slipped across the border into enhancement or has it simply done its job of maintaining athletes at peak performance? If this form of prevention is a legitimate part of sports medicine's mission, this will only accelerate the shifting "normal range" problem described above. Clearly, the normal-function approach will not be enough to distinguish acceptable from unacceptable genetic interventions in sports medicine, and the real ethical concern must lie elsewhere.

## Health and Disease

Probably the most common rejoinder to the problem of prevention is to focus on the problems to which prevention efforts respond. As Ljungqvist says, treatments "are intended for the prevention or cure of disease or alleviation of disease-related symptoms."[28] Performance enhancements, by contrast, are interventions aimed at improving healthy systems and normal traits. Thus, to justify an intervention as appropriate medicine means to be able to identify (or foresee) a pathological problem in the patient. If no medically recognizable malady can be diagnosed or predicted, the intervention cannot be "medically necessary" and is thus suspect as an enhancement. This would clear the way for safe and effective genetic "vaccines" against predictable muscle damage in sports medicine (even if they provided better than normal damage resistance) but would screen out as "enhancements" efforts to improve traits that were at no diagnosable risk of deterioration.

This interpretation has the advantages of being simple, intuitively appealing, and consistent with a good bit of biomedical behavior. Maladies are both objectively observable phenomena and the traditional target of medical intervention. They can be discovered through diagnosis, and it will be clear that one has gone beyond medicine when no pathology can be identified.[29] This interpretation is used by professionals working at the boundary, such as cosmetic surgeons, to justify their services in terms of relieving "diagnosable" psychological suffering rather than satisfying the esthetic tastes of their clients, as Morgan notes; it is also used when insurance companies insist on being provided with a diagnosis before providing coverage for surgery.[30]

However, this interpretation also faces two major difficulties as an approach to understanding what is wrong with gene doping within sports medicine. The first is biomedicine's nosological elasticity and its stigmatizing consequences for those suddenly diagnosed with medical problems. We have already seen that the legitimate domain of sports medicine is influenced by the goals of sport to focus professional attention on cultivating, preserving, and recovering the top of the species-typical functional range. If the problem with performance enhancement is that it is not combating disease, the logical response will be to medicalize the needs that gene doping can address and create new maladies to treat and prevent. The values of sport allow sports medicine to widen its domain to support performance, and supporting performance allows sports medicine to go beyond the normal functional range in preventing maladies. While an elite athlete's tolerance for fatigue, hypoxia, and pain during the extremes of physical endurance might already be well above species-typical, if it falls back into the normal range against a "diagnosable" pattern, it can become a bona fide malady for sports medicine. And if gene doping can correct or prevent such maladies, it similarly becomes legitimized. Unless there is something immoral about identifying new diseases in this way, this interpretation cannot explain the ethical problem of gene doping and would be a weak foundation for regulation.

On the other hand, this interpretation of enhancement does show how gene doping might lead us to view athletes as susceptible to a class of new maladies to which most of us are immune (either constitutionally or thanks to our good sedentary habits). In other medical specialties, the social risks of such medicalization are the concerns most often flagged by labeling interventions as "enhancements." For example, some argue that what makes the provision of human growth hormone to a normally short child a morally suspect "enhancement" is not the absence of a diagnosable disease or the "species-atypical" hormone level that would result. Rather, it is the intent to improve the child's social status by changing the child rather than by changing her social environment. Such enhancement interventions are almost always wrong-headed, because the source of the social problems they seek to avoid is, by definition, the social group's norms and not the individual's body. Attempting to address the issue by interpreting it as a medical problem for the individual amounts to a moral mistake akin to "blaming the victim": it misattributes causality, is ultimately futile, and, where the disadvantages are based on sheer prejudice, makes the physician "complicit with suspect social norms," as philosopher Margaret Little pointed out so well.[31]

Does this concern have any purchase with gene doping? A medicalized inability to compete at world-class levels is not likely to be socially stigmatizing in ordinary circumstances or to exacerbate serious social prejudices against the similarly disabled. Moreover, a key feature of sport is that it creates situations in which the athlete's social environment is fixed (by the rules of the game) precisely to compare physical abilities and inabilities. In a practice that gears access to opportunities and rewards to one's place in a hierarchy of performance, the more egalitarian principles of justice that animate our concerns over access to social opportunities in other spheres of life seem irrelevant. For the sports physician, medicalizing and operating on athletes' bodies to improve their performance is only being "complicit" with the social norms that structure the practice of sport and inform the physician's professional goals.

Nevertheless, it is instructive to note the limiting cases in which even sports physicians balk at their complicity with the norms of some sports. For example, consider this excerpt from a discussion of sports medicine's ethical dilemma of attending ringside at boxing matches: "Close physician involvement with hazardous sports has been shown to decrease the incidence of some serious injuries . . . However, given that the stated goal of boxing is to batter the opponent's brain into unconsciousness, one could easily argue that the physician has no place at ringside. The prospect of suturing lion wounds in the coliseum was not why Galen moved to Rome in the second century, and patching modern gladiators is no more a part of the physician's mission today."[32]

Although a "harm reduction" philosophy will obviously take sports physicians a long way in their willingness to participate in situations that put their patients in harm's way, even that apparently has limits. Part of what bothers these doctors about boxing and gladiatorial combat is the severe health consequences of such violence, of course. But there is something else at work as well: a concern for the social norms of sports that would, as their "stated goals," set athletes against each other (and against the lions!) in this violent way. As we shall see, it is the latter-day echo of those sporting norms that the gene-doping debate exposes to the critical light.

To summarize, it seems clear that attempting to distinguish, as Ljungqvist does, between "medicines for disease" and interventions in "healthy young bodies"[33] will also fail to provide a theoretical bulwark against gene doping in sports medicine—unless someone can show that medicalized gene doping exacerbates social norms so pernicious that they should not be tolerated even within the structured practice of sport. But even then, if that case were made and sports medicine took a righteous stand against gene doping on professional ethical grounds, a second major difficulty emerges for sports officials and athletes to which the boundary-marking concept of enhancement cannot speak—that is, the way in which all these efforts to interpret enhancement as a medical professional matter undercut the ability of sports medicine to be gene doping's gatekeeper and shift the policing problem to sports authorities and athletes themselves.

This problem emerges because most biomedical interventions that could become problematic as enhancement interventions will also have legitimate therapeutic applications in treating bona fide medical maladies in nonathletes. In fact, most biosynthetic biologicals and gene-transfer protocols with potential for enhancement uses in sport first emerge as therapeutic agents and are researched, developed, evaluated, and approved for clinical use well within the confines of mainstream medicine. Strength- and endurance-enhancement interventions, for example, are likely to be approved for use only in patients with wasting diseases such as muscular dystrophy.[34] However, once determined to be safe and effective in that clinical context, they will be in high demand by individuals seeking to use them for performance enhancement. Given the wide latitude that physicians legally enjoy to implement interventions "off-label" for unapproved uses, the availability of such therapies shifts the regulatory problem from medical gatekeeping to institutional policing and individual decision making.[35] Even if doctors eschew such use on professional ethical grounds, are there independent moral reasons why sports authorities, coaches, and athletes should turn away from their availability?

## Enhancement versus Achievement

For biomedicine, "enhancements" are interventions that transgress a boundary set by professional domains of practice, theories of "species-typical functioning," concepts of disease, or the medicalization of social prejudices. As we've seen, sports medicine seems to reside just where all of these line-drawing approaches are the weakest for the purpose of criticizing gene doping. Moreover, none of these interpretations of the concept illuminate concerns that are of special importance to athletes, coaches, or the institutions of sport.

In fact, in discussions of athletes' efforts to improve their performance in sports, the concept of enhancement does not even play the same kind of boundary-marking role. Although its invocation in the phrase "performance-enhancing drugs" has linked it to doping and thus to illegitimate forms of improvement, in sports ethics the concept functions normatively more like the medical ethical concept of "paternalism." Unlike "futility," paternalism does not mark a clear moral watershed, because we can think of medical situations in which it might be morally justified or even praiseworthy. But while identifying paternalism in a situation does not settle the matter morally, it does suggest that we should be careful to ask certain kinds of moral questions about the case: questions about coercion, decision-making capacity, and levels of benefit.[36]

Identifying enhancement in a case of athletic decision making functions similarly, to indicate the range of relevant moral question to pose in the circumstances at hand. For example, while Fastskin swimsuits were clearly performance enhancements when they were introduced in the Sydney Olympics, that did not immediately entail that their use should be prohibited as unethical. But it did alert Olympic officials to the problems that an inequitable distribution of these tools to athletes would create. In sports, in other words, enhancement is, like "paternalism," less a boundary marker than a warning sign to travelers of the risks of the moral road they are following. Thus, far from drawing a moral line against such enhancement, Olympic officials could legitimize the Fastskin suit by insisting that all competitors have equal access to these suits from their manufacturer. Whether gene doping might be similarly assimilated within sport depends similarly on what ethical questions this form of enhancement flags for sports and how they might be addressed.

In sports, the questions that "enhancement" most commonly seems to prompt (beyond safety concerns) are questions about the moral quality of an athlete's achievements: questions about fairness, natural achievement, and the spirit of sport as a social practice. Given the expense and technical complexity of current gene-doping scenarios, the fairness questions are probably the most pressing in practice. But the most powerful critiques of gene doping in principle flow from questions in the latter two areas—natural achievement and the spirit of sport— and it is in that context that the fundamental sports values at stake emerge, for better or worse.

## Fairness

At one level, gene doping would seem to be simply a problem of cheating. If the rules of sport forbid the use of genetic performance enhancements, then their use becomes illicit and confers an unfair advantage against athletes who either accept the rules of the game or do not have access to the enhancement interventions. That advantage, in turn, can create pressure for more athletes to cheat in the same way, undermining the basis for the competitions at stake and exacerbating the gap between athletes who can afford gene doping and those who cannot.[37] In fact, with WADA's addition of gene doping to the list of prohibited performance-enhancing activities for elite sports, this interpretation has already been operationalized, launching the difficult challenge of determining how to detect and police the practice.[38] But of course, this begs the question of why gene doping should be against the rules of sport in the first place. As the Fastskin example illustrates, novel forms of performance enhancement are routinely introduced into sports as athletic technology and expertise evolve. Where issues of athletes' equitable access arise, they can either be dealt with through policy, as in the Fastskin manufacturer's agreement, or accepted as unfortunate but not unfair, as in access of an underfunded equatorial country's skiing team to artificial (and thus year-round) snow. As long as gene-doping interventions can neither be distributed fairly nor reconciled as part of the inherent advantages that "come with the territory" for some fortunate elite athletes, then an argument based on fairness can support the current WADA ban on gene doping. But for those who can afford it, what would be ethically suspect about a mirror image of the "Special Olympics" for athletes with disabilities: a "Super Olympics," featuring athletes universally equipped with the latest modifications and enhancements?[39] For answers to that challenge, critics of gene doping must look to the other questions that "enhancement" flags: questions about the naturalness of athletic achievements and the meaning of sport.

## Natural Athletic Achievements

To explain why the rules of sport should not be rewritten to legitimize performance-enhancing interventions such as gene doping, most critics turn, at this point, from the consequences of gene doping to its intrinsic merits as a means for improving athletic achievements. Athletic achievements, they argue, are praiseworthy only to the extent that they are accomplished "naturally" by the athletes themselves, both because those are the achievements for which athletes can legitimately claim personal responsibility and credit and because only those achievements display the distinctly human excellences that sport celebrates.[40] Some methods of performance enhancement—training, nutrition, better equipment—are compatible with natural athletic achievements and are therefore unproblematic on this view. Other methods, however, such as gene doping, are unnatural shortcuts to achievement, producing gains the athlete has not earned and yielding hollow achievements that only cheapen the human excellences they are supposed to celebrate.[41]

As John Hoberman points out, this focus on the moral merits of the means that athletes use to improve their performance has meant that "the distinction between what is 'natural' and what is 'unnatural' is at the heart of the twentieth-century controversy over the use of performance-enhancing drugs in sport."[42] But how should this distinction be understood? Appeals to nature and to the "unnaturalness" of biomedical technologies are relatively common in bioethics, but they are used to signal at least three different kinds of moral concerns. They are concerns about the blurring of natural boundaries, or "abomination"; concerns about transgressing on the supernatural, or "blasphemy"; or concerns about undermining authenticity, or "fraud." Although invocations of unnaturalness in sports ethics focus on the third set of concerns, allusions to the first two also echo in the literature on performance enhancement in sport in instructive ways.

### ABOMINATION

Sometimes, accusations of unnaturalness are used in bioethics to express concern that biomedicine will undermine a given stability in the world by violating the categories that order it. Drawing from theological natural law traditions, Aristotelian essentialism, and nineteenth-century Romantic sensibilities, this concern gives high normative weight to the biological kinds produced by the "Wisdom of Evolution" and their relative ranking in a hierarchical "great chain of being." Like importing new species into an established ecosystem, "splicing life" in the creation of transgenic organisms, or interspecies tissue chimeras, or hybridized embryos is always dangerous enough on this view to justify the use of the "precautionary principle." For some, as philosophers Jeffrey Stout, Jason Robert, and Francois Baylis have pointed out, the creation of such "abominations" is also morally suspect, simply in its willful disregard for the natural order and the integrity of the species it crosses.[43]

In situations that involve the integrity of the human species, such as xenotransplantation or the creation of man-machine "cyborgs," this moral hazard can be explained as the danger of dehumanization: that polluting the constellation of traits that humans have inherited from our ancestors—our given "human nature"—with nonhuman attributes will inevitably degrade the elements of human identity we find morally important, such as human dignity, autonomy, and vulnerability. As Hoberman argues, "The scientization of the athlete, either through drugs or other techniques, also involves a crisis of identity. What sort of human being is competing? To what extent can the emotional experience of competition be truly shared by an athlete who has transformed himself with drugs? On this level, Ben Johnson revealed himself to be a modern reincarnation of Victor Frankenstein's artificial man."[44] One of the reasons that the Roman gladiatorial arena still resonates as a paradigm of sports that (even) sports physicians should eschew, for example, is its literal "*brutality*": the dehumanizing consequences of forcing humans to compete with other predators for their lives.

Moreover, it is not just the blurring of human-nonhuman lines that can be abominable: conflating the natural kinds of humans—as men and women, for example, or children and adults—evokes the same repugnance in sports ethics. For example, sports ethicists report that "while anecdotal, the members of our undergraduate Sport Ethics class were generally revulsed at the sight of the

Chinese women swimmers. These swimmers displayed a body type that did not fit into the socially constructed category of female . . . They looked like men, but were labeled 'women.' Interestingly, the class was not similarly disgusted with Ben Johnson . . . His sin was against a lesser god: he merely cheated. The problem with the Chinese swimmers was that they were gender freaks first, and cheaters a distant second."[45] Unfortunately, even female athletes who look like women can evoke similar reactions when they simply attempt to compete with men, and mixed-gender sports remain rarer than our bodies necessarily dictate.[46] In the past, competitions between athletes from different racial groups—or even different social classes—raised similar concerns about disturbing the natural order and its degrading effects on the most privileged players, dehumanizing the underprivileged in the process.[47]

Concerns about the degradation of human identity are also evident in discussions of gene doping, where images of identity-corrupting blends—"mortal engines,"[48] the cheetah-man,[49] and "bio-Amazons"[50]—seem apt ways to attract a reader's attention. For example, worries about the potential of gene doping to rob athletes of their humanity dominate the President's Council on Bioethics's discussion of the topic: "The runner with genetically enhanced muscles is still, of course, a human being who runs. But the doer of the deed is arguably less obviously himself and less obviously human than his unaltered counterpart. He may be faster, but he may also be on the way to becoming 'more cheetah' than man."[51]

The problem with this prospect becomes explicit in the following passage with which Hoberman ends his book on the "dehumanization of sport": "[J. B. S.] Haldane also dreamed of gene-grafting techniques that would permit the crossing of men and beasts, of legless astronauts and other specially adapted creatures—a vision perfectly suited to the development of athletes who would be monsters as well. The supreme biological question confronting mankind today is whether Haldane's vision of the pursuit of organismic efficiency will prevail over the human image that appeared in the Old Testament thousands of years ago."[52]

For all its dramatic appeal, however, it is hard for this critique to get a firm purchase on the kind of gene-doping possibilities that sports officials, sports physicians, and athletes will be confronted with first. As we've seen, these are most likely to take the form of prophylactic or "off-label" uses of human gene-transfer protocols developed for the treatment of disease. They will not involve interspecies gene transfer, suspicious intraspecies mixing, or even bodily pollution with exogenous drugs. In fact, as healthy people to start with, athletes will already carry the "enhanced" allele, compared with the patients for whom the intervention was developed. Gene doping will only give them more copies of the same gene or, even more likely, will simply "up-regulate" the replication and expression of the copies they were born with.[53] This may enhance their natural abilities but hardly makes them unnatural "monsters."

Moreover, as I think the allusions above to the history of sexism, racism, and social class bias in sport suggest, there are dangers in appealing to this interpretation of "unnatural." The notion that nature is normatively ordered into a hierarchy of natural kinds, each with its inviolable essence and fixed moral status, is a distinctly pre-modern view, increasingly rejected over the past two centuries by the natural sciences as a matter of fact, by the political sciences as a guide to human rights, and by theology as an adequate vision of creation. Maintaining this worldview for sport in the face of the history of oppression and intolerance that is fueling its rejection in other spheres of human activity would be an uphill challenge that most sports ethicists would rather avoid, particularly if there are other interpretations of "unnatural" to employ.

### BLASPHEMY

A second traditional way in which gene-doping interventions might be "unnatural" means for enhancing athletic performance is by attempting to be supernatural means. Miracles are the province of gods, and magic is the province of demons: attempts to perform either by ordinary mortals (saints and witches, by definition, excluded) reflect the moral vice of hubris and usually backfire in punishing ways. This, of course, is not just a pre-modern set of ideas, but positively ancient: it resonates with the lessons of Greek and Norse mythology and Old Testament Judaism. Interestingly, it remains alive in the rhetoric of gene doping, in which Prometheus, the Garden of Eden, and Ragnarok, the apocalyptic war of the Norse giants against the gods, are stock allusions.

Here the concern is not so much about violating or debasing natural categories as about ignoring our limits and attempting to transcend the natural. For theological writers, the distinction is often grounded in (or refuted by) views of the proper relation of humans and God: to use biomedical means to improve ourselves is to "play God" in a dangerously overreaching way, risking hubris in ways that humbly accepting the limits of natural achievement does not. As Michael Sandel says, "I do not think the main problem with enhancement and genetic engineering is that they undermine effort and erode human agency. The deeper danger is that they represent a kind of hyperagency—a Promethean aspiration to remake nature, including human nature, to serve our purposes and satisfy our desires . . . And what the drive to mastery misses and may even destroy is an appreciation of the gifted character of human powers and achievements."[54]

The best exposition of the roots and contours of this interpretation comes from Erik Parens, in his trenchant comparison of how both critics and proponents of enhancement technologies appeal to the moral ideal of authenticity. Parens contrasts two "ethical frameworks" in the debate, the "gratitude and creativity frameworks," which support different conceptions of what it means to be true to oneself or to human nature. Sandel's concerns exemplify the "gratitude framework": the view that "we human beings are not the creators of life; we are creatures, whose job is to remember that life is a gift. It is our responsibility to express gratitude for the mysterious whole, which we have not made."[55] In sports ethics, this is often rendered as the "admiration" and "celebration" of the talents of "gifted" athletes, and a criticism of the "ethic of willfulness," "mastery," or "striving" that would motivate a turn to performance-enhancing technologies.[56]

Yet, Parens's main point about the two "ethical frameworks" in the enhancement debate is that they inevitably live in tension with each other, as complementary expressions of the ideal of authenticity. Performance enhancement in sport is a perfect example of this tension, because so much of the spirit of sport is captured by the motto of the Olympic movement: *citius, altius, fortius*, "swifter, higher, stronger." It is not a coincidence that "Olympian" is used to describe both elite athletes and the Greek gods: to a large extent, as many have noted, sport does seem to be about transcending the "records" of human experience, about self-mastery, and about creative striving. As we have already seen in the context of sports medicine, sport seeks to press the upper limits of "species-typical functioning." Without a way to accommodate this Promethean dimension of sport, the "gratitude framework" is not going to suffice to ground a successful critique of gene doping.

Finally, it is interesting to note that the charge that gene doping is blasphemous is often invoked with apocalyptic overtones, as if our Promethean efforts at performance enhancement in sport had cosmological significance—at least for the universe of sport. For example, in criticizing the hubris they see motivating performance enhancement, the members of the President's Council on Bioethics write that "the desire to have a perfect body . . . is tantamount to a desire to transcend our embodiment altogether, to become as gods, to become something more-than-human . . . such longings risk becoming a full-scale revolt against our humanity altogether. Fueled in addition by a thirst not merely to excel but to defeat and surpass our rivals, the desire for superhuman powers easily becomes boundless."[57] Even more explicitly, the European editors of a recent volume on gene doping open their introduction with this declaration: "Present genetic technology poses a challenge to sport so serious that it is hard to overestimate. What is at stake is the very ethos of sport, nothing less than an epochal confrontation between a model of human identity as spelled out in the Book of Genesis and a science-based libertarian model. According to the former, sports is a means by which we explore human nature, admire it at its peak, and gain self-understanding. It is not up to us to play God, or, to put it in a more mundane and secular way, to meddle with our evolutionarily determined human nature."[58] This will be worth returning to when we consider the spirit of sport below, because they may be right: gene doping may provoke the Ragnarok that spells the beginning of the end for sport as we have known it.

FRAUD

The third way of interpreting enhancement to mean the use of "unnatural" means to improve athletic performance contrasts the natural with the *artificial.* This is probably the most commonly invoked interpretation in the rhetoric of sports ethics, in which problematic interventions are often labeled in ways that highlight the distinction, without much analysis. Thus, we are warned against "synthetic steroids,"[59] "designer doping,"[60] "the scientific manufacture of athletes,"[61] "artificially induced hypoxic conditions,"[62] and even "artificial genes"(!),[63] but seldom told precisely why these descriptors matter.

The distinction between the natural and the artificial is common in other bioethical debates as well, over issues ranging from the right to a "natural death" to the moral merits of "artificial reproductive technologies." Interestingly, however, it is usually invoked when the processes in question—death, conception, respiration, hydration, aging—are basic biological processes that we share with other living organisms. The distinction's point is to draw moral attention to biomedical attempts to "artificially" replicate, control, or improve on these processes, by emphasizing that these "natural" processes are not human inventions in the first place. As a call to arms in sport, unfortunately, this contrast falls flat, given that sport itself is, in the first place, a human invention, practiced with artificial rules and dependent on multiple technologies of human manufacture. This leads some to quickly dismiss this interpretation as incoherent[64]—perhaps too quickly, because it can point to the most plausible set of principled reasons to be concerned about "enhancement" in the sports context.

Some of those concerned to flesh out the moral meaning behind this distinction argue that explaining the unnaturalness of gene doping in terms of its artificiality is to express the concern that the achievements it would make possible would not be achievements authored by the athlete, for which he or she could legitimately take credit. Under this view, gene-doped victories would be fake, hollow, or inauthentic because they literally would not be the athlete's victory.[65] Even the WADA ethics committee takes this approach, when it argues, for example:

> Our analysis of artificially induced hypoxic conditions to modify performance alerted us to an important distinction: between technologies that operate on the athlete and in relation to which the athlete is a merely passive recipient, versus technologies with which the athlete actively engages and interacts as part of the process of training and competing in order to enhance performance. From the individual athlete's point of view, my responsibility for my performance is diminished by technologies that operate upon me, independent of any effort on my part . . . The human athlete utilizes, masters and controls the technology, not the other way round.[66]

The problem with this interpretation, of course, is the difficulty in disentangling the many conscious decisions athletes make that are accepted as legitimate, even praiseworthy contributors to their own responsibility for their accomplishments in the normal course of sport from a decision to undertake a gene-transfer intervention. If accepting a particular diet can be a legitimate feature of an athlete's "victory narrative," why not the decision to accept gene doping? A gene-doped victory may not be morally praiseworthy, but it would still be authored by the athlete. As Ronald Cole-Turner writes,

> The fact that I write at a computer makes writing easier by eliminating retyping and other frustrations, but writing itself is an intense struggle and it will remain so under any technological condition. The technological advance does not eliminate the struggle so much as relocate it; indeed, it makes it possible to eliminate secondary aggravations and focus attention on the core struggle at hand, namely, expressing new insights in just the right words. Even if technology increased our cognitive ability itself, . . . so that we could calculate or write or think more clearly, these activities would still be a struggle in the face of even greater intellectual challenges to which we human beings inevitably set ourselves.[67]

Claudio Tamburrini goes even further, to suggest that gene doping may even allow us to focus more explicitly on the features of athletic performance that do deserve our praise and admiration:

> We will no longer admire sport stars for their outstanding physical traits (they will be genetically designed). Rather, we will continue to admire them for all the sacrifices endured to actualize their genetic predisposition. In the same way that today's

natural talents cannot do without hard training, the genetically transformed athlete will have to devote herself to her discipline in a goal-directed and professional manner . . . Our admiration for sport heroes will, to a much higher degree than today, concentrate on their dedication and efforts, rather than on a fortuitous physiological predisposition. I cannot see anything unsound in such a development.[68]

Of course, unless the naturally talented are somehow prohibited from using gene doping (returning us to today's situation), the availability of such performance enhancements will never have this leveling effect. But even if it could, others can see, *contra* Tamburrini, something unsound in such a development. What makes a genetically engineered sport hollow, they argue, is not that it renders individual athletes frauds, but rather that it simply misses the point of sport as a social practice.[69]

In this view, even if the explicit rules of a sport are changed to allow new enhancements, their use would erode the value of the achievements they make possible, by undermining the practices that make the achievements valuable in the first place. These practices (disciplined training, graceful play, good teamwork, etc.) add value to the achievements because they are understood to be admirable social practices in themselves. Wherever a biomedical intervention is used to bypass an admirable social practice, then, the improvement's social value is weakened accordingly.[70] Interpreting enhancement interventions as those that short-circuit admirable human practices has special utility for sports ethics. To the extent that biomedical shortcuts allow specific accomplishments to be divorced from the admirable practices they were designed to signal, the social value of those accomplishments will be undermined. This line of thinking is becoming increasingly influential in sports ethics and seems to offer a stable moral platform from which to evaluate the gene-doping issue and the fundamental sports policy choice it raises. It means that for institutions interested in continuing to foster the social values for which they have traditionally been the guardians, choices will have to be made. Either they must redesign the game to find new ways to evaluate excellence in the admirable practices that are not affected by available enhancements, or they must prohibit the use of the enhancing shortcuts. However, knowing which way to go means having at least the sketch of a theory of sport as a social practice and of the values that animate it. Fortunately, the WADA ethics committee itself offers such a sketch, which is instructive to examine.

## The Spirit of Sport

If the problem with gene doping is that it misses the point of sport, what intrinsic values seem to be at stake? In a recent statement on hypoxic training chambers, WADA, echoing Sigmund Loland (see chapter 8 of this volume), Tom Murray (chapters 7 and 11), and others, says that the spirit of sport lies in "the celebration of natural talents and their virtuous perfection," which it explains in the following way:

> What is it that people around the world find honorable, admirable and beautiful about sport? In one important sense, sport is a celebration of human variation. Not all of us have the physiology or anatomy to be a great swimmer, hurdler, skier or discus thrower. Yet, biology is not all that matters: the most naturally gifted athletes must work to perfect their talents . . . The spirit of sport, as we understand it, celebrates natural talents and their virtuous perfection. We say "virtuous" in this context because virtues are qualities of character admirable in themselves, the qualities that outstanding athletes develop and embody in their quest for excellent performance. Some means we respect and want athletes to employ exemplify aspects of character that we admire in people more generally, such as fortitude, dedication, self-discipline, the willingness to suffer in the service of a worthy cause, courage, and strategic wisdom . . . So, for any particular means for enhancing performance . . . the crucial test will be whether it supports or detracts from sport as the expression of natural talents and their virtuous perfection.[71]

This sketch has several important features that bear scrutiny. First and foremost, sport celebrates human variation—that is, the differences between individual human bodies. But not all human differences are of interest in sport. Sport is concerned with celebrating differences in natural talents and the virtues that can be displayed in attempts to differentiate one's own talents even further. The virtues that sport celebrates are socially admirable habits and traits in themselves, and their promotion is what gives sport its social value as a practice. However, within the practice, the virtues are instrumental (either as side constraints or as facilitators) to the "perfection" of the athlete's natural talents (i.e., differentiation from other talents). Moreover, not all natural human talents are relevant in sport. Sport, we learn, is concerned with celebrating the variation in human natural talents that lead athletes to their goal of "excellent performance."

What constitutes excellent athletic performance? WADA's opening question offers three scales for judgment: a performance's moral virtues ("honorableness"), its esthetic qualities ("beauty"), and its place in a hierarchy of human accomplishments ("admiration"). Honorableness, as WADA suggests, is a necessary condition for performance excellence and, to a lesser extent, beauty may be as well. But neither seem sufficient conditions, alone or together. As other philosophers of sport have pointed out, an athletic performance can be beautiful and well played, but if it does not win, by beating either the athlete's own record or the competition, it is not as excellent as an equally beautiful, well-played event that does produce a champion. Performance excellence in sport, in other words, seems to be inevitably and intrinsically about the comparative ranking of performances. Thus, Loland concludes, "In spite of great diversity in sport-specific goals, then, it is possible to formulate a general goal that characterizes sports competitions as such: the goal of sports competitions is to measure, compare and rank two or more competitors according to athletic performance. This goal seems to be common to all sports however diverse their ethos. It defines sport's characteristic social structure and I shall therefore call it the structural goal of sport competition."[72]

The key role of hierarchical ranking in sport is often ignored in the official rhetoric of sports organizations, but as sports ethicist J. J. Coakley acknowledges, fixation with hierarchical ranking—with competition, contest, scorekeeping, record breaking, championship, victory, and defeat—is pervasive in the everyday practice of sport.[73] In ordinary discourse, sport remains true to its historical roots in the war games of ancient and medieval "arenas," "tournaments," and "(battle) fields." As Torbjorn Tännsjö provocatively pointed out, the admiration of champions can easily become contempt for the losers: to "beat," to "own," to "dominate" the competition is to metaphorically subjugate them, just as conquering champions have always enslaved those they overcome.[74] While the hierarchies established by sport are usually more benign than the language of sport (and of Tännsjö, for that matter) suggests, the aptness of our bellicose metaphors shows a similar human urge at work: the urge to establish interpersonal and intergroup hierarchies and locate ourselves within them.

Perhaps most ordinary sports metaphors also miss the point of sport and betray its true spirit. But the value of comparative ranking also insinuates itself into careful attempts to reason about ethical issues in sport, such as gene doping, as our tour of the debate has shown, and that is even more telling.

Thus, as we saw above, the athletic imperative to perform better than others (or oneself) expands the traditional goals of medicine for sports physicians, making it more difficult to rule out performance-enhancing interventions as unprofessional crossing of a medical boundary by undermining the "normal-function" account of that boundary and medicalizing suboptimal performance—and even risks for suboptimal performance—as pathological. At the same time, it is a concern for complicity with suspect social tendencies to use hierarchical human ranking in stigmatizing and oppressive ways that, in limiting cases, causes physicians to eschew particularly brutal forms of sport (boxing, say, or feeding Christians to lions) and to worry about the social consequences of performance enhancement. Similarly, the value of hierarchical taxonomies for sport echoes through the worries that the achievements of gene doping may be "unnatural" because they "degrade" or dehumanize athletes by infecting their identities with the attributes of lower classes of entities—such as machines, chemicals, or animals; or because they violate "our place in nature" in the other direction, by willfully encroaching on the gods' domain; or because gene doping enables victories that athletes cannot authentically claim as their own.

Returning to WADA's description of the spirit of sport, then, this analysis suggests an important clarification to WADA's claim that sport "celebrates human diversity." Perhaps one could say that the many different forms of sport accommodate the diversity of human body types in an appreciative and equitable way. But within any one sport, the "celebration of human variation" is always comparative and hierarchical. The spirit of sport, then, is the celebration of the differences in the human talents and virtues that allow athletes to honorably and beautifully accomplish achievements that place them higher in a hierarchy of human excellence than their competition.

Again, the point of analyzing WADA's description of the spirit of sport was to determine if that spirit is betrayed by gene doping so badly that any achievements facilitated by gene doping would be hollow victories, artificial in the sense of inauthentic, and therefore "unnatural" in a way that is morally problematic. So far, nothing about this spirit of sport would seem to be betrayed by the prospect of safe and openly available gene doping. As the apologists for gene doping insist, genetic interventions would not diminish the need for effort, courage, or self-discipline in sport, because the bar to victory would simply be lifted higher and these traits would still be required. In fact, genetic interventions could help produce even greater champions to celebrate by elevating the starting points for their accomplishments: the physical and mental talents that, as athletes, they set about to virtuously perfect.[75]

But there is still another feature of WADA's description that has not been examined: that in its invocation of the spirit of sport, WADA's ethics committee restricts the kinds of talent that sport celebrates to "*natural* talents." I think this is a new use of the word *natural* yet again, and it is where the problem lies for gene doping.

The term is being used here to qualify the kinds of talent that athletes attempt to virtuously perfect and that authentically excellent (honorable, beautiful, and admirable) athletic performances celebrate. We have already put aside the possibilities that this use of "natural" might be intended to exclude monstrous or blasphemous talents or talents aided by technological artifice per se, for the same reasons that brought us to this point in the analysis. Only one other plausible interpretation of "natural" in this phrase presents itself: "natural talents" are the talents we are born with (i.e., inherited characteristics over which athletes have no control and which are ultimately traceable to particular combinations of ancestors and their genes). As Loland concludes, "Now I can say more precisely what I mean by talent in sport. It is an individual's genetic predisposition to develop phenotypes of relevance to performance in the sport in question. The distribution of talent in the natural lottery is a random process."[76]

In WADA's interpretation, in other words, the spirit of sport is in part a celebration of differential genetic endowments, distributed through the "natural lottery" of genealogy. Sport creates a system of values, virtues, and practices designed to hierarchically grade people in terms of their (virtuously perfected) inherited traits and glorify the best specimens as champions. This is a turning point for our analysis: biomedical interventions at the genetic level would miss the point of the sport if this view is correct, because gene doping would undermine the ability of sport to distinguish those who passively inherited their talents from their progenitors from those who actively acquired them from their physicians. As Sandel says:

> Which aspect of the athletic ideal—effort or gift—would be more deeply offended? Some might say effort: the problem with drugs is that they provide a shortcut, a way to win without striving. But striving is not the point of sports; excellence is. And excellence consists at least partly in the display of natural talents and gifts that are no doing of the athlete who possesses them . . . No one believes that a mediocre basketball player who works and trains even harder than Michael Jordan deserves greater acclaim. The real problem with genetically altered athletes is that they corrupt athletic competition as a human activity that honors the cultivation as display of natural talents"[77]

At last, our map of enhancement concepts has brought us to an interpretation of the problem of gene doping that WADA might use to theoretically ground its prohibition and motivate the search for detection techniques. For all the ways in which our discussions of "enhancement" in applied ethics are challenged by the gene-doping case, here is one rationale that can provide a definitive answer. Gene doping is wrong for athletes to pursue and sports medicine to provide because it compromises the ability of sport to segregate and elevate genetically advantaged athletes from their disadvantaged competitors, which is a key element of the spirit of sport and one of the intrinsic values of the enterprise. This will be true even if gene doping is proven safe and effective, and even if it could be provided equitably to every competitor in noncoercive ways.

## Conclusion

After all our conceptual orienteering, why is reaching this destination so disturbing? Perhaps it is because of the uncomfortable light that the problem of gene doping throws back on the spirit of sport itself and the broader questions it raises for sports ethics. The very prospect of gene doping forces sport to notice that the "natural lottery" of genetics is getting less "random" all the time as our knowledge of human genetics grows, and as that happens, the moral justification for celebrating human genetic hierarchies as facts of nature begins to falter. It is one thing to acknowledge as perhaps unfortunate but not unfair that human talents vary across individuals in ways that allow some to do some things that others cannot. To admire those inborn differences as beautiful and to reward those who seek to (virtuously) perpetuate and increase them seems arbitrary, but no less pernicious than other idiosyncrasies of social taste, such as celebrity worship. But to glorify those genetic disparities to the extent of prohibiting their abatement when biomedicine provides the ability to do so exposes a fundamental tension with the spirit of sport itself: while the variable genetic distribution of human talent may be a natural fact, the creation of social hierarchies out of that distribution is a distinctly human project, and never a random one. For sports ethicists, this raises a challenging question for further discussion. As a human project, what differentiates the hierarchical ranking of genetic talents by sports institutions from the reciprocal devaluing of genetic defects by insurance risk underwriters? In both cases, the internal logic of the practice is clear, but their use of inherited genetic identity as a social ranking criterion raises large questions about the fairness of the enterprise as a whole.

This may be the reason for the apocalyptic tone with which sports authorities frame the issue of gene doping. After all, in most discussions of the ethics of genetic enhancement outside the sports context, a key concern is to avoid the creation of a "genobility" and the errors of genetic essentialism and risks of genetic discrimination this would entail.[78] Even within medicine, the strongest case against going "beyond therapy" with genetic interventions is the danger of exacerbating invidious social divisions by reducing them to individual genetic advantages and disadvantages. In a world that is struggling to realize a commitment to treating people as moral equals despite their biological differences, a social practice that creates and glorifies hierarchies of genetic endowment seems anachronistic and slightly ominous. As Sandel acknowledges about his defense of the role of sport's commitment to genetic stratification, "This is an uncomfortable fact for democratic societies. We want to believe that success, in sports and in life, is something we earn, not something we inherit. Natural gifts, and the admiration they inspire, embarrass the meritocratic faith; they cast doubt on the conviction that praise and reward flow from effort alone."[79]

To discover that the principal problem with gene doping is that it threatens sport's commitment to the creation and promotion of human genetic stratification should give us pause. On the one hand, of the many ways that humans use inherited traits to create interpersonal hierarchies, athletic competition is among the most benign. When it is "just a game," comparative interpersonal ranking in terms of genetic identity in sports is a welcome substitute for blood feuds, racism, and genocide. What the gene-doping debate suggests, however, is that sport may have more in common with these extreme human vices than we would like to think. Being one's peers' last choice as a teammate hurts enough in a friendly pickup game. But when sport becomes a matter of national pride and a source of economic opportunity, athletic losers risk more than simply admiration and social status: like insurance applicants with genetic susceptibilities, less naturally talented athletes risk access to important social benefits and potential life plans. In this regard, the apocalyptic challenge that genetic engineering poses to sport reduces to a simple question that echoes Cole-Turner's concern to "relocate the struggle" of human achievement on what matters.[80] Are there ways to enjoy, appreciate, and even show off our bodies and abilities without requiring someone else to lose social standing on genetic grounds?

ACKNOWLEDGMENTS

Support for the development of this chapter was provided by the USADA (U.S. Anti-Doping Agency) grant "Ethical, Conceptual and Scientific Issues in the Use of Performance Enhancing Technologies in Sports" (Thomas Murray, P.I.), NIH grant R01 HG003879 (Maxwell Mehlman, P.I.), and NIH grant P50 HG03390 (Eric Juengst, P.I.). I am grateful for helpful readings by Robert Binstock and Tom Murray and for useful comments by the Enhancement Research Group of the Case Western Reserve University Center for Genetic Research Ethics and Law.

## NOTES

1. E. Parens, ed., *Enhancing Human Traits: Ethical and Social Implications* (Washington, DC: Georgetown University Press, 1998).
2. N. Daniels, "Growth Hormone Therapy for Short Stature: Can We Support the Treatment/Enhancement Distinction?" *Growth, Genes and Hormones* 8, suppl. 1 (1992): 46–48; G. White, "Human Growth Hormone: The Dilemma of Expanded Use in Children," *Kennedy Institute of Ethics Journal* 3 (1993): 401–9.
3. W. F. Anderson, "Human Gene Therapy: Why Draw a Line?" *Journal of Medicine and Philosophy* 14 (1989): 681–93; P. Baird, "Altering Human Genes: Social, Ethical and Legal Implications," *Perspectives in Biology and Medicine* 37 (1994): 566–75.
4. President's Council on Bioethics, *Beyond Therapy: Biotechnology and the Pursuit of Happiness* (Washington, DC: President's Council on Bioethics, 2003); S. Rothman and D. Rothman, *The Pursuit of Perfection: The Promise and Perils of Medical Enhancement* (New York: Pantheon Books, 2003).
5. T. H. Murray, "Drugs, Sports, and Ethics," in *Feeling Good and Doing Better: Ethics and Nontherapeutic Drug Use*, ed. T. H. Murray, W. Gaylin, and R. Macklin, 107–26 (Clifton, NJ: Humana Press, 1983); T. H. Murray, "The Ethics of Drugs in Sport," in *Drugs and Performance in Sports*, ed. Richard Strauss, 11–21 (Philadelphia: W. B. Saunders, 1987).
6. S. Loland, *Fair Play in Sport: A Moral Norm System* (New York: Routledge, 2002).
7. R. L. Simon, *Fair Play: Sport, Values and Society* (Boulder, CO: Westview Press, 1991); A. Schneider and R. B. Butcher, "A Philosophical Overview of the Arguments on Banning Doping in Sport," in *Values in Sport: Elitism, Nationalism, Gender Equality and the Scientific Manufacture of Winners*, ed. T. Tännsjö and C. Tamburrini, 185–99 (New York: Routledge, 2000).
8. J. Hoberman, *Mortal Engines: The Science of Performance and the Dehumanization of Sport* (Caldwell, NJ: Blackburn Press, 1992).
9. World Anti-Doping Agency, "The World Anti-Doping Code: The 2007 Prohibited List, International Standard," effective January 1, 2007, www.wada-ama.org/rtecontent/document/2007_List_En.pdf.
10. E. Juengst, "What Does Enhancement Mean?" in *Enhancing Human Traits: Ethical and Social Implications*, ed. E. Parens, 29–47 (Washington, DC: Georgetown University Press, 1998).
11. A. Ljungqvist, "The International Anti-Doping Policy and Its Implementation," in *Genetic Technology and Sport: Ethical Questions*, ed. C. Tamburrini and T. Tännsjö, 13–19 (New York: Routledge, 2005).
12. Ibid.; F. Miller, H. Brody, and K. Chung, "Cosmetic Surgery and the Internal Morality of Medicine," *Cambridge Quarterly of Healthcare Ethics* 9 (2000): 353–64.
13. L. Kass, *Toward a More Natural Science: Biology and Human Affairs* (New York: Free Press, 1985).

14. B. Good, *Medicine, Rationality, and Experience: An Anthropological Perspective* (New York: Cambridge University Press, 1994).

15. H. T. Engelhardt, "Human Nature Technologically Revisited," *Social Philosophy and Policy* 8 (1990): 180–91.

16. J. Bernstein, C. Perlis, and A. Bartolozzi, "Ethics in Sports Medicine," *Clinical Orthopaedics and Related Research* 378 (2000): 50–60.

17. Hoberman, *Mortal Engines.*

18. E. Juengst, R. Binstock, M. Mehlman, S. Post, and P. Whitehouse, "Biogerontology, 'Anti-Aging Medicine,' and the Challenges of Human Enhancement," *Hastings Center Report* 33, no. 4 (2003): 2–10.

19. J. Sabin and N. Daniels, "Determining 'Medical Necessity' in Mental Health Practice," *Hastings Center Report* 24, no. 6 (1994): 5–13; N. Daniels, *Just Health Care* (Cambridge: Cambridge University Press, 1986).

20. E. Berger and B. Gert, "Genetic Disorders and the Ethical Status of Germ-Line Gene Therapy," *Journal of Medicine and Philosophy* 16 (1991): 667–85.

21. See A. Buchanan, D. Brock, N. Daniels, and D. Wikler, *From Chance to Choice: Genetics and Justice* (New York: Cambridge University Press, 2000).

22. J. L. Scully and C. Rehmann-Sutter, "When Norms Normalize: The Case of Genetic 'Enhancement,'" *Human Gene Therapy* 12 (2001): 87–95; A. Silvers, "A Fatal Attraction to Normalizing: Treating Disabilities as Deviations from 'Species Typical' Functioning," in Parens, *Enhancing Human Traits*, 95–123.

23. Silvers, "Fatal Attraction."

24. Ljungqvist, "International Anti-Doping Policy"; Bernstein, Perlis, and Bartolozzi, "Ethics in Sports Medicine."

25. P. Whitehouse, E. Juengst, T. H. Murray, and M. Mehlman, "Enhancing Cognition in the Intellectually Intact," *Hastings Center Report* 27, no. 3 (1997): 14–22.

26. E. Juengst, "Can Enhancement Be Distinguished from Prevention in Genetic Medicine?" *Journal of Medicine and Philosophy* 22 (1997): 125–42.

27. See J. Hall, J. Dunlap, T. Friedman, and V. van Hyningen, "Gene Transfer in Sports: An Opening Scenario for Genetic Enhancement of Normal Human Traits," *Advances in Genetics* 51 (2006): 37–49.

28. Ljungqvist, "International Anti-Doping Policy."

29. Juengst, "Can Enhancement Be Distinguished?"

30. K. Morgan, "Women and the Knife: Cosmetic Surgery and the Colonization of Women's Bodies," *Hypatia* 6 (1991): 25–53; Sabin and Daniels, "Determining 'Medical Necessity.'"

31. M. Little, "Suspect Norms of Appearance and the Ethics of Complicity," in *In the Eye of the Beholder: Ethics and Medical Change of Appearance*, ed. I. de Beaufort, M. Hilhorst, and S. Holm, 151–67 (Stockholm: Scandinavian University Press, 1997).

32. Bernstein, Perlis, and Bartolozzi, "Ethics in Sports Medicine," 55.

33. Ljungqvist, "International Anti-Doping Policy."

34. Hall et al., "Gene Transfer in Sports."

35. M. Mehlman. "How Will We Regulate Genetic Enhancement?" *Wake Forest Law Review* 34 (1999): 671–714.

36. J. Childress, *Who Should Decide: Paternalism in Health Care* (New York: Oxford University Press, 1982).

37. Murray, "Ethics of Drugs in Sport."

38. Hall et al., "Gene Transfer in Sports."

39. C. Munthe, "Selected Champions: Making Winners in the Age of Genetic Technology," in Tännsjö and Tamburrini, *Values in Sport*, 217–21.

40. Hoberman, *Mortal Engines*.

41. Cf. President's Council on Bioethics, *Beyond Therapy*; Schneider and Butcher, "Philosophical Overview."

42. Hoberman, *Mortal Engines*, 104.

43. J. Stout, *Ethics after Babel: The Languages of Morals and Their Discontents* (Princeton: Princeton University Press, 1988); J. S. Robert and F. Baylis, "Crossing Species Boundaries," *American Journal of Bioethics* 3, no. 3 (2003): 1–14.

44. Hoberman, *Mortal Engines*, 21.

45. M. Burke and T. Roberts, "Drugs in Sport: An Issue of Morality or Sentimentality?" *Journal of the Philosophy of Sport* 24 (1997): 99–113.

46. L. Davis and L. Delano, "Fixing the Boundaries of Physical Gender: Side Effects of Anti-Drug Campaigns in Athletics," *Sociology of Sport Journal* 9, no. 1 (1992): 1–19.

47. Hoberman, *Mortal Engines*.

48. Ibid.

49. A. Miah, *Genetically Modified Athletes: Biomedical Ethics, Gene Doping and Sport* (New York: Routledge, 2004).

50. S. Sherwin and M. Schwartz, "Resisting the Emergence of Bio-Amazons," in Tamburrini and Tännsjö, *Genetic Technology and Sport*, 199–205.

51. President's Council on Bioethics, *Beyond Therapy*, 144.

52. Hoberman, *Mortal Engines*, 290.

53. Hall et al., "Gene Transfer in Sports."

54. M. Sandel, "The Case against Perfection: What's Wrong with Designer Children, Bionic Athletes and Genetic Engineering," *Atlantic Monthly*, April 2004, 51–62.

55. E. Parens, "Authenticity and Ambivalence: Toward Understanding the Enhancement Debate," *Hastings Center Report* 35, no. 3 (2005): 34–41; comment on Sandel on p. 37.

56. Cf. President's Council on Bioethics, *Beyond Therapy*; Sandel, "Case against Perfection."

57. President's Council on Bioethics, *Beyond Therapy*, 150.

58. Tamburrini and Tännsjö, *Genetic Technology and Sport*, 2.

59. Hoberman, *Mortal Engines*.

60. M. Joyner, "Designer Doping," *Exercise and Sport Science Reviews* 20 (2004): 81–82.

61. T. Tännsjö, "Is Our Admiration for Sports Heroes Fascistoid?" in Tännsjö and Tamburrini, *Values in Sport*, 24–38.

62. World Anti-Doping Agency, "WADA Note on Artificially Induced Hypoxic Conditions," www.wada-ama.org/rtecontent/document.

63. M. Unal and U. Durisehvar, "Gene Doping in Sports," *Sports Medicine* 34 (2004): 357–62.

64. Cf. M. Mehlman, *Genetic Enhancement and the Future of Society* (Bloomington: Indiana University Press, 2003), 95–101.

65. President's Council on Bioethics, *Beyond Therapy*, 124–34.

66. World Anti-Doping Agency, "WADA Note."

67. R. Cole-Turner, "Do Means Matter?" in Parens, *Enhancing Human Traits*, 151–61.

68. C. Tamburrini, "After Doping, What? The Morality of the Genetic Engineering of Athletes," *Sport Technology: History, Philosophy and Policy* 21 (2002): 243–68.

69. Murray, "Ethics of Drugs in Sport."

70. Ibid.; Schneider and Butcher, "Philosophical Overview"; Loland, *Fair Play in Sport*.

71. World Anti-Doping Agency, "WADA Note."

72. Loland, *Fair Play in Sport*, 10.

73. J. J. Coakley, *Sport in Society: Issues and Controversies*, 6th ed. (Boston: McGraw-Hill, 1998).

74. Tännsjö, "Is Our Admiration for Sports Athletes Fascistoid?"

75. Miah, *Genetically Modified Athletes*; Tamburrini, "After Doping, What?"

76. Loland, *Fair Play in Sport*, 69.

77. Sandel, "Case against Perfection," 55.

78. Mehlman, *Genetic Enhancement and the Future of Society*.

79. Sandel, "Case against Perfection."

80. Cole-Turner, "Do Means Matter?"

# CHAPTER TEN

# Genetic Enhancement in Sport

## Ethical, Legal, and Policy Concerns

MAXWELL J. MEHLMAN, J.D.

The efforts of organized sport to combat the use of performance-enhancing drugs will soon be confronting new challenges, as interventions emerge from discoveries in human genetics. This chapter begins by defining *genetic enhancement* and describing the different types of genetic enhancements that are currently available or might be developed in the future. I then discuss whether these interventions differ in relevant ethical, legal, or policy respects from performance-enhancing drugs and make some recommendations on how sport should respond to the challenges presented by these emerging genetic technologies.

## The Meaning of Genetic Enhancement

To understand the issues raised by the use of genetic enhancement in sport, we must first understand what is meant by *genetic* and *enhancement*. Neither of these terms is easy to define. *Genetic* could refer only to an intervention that involves actively manipulating human genes, such as inserting exogenous DNA into a viral vector and injecting this into the target organism or tissue. Alternatively, the term could be used broadly to apply to any intervention based in some respect on genetic science and technology. This definition would include drugs made with recombinant DNA technology, reproductive decisions about which embryos to implant following in vitro fertilization (IVF) and preimplantation genetic testing, and tailoring performance-enhancing drugs to an athlete's personal pharmacogenetic profile. For several reasons, it seems appropriate to adopt the broader approach. First, this allows for the most complete discussion of the topic. Second, there is no obvious basis for excluding some interventions and not others.

Third, different types of intervention raise different concerns and invite different responses: if the attitude that sport has adopted toward performance-enhancing drugs is appropriate for some genetic enhancements, it may not be appropriate for all. Finally, the broader definition increases the immediacy of the inquiry; although gene transfer to improve athletic performance may not be available for some time, athletes already are using genetically engineered drugs.

Under this broad definition, then, six kinds of genetic intervention might be used to enhance athletic performance.

1. *Genetic testing to identify innate athletic ability.* Recently, researchers in Australia announced that they had identified a genetic variation, ACTN3, associated with different types of athletic ability.[1] Discoveries like this could lead to genetic testing that could pinpoint promising candidates for intensive coaching and training. Testing could occur at any point but might be especially useful in childhood or early adolescence, when individuals could maximize their future athletic potential.

2. *Performance-enhancing drugs developed with genetic science and technology.* Performance-enhancing substances that occur naturally in the body can be manufactured artificially by inserting the substance-producing genes into bacterial DNA, a process known as recombinant DNA. Synthetic erythropoietin (EPO) and human growth hormone (HGH) are among the recombinant DNA performance-enhancing drugs currently used by athletes. New knowledge about the human genome also could make possible the design of drugs that supplement or block the effects of proteins associated with certain forms of athletic ability.

3. *Pharmacogenetics.* Researchers are learning that certain genetic variations are associated with different responses to drugs. This opens the door to the development of drugs targeted at specific population groups or individuals and to more efficient drug prescribing that maximizes efficacy and minimizes adverse effects, without the need for so much trial and error.[2] Similarly, researchers could find genetic variations that make athletes react differently to various performance-enhancing drugs, so that athletes could use the safest and most effective enhancement interventions.

4. *Reproductive enhancement.* The development of genetic tests to detect innate athletic ability would make possible a range of reproductive actions to produce athletically gifted offspring. Individuals could get tested before marrying and conceiving children, then proceed only if the match would yield genetically favorable results. Similar tests could be performed on donor eggs or sperm. Through the process of preimplantation genetic testing, embryos fertilized in the laboratory could be tested and only those with desirable genes implanted in the uterus.

This is now being done not only to screen for genetic diseases but also to select gender.[3]

Fetuses could be tested and aborted if they did not come up to genetic expectations. This is unlikely to occur frequently, given the attendant health risks and emotional toll of abortion, but there are reports of fetuses being aborted because of gender, especially in Asia. Moreover, it is conceivable that rapid genetic tests could be developed that would generate test results in time to terminate pregnancies at a very early stage, perhaps with the use of something akin to a "morning-after pill." Finally, parents could have their children tested and continue to reproduce until they produced a child with the desired athletic abilities, or they could adopt a child with a favorable genetic test result.

Genetic testing in the course of reproductive decision making can only enable parents to select embryos or fetuses based on their naturally occurring genetic endowments for athletic ability. An alternative form of genetic enhancement would be to install genes into individuals that they would not naturally have possessed. These may be genes found naturally in the genomes of other persons or completely new genes, not found in nature. This approach is described next.

5. *Somatic gene transfer.* Numerous trials are under way to treat genetic disorders by injecting corrected genes into the body. So far they have had limited success; in 1999, 18-year-old Jesse Gelsinger died in one such experiment, and several infants who underwent gene therapy in France contracted leukemia.[4] However, substantial progress is likely in the future, leading to the possibility of inserting genes that code for proteins associated with athletic ability or resistance to athletic injury. Gene-therapy experiments are currently in progress to treat muscle-wasting diseases such as muscular dystrophy. If successful, these could yield interventions that enhance musculature or vascularization, which could improve athletic performance.

6. *Germ-line gene transfer.* Somatic gene transfer does not affect reproductive cells (sperm and eggs), and therefore enhanced characteristics would not be inherited by offspring. However, if gene transfer took place at an early enough stage of development—for example, before fertilization or at the embryonic or early fetal stage—altered DNA could find its way into reproductive cells. Already there have been reports of inadvertent germ-line changes resulting from an infertility treatment called ooplasmic transfer.[5] Parents might seek to alter the germ line of their children deliberately to enhance athletic ability, so that the changes could be passed on to future generations.

With this idea of which performance-related interventions might be considered genetic, we now need to consider what is meant by *enhancement.* Many scholars have struggled with the distinction between an "enhancement" and a "treatment" or "remedy," including Eric Juengst (see chapter 9). They have pointed out the difficulty of considering something to be an enhancement if it gives someone more than "normal" abilities, because the notion of "normality" is based on population characteristics that vary by time and place. For example, increasing an adult's height from 4 to 6 feet might be considered therapeutic, because 4 feet is below normal, and an increase from 6 to 7 feet might be deemed an enhancement, because 7 feet is above normal. But what about within the population of professional basketball players? In that context, being only 6 feet tall might be considered abnormal, so it could be argued that increasing height to 7 feet would be therapeutic. Moreover, as Juengst observes, some already well-accepted preventive measures, such as immunizations, are intended to give people capacities they do not normally possess.[6] Juengst argues that immunizations should not be regarded as enhancements, because they are intended to combat disease. But he acknowledges that the concept of disease itself is uncertain. Before 1973, for example, the American Psychiatric Association regarded homosexuality as a mental disorder.[7]

In the context of sport, the distinction between enhancement and therapy or remediation may be less important. The international Olympic movement bans certain interventions, for example, even if, arguably, they are being used for therapeutic or remedial purposes. A Romanian gymnast was stripped of her gold medal in the 2000 Olympics for using an over-the-counter cold remedy, even though she had a cold.[8] This points to a crucial feature of sport that we will return to later: a sport can adopt any rules that it wishes. Nevertheless, advances in genetics could present difficult choices for rule makers. For instance, if it becomes possible to test people to determine their innate athletic ability, could people whose ability is below the population mean argue that they are genetically impaired, so that gene insertion to improve their athletic ability should be considered a remedy rather than an enhancement? Another dilemma would arise, which Juengst also addresses in chapter 9, if scientists developed genetic interventions that could reduce the likelihood that athletes will be injured. Work is under way, for example, on genetically engineered therapeutic antibodies and cytokines, which could reduce susceptibility to injury.[9] Should this be regarded as preventive therapy or as enhancement?

For the same reasons that a broad definition of "genetic" was adopted earlier, it seems appropriate to employ a broad definition of what counts as an enhancement. Rather than deciding a priori that something is or is not an enhancement, it makes more sense to admit that it may be an enhancement and then ask what response it should trigger from sport. Therefore, for the purposes of this discussion, a genetic intervention—that is, any of the genetic techniques listed earlier—will be considered an enhancement if it improves athletic ability or confers a competitive advantage in sport. Under this definition, even genetic testing to identify innate athletic ability can be considered an enhancement, because it can confer competitive advantage by concentrating scarce coaching and training resources on certain individuals.

## Are Genetic Enhancements Like Performance-Enhancing Drugs?

Sport bans the use of performance-enhancing drugs for several reasons, related to their nature and effect. The question is whether genetic enhancements are sufficiently similar to performance-enhancing drugs that these reasons apply to them as well.

The basic rationales for banning performance-enhancing drugs were laid down by the International Olympic Committee in 1967: (1) "protection of the athletes' health"; (2) "respect for medical and sports ethics"; and (3) "ensuring an equal chance for everyone during competition."[10] The first of these focuses on the health dangers posed by the drugs. In some cases, the dangers are well-known. Anabolic steroids, for example, can cause heart attacks and liver cancer.[11] In other instances, athletes may use drugs for which little safety information is available. Some drugs that are used to enhance athletic performance, such as EPO and HGH, are approved only for therapeutic purposes. To obtain this approval, the manufacturers submitted data to the U.S. Food and Drug Administration (FDA) that included a catalogue of the adverse effects occurring in the course of clinical trials on defined patient populations, and convinced the agency that these risks were outweighed by the therapeutic benefits that the study participants received. Although this information can give some indication of the toxicity that can be expected from the drug when used for unapproved purposes, it does not disclose the effects the drug might have in populations different from those in which it was tested or what interactions it could cause when taken with other substances. The FDA requires drug manufacturers to notify the agency of any adverse effects they become aware of after their drugs are already approved and in use, regardless of the purpose for which the drugs are used, but reporting is generally acknowledged to be unsatisfactory.[12] Other performance-enhancing drugs may be produced entirely on the black market, with no safety information available whatsoever. In the fall of 2003, for example, some athletes were caught using a so-called designer steroid that had been concocted by a black-market chemist to thwart standard drug tests.[13] For all of these reasons, athletes who use performance-enhancing drugs may not know how dangerous they are.

Similar concerns about safety risks and lack of safety information would be raised by genetic enhancements. There is no reason to believe that genetically engineered drugs are safer than other drugs. As the death of Jesse Gelsinger illustrates, gene transfer can be lethal. Not only may these drugs and techniques be dangerous, but they may be approved for therapeutic use only because the risks are deemed to be outweighed by the seriousness of the conditions of patients for whom they are prescribed. The gene therapy study in which Gelsinger died, for example, was aimed at treating an inherited metabolic disorder that severely damages the brain of newborns and kills half of affected infants before they are six months old.[14] In contrast, it may be difficult to evaluate nontherapeutic benefits and to balance them against risks. Furthermore, the risks may be unknown. Approved genetically engineered drugs and somatic and germ-line gene-transfer techniques may be employed for unapproved, enhancement purposes. Germ-line gene transfer raises special concerns because the hazards may not become apparent until subsequent generations have matured and reproduced. Finally, there is the possibility that unscrupulous entrepreneurs will offer dangerous somatic or germ-line gene transfer on the black market without any regulatory oversight.

At the same time, there is no reason to expect that drugs made with recombinant DNA techniques or by methods based on a knowledge of genetic science would be any more dangerous than drugs produced in other ways. Drug companies have used recombinant DNA manufacturing since the mid-1980s, and the FDA has long maintained that products made with this technique do not require any different or greater scrutiny than drugs manufactured by other processes.[15]

Genetic testing presents a somewhat different set of safety concerns than drugs or gene transfer. Genetic testing is a diagnostic technique rather than a treatment, so it does not introduce active drugs into the body, and unlike some types of diagnostic imaging, which employ potentially dangerous contrast media, the only physical invasion required for genetic testing is a blood draw or cheek swab. Genetic testing can still cause harm, however. Like other diagnostic testing, it can produce inaccurate results, due either to inherent limitations in the test methodology or to laboratory error. A false positive result for athletic prowess could subject the person who was tested to physically and emotionally taxing training and to the mental anguish of inexplicably failing to make adequate progress. False negative results could deprive people of the opportunity to fulfill their true athletic potential. Moreover, genetic test information may stigmatize the individuals tested, as well as members of their family and those who share their genetic heritage. For example, it might turn out that certain families or genetically related populations test poorly for athletic ability, leading to discrimination and ridicule. Or health insurers might want to charge people with genetic athletic ability higher premiums to cover the risk of sports injuries. Finally, testing children for athletic potential could cause various harms to the children, such as decreased control over their destinies and loss of self-esteem if the test results are negative. Testing also could harm the parent-child relationship. Parents might be disappointed if children who test positive refuse to play sports or do not become star performers, or they might give less affection to children who test negative.

Pharmacogenetics would involve performing genetic tests on athletes to ascertain their genetic susceptibility to certain drug interactions, both positive and negative. Hence, it would carry the same risks as testing for genetic athletic potential. But one function of pharmacogenetic testing is to identify individuals who may react badly to certain chemical compounds so that they can avoid taking them. Pharmacogenetic testing before use of a performance-enhancing drug could promote safety by reducing the risk of adverse effects. For example, it may be possible to identify certain athletes who will not suffer serious harm from the use of anabolic steroids.

The final set of genetic enhancements involves reproductive decision making to produce athletically optimum offspring. This entails genetic testing—of potential parents, gametes, embryos, fetuses, or children—and therefore creates the same testing risks discussed above. Reproductive decisions to refrain from implanting embryos or to abort fetuses prevent live births, which might be considered a form of harm. IVF employs fertility drugs that have safety risks and sometimes leads to multiple births, which can compromise the health of the offspring.[16]

In summary, all genetic enhancements carry some degree of risk. If sport is entitled to prohibit performance-enhancing drugs to avoid harm, the same justification could be applied to prohibit the use of genetic enhancements. However, genetic enhancements also could yield significant benefits, including improved athletic performance, the safer use of performance-enhancing drugs, more focused development of athletic potential, and more informed reproductive decisions. This raises the question of whether the benefits outweigh the risks. Sports that ban the use of performance-enhancing drugs answer the question in the negative. Their position seems to be based not so much on a conclusion that the risks outweigh the benefits as on a conviction that there are no legitimate benefits at all to the use of performance-enhancing drugs. This attitude stems from the other two rationales that sport asserts in defense of its antidrug position: respect for medical and sports ethics and ensuring an equal chance for everyone during competition. The question is whether these rationales apply as well to genetic enhancement.

The "equality" rationale is premised on the notion that performance-enhancing drugs could give athletes who use them an unfair advantage over others who do not. This would be a valid concern if the drugs were not available to everyone, which may be the case, because rogue chemists continue to develop new drugs to defeat existing tests and many athletes may not be in the distribution loop, especially when the drugs are first developed. But athletes do not seem to have great difficulty obtaining most commonly used performance-enhancing drugs. If the drugs are readily available, the "inequality" objection becomes a concern about freedom of choice. The problem is that for everyone to have an equivalent chance of winning, if anyone uses performance-enhancing drugs, everyone must. Thus, when Ben Johnson was stripped of his 1988 Olympic gold medal, his coach repeatedly stressed that athletes cannot survive in highly competitive environments without the use of drugs.[17] As this statement suggests, the athletes' own compulsion to use drugs can be exacerbated by the pressure placed on them by coaches and trainers. Opponents of drugs in sport go on to assert that universal use of drugs makes the practice futile: if everyone uses the drugs, then the effect on winning is the same as if no one used them—except that everyone now has to suffer the adverse health effects. This argument may be erroneous, because it assumes that drugs affect all athletes in the same way; more likely, the effects vary somewhat from person to person. But this merely brings us back to the initial objection that drugs foster inequality.

If anything, the inequality objection applies with even greater force to genetic enhancements. Genetic enhancements may be harder to obtain than performance-enhancing drugs. Gene transfer and preimplantation genetic manipulation, for example, may require technical skills and equipment that are not widely available. IVF, the precursor to many forms of genetic enhancement, is expensive, costing as much as $58,000 per live birth.[18] Moreover, individuals may have even less freedom to choose whether or not to become genetically enhanced than whether or not to use performance-enhancing drugs. Parents who base reproductive decisions on genetic test results, such as selecting embryos for implantation for their superior athletic ability, or who undergo procedures to manipulate DNA at an early stage of a child's development, would be making choices without the input of the offspring who will be affected. Finally, if genetic enhancement reaches its full potential, it could give a decisive advantage to those who gained access to it.

Yet, in a sense, all of these arguments beg several questions. Why are performance-enhancing drugs prohibited, when athletes are permitted, indeed encouraged, to train hard, which may carry comparable risks of physical injury? Why should competitors be punished for supplementing their natural talent with biochemical adjuncts, when natural talent itself is something they have done nothing to deserve? Is there something fundamentally wrong with using performance-enhancing drugs?

The answers lie in the remaining rationale asserted by the International Olympic Committee: that performance-enhancing drugs violate the ethics of medicine and sport. Sport holds that athletes who win because they are driven to succeed, put in endless hours of training and practice, have innate athletic ability, and enjoy the good fortune, say, of having wealthy, supportive parents and of avoiding injury are entitled to their medals. Their victory is worthwhile, "authentic." By contrast, accomplishments by athletes who use drugs are "inauthentic." In short, the argument goes, sport necessarily values only certain inputs: determination, effort, natural talent, and luck.

But it is hard to see why sport values all of these inputs. Neither natural talents nor good fortune are earned or deserved. Indeed, the fact that—before genetic engineering, at least—they could not be manipulated may be what gave them their appeal. Opponents of drug use might argue that a sport cannot permit the use of drugs and still count as a sport, but some strength competitions, including certain powerlifting events, are conducted without drug testing. These events may not be to everyone's taste, such as Jan and Terry Todd's, who criticize the proliferation of powerlifting federations (see chapter 3). Few people may compete in or attend these events. But it is difficult to maintain that they are not sport.

So what is it that defines a sport? Arguably, a sport involves substantial physical activity. (Otherwise, like chess, it would merely be a game.) But beyond that, a sport is an activity that is conducted according to a set of rules, including rules that define an ultimate objective (e.g., to score the most runs, lift the heaviest weight) and the manner in which the objective is to be attained. The rules may be based on historical accident (such as the decision that baseball would be played with nine players on a side), or on a sense of propriety or esthetics (people might complain if weightlifters were naked), or, like the designated-hitter rule in baseball, on an estimate of what would attract more spectators.[19] Also, the rules can be changed. For example, pole-vault poles originally were made of bamboo, but the sport decided to permit the use of fiberglass poles when they were invented in the early 1960s.[20] Furthermore, as is borne out by the foregoing examples, the rules of a sport can be completely arbitrary. Indeed, they often are. Why 9 players on a baseball team, for instance, instead of 11? But the crucial point is that a sport must be played according to its rules for it to have meaning as a sport. (You may remember, as a child, the pointlessness of trying to play a game in which the individual players could make up the rules to suit themselves as they went along.) Sport can make a rule that a batter may not use a corked bat, or that a skater must perform certain obligatory moves on the ice, or that athletes forfeit their medals if they are caught using banned substances. Sport even can adopt rules that seem hard to justify, such as disqualifying Olympic athletes who use perfectly safe, over-the-counter cold medicines when they have colds. The point is that obedience to the rules is the central ethic of sport. The key question here, then, is whether genetic enhancement should be against the rules.

## Should Sport Ban Genetic Enhancement?

To answer this question, we must begin by considering whether there is something about an enhancement being "genetic" that justifies banning it on that basis alone. Something that is "genetic," it might be said, belongs to a fundamental, perhaps even an elemental, domain of biology. Until recently, the only way to alter the human genome deliberately was through the slow processes of reproduction and evolution or by committing abominable acts of genocide. The ability to rapidly and directly manipulate human DNA smacks of hubris. These techniques are powerful and frightening. Their consequences are unforeseeable. They unleash a primal force of nature that should be used sparingly, if at all, and then only for therapeutic purposes.

This attitude toward genetics may be too alarmist. Arguably, it overestimates the impact of genes on human abilities and behavior and underestimates the role of the environment. This can lead to bad public policies such as reducing funding for programs to help the disadvantaged on the ground that these people are genetically programmed to fail, or to unfortunate behavior such as expecting too much from one's children because of their genetic pedigree. It is a view that has led legislatures to scurry to enact laws protecting the privacy of genetic information, when *all* sensitive, personal information needs better protection. People who think this way are accused of being "genetic exceptionalists."[21]

Regardless of which view is correct, it clearly is a mistake to lump all genetic enhancements together for purposes of ethical or public policy analysis. Some, such as gene transfer, are novel. Others are applications of, by now, familiar technology such as recombinant DNA manufacturing, IVF, and abortion. These technologies differ in important moral and legal respects, and therefore, to begin to answer the question of what attitude sport should adopt toward them, we must consider each type of genetic enhancement separately.

As described above, there are several reasons that sport might take an actively hostile approach to genetic enhancements: to prevent physical and psychosocial harm, to promote equality, and to uphold the ethics of sport and the rules of the game. But there are also important reasons that the use of genetic enhancements might be tolerated. In the first place, as the experience with performance-enhancing drugs has shown, a ban may be difficult to enforce. It may be hard, for instance, to determine whether or not an athlete has employed a genetic enhancement. Detection may require sophisticated testing programs that are intrusive and expensive. Even then, athletes may stay one step ahead of the tests by switching to new chemical or biological variations. And even if users of genetic enhancements could be identified, it might be costly to punish them. Not only would imposing sanctions require the use of expensive scientific and legal resources, but it could exact a high price in terms of conflicting with accepted notions of privacy and autonomy. Finally, organizers of sport would have to justify why genetic enhancements should be banned while other inputs that affect performance are permitted or ignored. In short, as sport evaluates each type of genetic enhancement for the purposes of deciding what approach it should adopt, it must consider both the costs and benefits of its options.

## Genetic Testing to Identify Innate Athletic Ability

Sport might oppose genetic testing because it confers unfair advantages on those who test positive for athletic talent (leading to inequality) and stigmatize those who test negative (causing harm). The question is whether the costs of attempting to prevent this type of testing are worth paying. As a practical matter, it would be extremely difficult to prevent people from getting tested. Sport could pressure the government to make this type of testing illegal, but the government has only limited control over genetic testing practices.[22] Hospital laboratories, in particular, could provide this testing with little legal exposure. The government might tighten the rules governing genetic testing, but it is doubtful that it would do so because of enhancement testing in particular. Sport could prevail upon physicians, genetic counselors, and laboratories to refuse voluntarily to offer this type of testing. There is precedent for this in the position adopted by the American College of Medical Genetics and the American Society of Human Genetics against offering people genetic testing for the ApoE mutation associated with Alzheimer disease.[23] But if the advantages conferred by testing were perceived as substantial, a black market would emerge to provide access. Because all that people would have to do to be tested is to swab the inside of their cheek, mail the swab away, and wait to receive the results by phone, mail, or over the internet, the black market could operate domestically or overseas. No direct involvement of health professionals would be necessary, so it would be virtually impossible to stop.

Moreover, a powerful argument can be made that individuals should have the right to learn their genetic makeup. They should be fully informed of the potential risks of testing, such as mistakes, misinterpretations, and psychological distress, but once made aware of these considerations, they should be free to decide for themselves if the risks are outweighed by the benefits. Thus, the position of various medical groups against offering predictive genetic testing for breast cancer to certain patients has been criticized as overly paternalistic.[24] The courts even might recognize a constitutional right to be tested, particularly if, as discussed later, one purpose of the testing can be said to be to facilitate reproductive decision making.

Opponents of genetic testing might make a stronger case against testing minors, because minors are presumed to be unable to give their informed consent to the risks involved, such as psychological harm and reduced control over their destinies. The government might step in to protect child welfare. Medical organizations might declare it unethical to provide testing for minors. For example, they commonly oppose testing children for nonpreventable or late-onset genetic disorders such as Huntington disease.[25] But even then, it can be argued that parents ought to be allowed to decide what information they want to obtain concerning their children, especially when collecting the test sample itself is safe and noninvasive. It is hard to believe that the government would take the position that testing children for their innate athletic ability amounted to child abuse or neglect. Furthermore, minors often are permitted to make medical decisions for themselves. They are asked to give their "assent" to treatment or to enroll in clinical trials, and they are treated as adults under the law if they are deemed to be "mature" or "emancipated." Even genetics organizations that oppose genetic testing for minors except for treatable disorders make an exception if the minor is likely to be sexually active.[26]

Yet it would seem to be appropriate for sport to take the position that children should not be tested without the knowledge and voluntary consent of both the children and the parents. Schools and sports teams should not be allowed to require children to be tested for athletic ability as a condition of participation. Sport can support this position by an appeal to its desire to prevent the harm from unwanted testing, including the loss of decision-making autonomy.

## Performance-Enhancing Drugs Developed with Genetic Science and Technology

If the argument described earlier—that there is no reason to single out genetic enhancements *qua* genetic for disapproval—is valid, then there seems to be no reason for sport to adopt a different approach to performance-enhancing drugs made with genetic knowledge or technology than to drugs made with other knowledge bases or manufacturing techniques. In either case, sport has to decide whether the potential harms from drug use justify the costs of attempting to interdict it. Genetic enhancement drugs may be particularly difficult to detect if they are synthetic versions of substances that occur naturally in the body. This already has created problems for the Olympics in catching athletes who use substances such as synthetic EPO and HGH.[27] But it does not necessarily mean that sport should take a different approach to genetic products than to others.

### Pharmacogenetics

The development of genetic tests that would make the use of performance-enhancing drugs safer and/or more effective would create an ethical dilemma for sport. On the one hand, pharmacogenetic testing would decrease the risks to athletes, thereby weakening one of the primary objections to performance-enhancing drugs. On the other hand, athletes would feel freer to use performance-enhancing drugs and to resist efforts by sport to prevent their use. If sport prohibited pharmacogenetics, it could be accused of endangering athletes' health. If sport accepted pharmacogenetics, it would appear to be condoning the use of performance-enhancing drugs.

Resolving this dilemma may not be too difficult, however. Pharmacogenetic testing is a type of genetic testing. Therefore, the ethical and policy analysis is similar to that in the foregoing discussion of genetic testing for athletic prowess, which favored a generally permissive attitude because of the relative safety of the testing process and the value of providing information to individuals to promote their autonomy. Moreover, as a practical matter, it may be impossible to prevent people from obtaining pharmacogenetic testing. Not only would it be difficult to prevent black-market access—because, as in genetic testing generally, samples could be taken at home and mailed to laboratories without the need for professional intermediaries—but many performance-enhancing drugs, including anabolic steroids, EPO, and HGH, are approved for therapeutic use. In a likely future scenario for pharmacogenetic testing, individuals will be tested routinely for reactions to drugs when they first enter the health care system, perhaps even at birth, rather than undergoing targeted tests only when treatment is needed. Therefore, individuals are likely to learn, or have access to, pharmacogenetic information without the information being gathered specifically for sports enhancement purposes.

## Reproductive Enhancement

If genetic testing for athletic ability becomes a reality, it is hard to predict whether many people would base their reproductive decisions on a desire to produce athletic children. Athletic ability might seem to be a low priority compared with intellectual ability, good looks, or good health, all of which may be amenable in some degree to genetic testing and manipulation. But the rewards of a successful athletic career no doubt will prompt some people to make sport-oriented reproductive choices. More importantly, the same reproductive techniques that allowed parents to affect their offspring's health, appearance, and cognitive genetic capacities would enable them to influence the children's athletic abilities, perhaps even at the same time. All that would be necessary would be genetic tests that could identify genomes particularly well-suited to sport, as well as possessing other desired attributes. As described earlier, couples could get tested to determine whether or not to marry and beget children. They could employ IVF using either their own zygotes or donor eggs or sperm that matched their specifications, and then could select embryos for implantation after further testing. Individuals choosing not to avail themselves of IVF, perhaps because of the cost or attendant discomfort and health risks, could get pregnant the old-fashioned way and then decide whether to continue the pregnancy based on the results of tests of the embryo or fetus. Finally, parents could test their children and continue to reproduce until they gave birth to a child with the desired abilities. Alternatively, they could decide to adopt, with genetic testing for athletic prowess part of the screening method used to select the child.

As detailed earlier, the same objections that can be made against the use of performance-enhancing drugs apply to many types of enhancement through reproductive decision making. IVF can cause harm to both mothers and children.

If being conceived and not brought to term is a harm, as many would contend, then discarding undesirable embryos and aborting fetuses causes harm. Test results that reveal one's own genetic makeup, or that of potential mates or of one's children, could have adverse psychosocial effects. Some of these reproductive techniques would be inaccessible to many people because of their cost, so those individuals whose parents gained access to such techniques could obtain an unfair advantage over competitors. Finally, these reproductive actions may be repugnant to those who hold to the ethics of sport.

Yet, reproductive decision making differs in important respects from other types of genetic enhancement. Reproductive decisions are made by parents, not by the athletes themselves. Disqualifying athletes because of their parents' actions would punish the wrong parties, and for something over which they had no control. From the position of the enhanced athlete, reproductive enhancements might be said to resemble naturally acquired talents and good luck, which are rewarded even though they are undeserved. Furthermore, penalizing athletes on account of their genetic endowment, whether manipulated or not, could run afoul of laws prohibiting genetic discrimination or protecting the privacy of genetic information. Current antidiscrimination laws are aimed at employers and insurers, but in the future their targets might be expanded to include other types of private actor, including private sports organizations, by adding "genetic endowment" to classifications based on race and gender, which under the Civil Rights Acts are illegal bases for discrimination.

Reproductive decisions also enjoy special protection from government interference. This is true of decisions not only to avoid reproduction but also to engage in reproduction. In striking down a compulsory sterilization law in *Skinner v. Oklahoma*, for example, the U.S. Supreme Court in 1942 stated that reproduction "involves one of the basic civil rights of man. Marriage and procreation are fundamental to the very existence and survival of the race." More recently (1992), in *Planned Parenthood v. Casey*, the Court reiterated its recognition of "the right of the individual, married or single, to be free from unwarranted government intrusion into matters so fundamentally affecting a person as the decision whether or not to beget a child."[28] There is some question about whether, or to what degree, these protections extend to reproductive techniques such as IVF.[29] But absent a compelling reason for interfering with reproductive decisions, it is unlikely that the courts would uphold government intrusion.

Even if the laws were interpreted to permit the government, or private sports organizations acting on their own behalf, to penalize reproductive enhancements, it would be extremely difficult to prevent their use. In the first place, as noted earlier, the government would have great difficulty preventing people from testing themselves, their products of conception, or their children to measure athletic ability. Assuming people could get tested, there would be no way to prevent them from incorporating the test results into their reproductive decision making. Determining whether an athlete had been enhanced through parents' reproductive decisions would be even more problematic. There would be no way to tell whether their parents decided to conceive, implant, or bring them to term based on the results of genetic testing. As a consequence of all these factors, reproductive enhancement is likely to remain viable and legal.

## Somatic Gene Transfer

From an ethical standpoint, somatic gene transfer to enhance athletic ability raises the same objections as the use of performance-enhancing drugs. But it is likely to be even harder to detect. If the intervention left some sort of biological footprint, it would be possible to know that it had taken place. Modified DNA can be "tagged" so that it can be detected when present in an organism; this is how agricultural firms attempt to prevent the unlicensed use of genetically modified seeds.[30] Tests could be administered to athletes that would identify the presence of the modified DNA. But this would work only if athletes used ethically manufactured DNA products. The history of steroid use shows that they may turn to black-market products to thwart the tagging tests. Absent an effective tagging system, the only way to discover the presence of transferred genes would be to compare the athlete's genome with a genetic profile obtained before the transfer took place. But there may be strenuous objection to conducting these tests, which could reveal all sorts of personal information aside from whether or not the individual had employed somatic gene transfer. In this connection, it might be noted that the DNA testing conducted by law enforcement officials and recorded in the FBI's CODIS database supposedly is performed on portions of DNA that do not code for phenotype.[31]

Furthermore, the baseline testing might have to be performed at an early age to detect gene transfers that have long-lasting effects. If the technology advanced to the point that genes could be inserted at an early enough stage of development, testing might have to take place at birth or even before. As I have argued elsewhere, it might be necessary for society to mandate baseline genetic testing prenatally or at birth to deter parents from using gene-transfer technology to achieve socially unacceptable enhancement goals.[32] These schemes would raise major objections about the loss of genetic privacy and the risk of genetic discrimination, but unless something like this is done, interdicting the use of somatic gene transfer, as a practical matter, is likely to be impossible.

## Germ-Line Gene Transfer

Intentional germ-line gene transfer to enhance athletic ability is especially objectionable because it would be designed to transmit the enhancement effect to future generations. This could exacerbate the inequality problem by creating dynasties of genetically enhanced athletes against whom no unenhanced athlete could successfully compete. Moreover, serious, unforeseen health risks may emerge only in later generations. Unintentional germ-line enhancement—which could occur when, to obtain a significant degree of enhancement, DNA transfer was performed at such an early stage of development that the modified DNA became incorporated in the individual's reproductive cells—would raise the same issues, despite the lack of intent. However, it may seem even more unfair to penalize athletes for decisions made by even more remote ancestors than their parents. A ban on germ-line transfer would also encounter the same practical difficulties as a ban on somatic transfer. It is unlikely that a prohibition on germ-line transfer to enhance athletic ability could be successfully implemented, unless a database of baseline genetic pedigrees were created with which the genomes of subsequent generations could be compared. Given concerns over genetic privacy and discrimination, this would require a major change in policy, and possibly even an amendment to the U.S. Constitution.

## Summary

As these discussions show, any attempt by sport to prevent people from testing themselves or their children for innate athletic ability or basing reproductive decisions, in whole or in part, on the results of such testing would be inadvisable. It is also likely to be a mistake to try to block athletes' use of pharmacogenetic testing. These genetic interventions essentially are based on information, and it is impractical and arguably unethical to try to prevent informed individuals from voluntarily obtaining genetic information about themselves or their offspring. Yet, genetically engineered performance-enhancing drugs and somatic gene transfer to improve performance are sufficiently similar to performance-enhancing drugs generally that sport may well want to prohibit them, although detecting when they have been used may prove difficult. Finally, although germ-line gene transfer may be highly objectionable, sport may have difficulty in preventing it or in identifying athletes whose genomes have been altered in this fashion, and in justifying punishing athletes for the actions of their progenitors.

## Conclusion

Given the difficulties of successfully prohibiting reproductive and gene-transfer enhancements, the future of sport conducted according to the ethical principles of the international Olympic movement may appear dismal. Sports organizations may find themselves calling for radical, unpopular changes in norms of genetic privacy to mount increasingly expensive and intrusive testing programs that fail to stay ahead of advances in genetic technology. Alternatively, sport could abandon its ethical ideals. Or it could just pay lip service to them, adopting symbolic but unenforceable prohibitions.

There may be another option, however. That would be for sport to reject talent as an acceptable basis for differences in performance, regardless of how the talent was acquired. Athletes would be tested before competing and handicapped according to their native ability. This would not be performance testing, because that would conflate talent with effort, thereby handicapping athletes who worked hard at the same level as those with inherited or installed ability. Instead, some method would have to be found to measure pure ability—most likely a sophisticated combination of phenotypic and genetic markers.

If such a system could be devised, it would have several benefits besides responding to genetic enhancement. It would elevate determination and hard work above native talent and good fortune, making victories more earned and therefore more deserved. (This assumes that the handicapping system also would correct for an innate ability to work hard.) It also could eliminate discrimination against athletes with severe disabilities, who are not now able to compete in regular events. Crude versions of this approach in the form of weight and age classes already are incorporated into some sports.

Converting to such a system for all major sporting competitions would not be easy. Genetic testing for athletic ability would raise serious privacy concerns. It would be difficult to keep the results confidential. Sport would have to decide whether to allow any events to be conducted without testing. Suitable handicapping methods would have to be developed. The rules of sport would have to change, and the public might object to the loss of cherished traditions. But this may the price that sport has to pay to cope with genetic enhancement.

NOTES

1. N. Yang, D. G. MacArthur, J. P. Gulbin, A. G. Hahn, A. H. Beggs, S. Easteal, and K. North, "ACTN3 Genotype Is Associated with Human Elite Athletic Performance," *American Journal of Human Genetics* 73, no. 3 (2002): 627–31.

2. M. Rothstein and P. Epps, "Ethical and Legal Implication of Pharmacogenomics," *Nature Review Genetics* 2 (2001): 228.

3. S. Roan, "A Way to Choose a Baby's Gender," *Los Angeles Times*, March 3, 2003.

4. S. Stolberg, "The Biotech Death of Jesse Gelsinger," *New York Times Sunday Magazine*, November 28, 1999; American Society of Gene Therapy, "American Society of Gene Therapy Responds to a Second Case of Leukemia Seen in a Clinical Trial of Gene Therapy for Immune Deficiency," press release, January 14, 2003, www.asgt.org/news_releases/01132003.html.

5. E. Parens and E. Juengst, "Inadvertently Crossing the Germ Line," *Science* 292 (2001): 397.

6. E. Juengst, "The Meaning of Enhancement," in *Enhancing Human Traits: Ethical and Social Implications*, ed. E. Parens, 29–47 (Washington DC: Georgetown University Press, 1998).

7. American Psychiatric Association, "Healthy Minds, Healthy Lives: Gay, Lesbian, and Bisexual Issues," www.healthyminds.org/glbissues.cfm.

8. R. Sandomir, "Sydney 2000: Gymnastics; Despite Losing Appeal, Romanian Says Her Heart Is at Peace," *New York Times*, September 29, 2000.

9. C. Lamsam, F. Fu, P. Robbins, and C. Evans, "Gene Therapy in Sports Medicine," *Sports Medicine* 25, no. 2 (1998): 73–77.

10. International Olympic Committee Medical Commission, http://multimedia.olympic.org/pdf/en_report_6.pdf.

11. National Institute on Drug Abuse, "Research Report Series: Anabolic Steroid Abuse," http://165.112.78.61/ResearchReports/Steroids/anabolicsteroids3.html.

12. J. Lazarou, B. H. Pomeranz, and P. N. Corey, "Incidence of Adverse Drug Events in Hospitalized Patients: A Meta-analysis of Prospective Studies," *JAMA* 279 (1998):1200–1205.

13. J. Curry, "Four Indicted in a Steroid Scheme That Involved Pro Athletes," *New York Times*, February 13, 2004.

14. Stolberg, "Biotech Death of Jesse Gelsinger."

15. U.S. Food and Drug Administration, Statement of Policy for Regulating Biotechnology Products, 49 Fed. Reg. 50,878 (1984).

16. American Society for Reproductive Medicine, "Patient's Fact Sheet: Complications of Multiple Gestation," 2004, www.asrm.org/Patients/FactSheets/complications_multiple births.pdf.

17. R. Starkman, "Can Johnson Come Back?" *Toronto Star*, January 5, 1991.

18. K. Greif and J. Merz, *Current Controversies in the Biological Sciences: Case Studies of Policy Challenges from New Technologies* (Cambridge, MA: MIT Press, 2007), 87.

19. S. Wulf, "Distinguished History," *Sports Illustrated*, April 5, 1993.

20. J. Jerome, "Physics at the Bar: Pole Vaulting," *Science* 5 (1984): 84.

21. T. H. Murray, "Genetic Exceptionalism and Future Diaries: Is Genetic Information Different from Other Medical Information," in *Genetic Secrets: Protecting Privacy and Confidentiality in the Genetic Era*, ed. M. A. Rothstein (New Haven: Yale University Press, 1997), 60.

22. L. Andrews, M. Mehlman, and M. Rothstein, *Human Genetics: Ethics, Law, and Policy* (Minneapolis: West Group, 2003).

23. American College of Medical Genetics and American Society of Human Genetics, "Points to Consider: Ethical, Legal, and Psychosocial Implications of Genetic Testing in Children and Adolescents," *American Journal of Human Genetics* 57 (1995): 1233.

24. R. Kodish, G. Wiesner, M. Mehlman, and T. H. Murray, "Genetic Testing for Cancer Risk: How to Reconcile the Conflicts," *JAMA* 279, no. 3 (1998): 179–81.

25. American Medical Association, Council on Ethical and Judicial Affairs, Current Opinion 2.138 (1995).

26. American College of Medical Genetics and the American Society of Human Genetics, "Working Group on ApoE and Alzheimer Disease," *JAMA* 274, no. 20 (1995): 1627.

27. J. Longman, "Backtalk: Lifesaving Drug Can Be Deadly When Misused," *New York Times*, July 26, 1998.

28. *Skinner v. Oklahoma*, 316 U.S. 535, 541 (1942); *Planned Parenthood v. Casey*, 505 U.S. 833, 857 (1992).

29. J. Robertson, "Procreative Liberty in the Era of Genomics," *American Journal of Law and Medicine* 29, no. 4 (2003): 439–87; L. Andrews, "Is There a Right to Clone? Constitutional Challenges to Bans on Human Cloning," *Harvard Journal of Law and Technology* 643 (1998): 643–67.

30. M. Pollan, "Playing God in the Garden," *New York Times Sunday Magazine*, October 25, 1998, 44.

31. Andrews, Mehlman, and Rothstein, *Human Genetics*, 2003.

32. M. Mehlman, *Wondergenes: Genetic Enhancement and the Future of Society* (Bloomington: Indiana University Press, 2003); M. Mehlman, "The Law of above Averages: Leveling the New Genetic Enhancement Playing Field," *Iowa Law Review* 85 (2000): 517–93; M. Mehlman, "How Will We Regulate Genetic Enhancement?" *Wake Forest Law Review* 34 (1999): 671–714.

# CHAPTER ELEVEN

# In Search of an Ethics for Sport

## Genetic Hierarchies, Handicappers General, and Embodied Excellence

THOMAS H. MURRAY, PH.D.

While each of the chapters in this book contributes significantly to the ethics of sport, three in particular caused me to reconsider and refine my understanding of the meaning and value of sport. In chapter 8, Sigmund Loland defends a "fair opportunity principle" as applied to sport. In chapter 9, Eric Juengst follows the trail laid down by Loland's fair opportunity principle only to discover, he believes, that it leads to the creation of genetic hierarchies. We are troubled by other uses of genetic information to construct rankings of social desirability—as in health insurance, for example. Juengst worries that "in a world that is struggling to realize a commitment to treating people as moral equals despite their biological differences, a social practice that creates and glorifies hierarchies of genetic endowment seems anachronistic and slightly ominous." For Max Mehlman (in chapter 10), the power and ubiquity of genetic interventions, which he defines broadly, combined with the unavoidable difficulties that societies encounter in attempting to regulate their use, underscore a deep pessimism about the future of sport without genetic enhancement. His solution? "Reject talent as an acceptable basis for differences in performance, regardless of how the talent was acquired." Mehlman proposes that we test athletes' native abilities and handicap them accordingly. Then, he claims, victory would belong to the truly worthy.

## What Does "Fair Opportunity" Mean for Sport?

Sigmund Loland is an accomplished athlete who understands sport from the inside, as it were. He is also a thoughtful philosopher who wants to develop an account of fairness in sport. A brief recap of his account is helpful. He offers two principles. The first, *equality of opportunity to perform*, is a purely formal principle, like Aristotle's account of distributive justice. According to Aristotle, justice consists in treating like cases alike and different cases differently. So far, so good. But what makes cases relevantly alike or different? The principle is a formal structure, stripped of the details needed to give it life. It is useful, nonetheless, in pointing us toward the intellectual task we face and the test we must perform as we ponder justice and try to avoid injustice. Should the fact that one person has a genetic predisposition to breast cancer while another person lacks that risk count as a relevant difference in access to health insurance, so that it is fair to deny coverage to the first person but offer it to the second? Or is that a case of rank injustice? The principle tells us where to look for the answer, in relevant similarities and differences, but we need to fill in the blanks ourselves. The ever-present challenge lies in identifying, among all the things that make us similar or different, what counts as *relevant*.

So it is with Loland's "equal opportunity to perform" principle, as he acknowledges: "as a formal principle, this is of little help in resolving dilemmas arising from the various procedures for evaluating performance in practice. For instance, where are we to draw the line in outdoor sports for degree of climatic inequalities? What is a fair classification of competitors in golf? To what extent are inequalities in technology and equipment acceptable in sport? There is a need here for substantial criteria for what should count as relevant and nonrelevant equalities and inequalities."

There are a multitude of potential difference-making factors in sport. Loland notes that "challenges to fairness can come from rule violations and cheating and from inequalities in external conditions, in competitors' individual characteristics, and in the strength of their support systems." But, as with Aristotle's formal principle of distributive justice, the "equal opportunity to perform" principle requires us to make judgments about which factors should and should not be permitted to make a difference.

Loland's description of the fair opportunity principle (FOP) attempts to give some guidance about deciding what should count as relevant differences: "we should eliminate or compensate for essential inequalities between persons that cannot be controlled or influenced by individuals in any significant way and for which individuals cannot be deemed responsible." We are not in any morally meaningful way responsible for being tall or short, inheriting a body favorable or not to running fast, leaping high, or throwing heavy objects. Loland's statement of FOP leaves the door wide open to Mehlman's claim that differences in physical talents should not count. We don't earn or deserve our natural talents. The leap from a narrow interpretation of Loland's FOP to Mehlman's call for leveling the impact of natural talents is a short one.

Yet Loland reminds us that treating people as equals "by no means indicates equal or identical treatment in all settings. On the contrary, in most human practices, certain inequalities are considered relevant, acceptable, and even admirable, whereas others are considered nonrelevant and/or problematic and should be eliminated or compensated for." We come, then, to two crucial questions. First, should differences in natural talents be the sort of difference-making factors that ought to be permitted under FOP in sport? Second, how should we understand the meaning of those differences in natural talent? I turn now to Mehlman's answer to the first question.

## Max Mehlman and the Apotheosis of Pure Talent

Mehlman is pessimistic about the future of sport as understood in the Olympic movement. Genetic and reproductive interventions, he argues, will make enhancement impossible to prohibit. He proposes a different future for sport: "That would be for sport to reject talent as an acceptable basis for differences in performance, regardless of how the talent was acquired. Athletes would be tested before competing and handicapped according to their native ability. This would not be performance testing, because that would conflate talent with effort, thereby handicapping athletes who worked hard at the same level as those with inherited or installed ability. Instead, some method would have to be found to measure pure ability—most likely a sophisticated combination of phenotypic and genetic markers."

This is, to say the least, a bold proposal. I see three major problems with Mehlman's alternative future of sport. First, we would have to learn how to measure "pure ability." Second, we would have to clarify what factors should be permitted to count—Mehlman proposes "effort"—and we'd have to make certain that they were uninfluenced by "inherited or installed" factors for which the athlete could not justly claim credit. Third, we would have to devise elaborate handicapping schemes to neutralize natural talents, and we'd have to do this in such a manner that whatever we valued about sport was not demolished along the way.

I don't have much to say about the first problem, measuring "pure ability." It is not difficult to imagine endless squabbles over what counts as a "pure" talent or to see a new kind of cheating bursting forth, a species of "reverse doping." Here, athletes will try to disguise or diminish their natural talents, the way Little Leaguers sometimes present phony birth certificates so that they can compete against younger, less mature players. Measuring pure talent will be technically daunting, open to endless conceptual and ethical quarrels, and susceptible to its own forms of cheating.

What should be allowed to make a difference? Mehlman suggests effort. We could add, I suppose, perseverance, the willingness to suffer through arduous training, the patience to acquire technique, and attentiveness to coaching. These are all examples of what I've called "virtuous perfection" (see chapter 7)[1]—doing what needs to be done to hone one's natural talents toward the goal of excellent performance. But if we take Mehlman at his word, that "inherited or installed ability" should be thoroughly neutralized, we run into a problem. Without lapsing into simplistic ideas about the genetic determination of complex traits, we must nevertheless acknowledge that some aspects of effort and other morally praiseworthy factors may also reflect underlying individual differences for which persons deserve neither moral credit nor blame.

Effort, for example, includes persevering through pain, as anyone can attest who has repeated an exercise until muscles ached, or run, swam, skied, or cycled long distances until their lungs were ready to burst. What would Mehlman have us do if evidence accumulates that people differ biologically in their sensitivity to pain, such that it's just easier and less painful for some people than others to push themselves harder? The capacity for effort, itself, may be affected by morally unearned differences. The line between natural talents and our capacities to strive for their virtuous perfection is less clear than Mehlman assumes.

But suppose, for a moment, that we could successfully measure pure ability and that we could parcel out that part of effort for which people did not deserve moral credit: what would a sport that neutralized these factors look like? We might be treated to some ugly contests. High-jumpers with strong legs and high proportions of fast-twitch muscle fibers might have weights strapped around their ankles and waists. Strong shot-putters would be given heavier balls to throw. Lithe marathoners might have to wear wide vests to increase wind resistance. And what on earth do we do with tall people in basketball? Coaches are fond of saying that you can't coach height; so how do you handicap for it? Perhaps we could install special spikes in the shoes of tall players that lacerated their feet when they touched down after jumping. If we can't make them shorter, at least we can discourage them from leaping.

Handicapped contests like these seem to miss something crucial about sport. Fairness requires diminishing the impact of those factors we believe should not affect the outcome. We still need to decide what factors should count. Step outside the arena of sport for a moment. What other important spheres of human practice insist that earned virtue alone should prevail? Do we insist that employers should ignore talent and ability, hiring and promoting people based solely on how many hours they are willing to work? The abuses in awarding ecclesiastical office include simony, paying for a position; but can anyone seriously argue that competence and intelligence shouldn't be criteria, only pure virtue? The very law schools, medical schools, and other university programs that the contributors to this volume inhabit are forced to choose among applicants for admission. In making that choice, virtuous character figures in, but so do natural talents such as mental agility. Why should sport be expected to zero out the effect of unearned talent when other social practices accept it as legitimate? Singling out sport for criticism on the grounds that people with physical talents are favored—and that not taking differences in talent into account is somehow unfair—alerts us to an underlying uneasiness with the reality that we have bodies and that those bodies are different from one another in their capacities for various sports. This uneasiness leads to suggestions such as Mehlman's that those differences should be effaced and to accusations such as Juengst's that sport contributes to identifying and reinforcing morally suspect genetic hierarchies.

## Eric Juengst and the Quest for Suspect Genetic Hierarchies

Juengst takes the notion that sport is about determining hierarchies from Loland, who writes: "The characteristic, structural goal of sports competitions is to measure, compare, and rank competitors according to performance of relevant skills within the framework of the rules." Those rankings lead directly to hierarchies, just as Juengst infers. But Juengst's account moves too quickly from the notion of hierarchies in sport to the conclusion that these particular hierarchies are genetic, and to what such hierarchies signify. Neither does Juengst consider the relationship of *competitive* sport—the subject of Loland's FOP—to the great mass of sporting activity, most of which is not structured as formal competitions. Looking at that relationship yields insights into the meaning of sport.

In response to the World Anti-Doping Agency's brief description of the "spirit of sport," Juengst concludes that the spirit of sport must be "the celebration of the differences in the human talents and virtues that allow athletes to honorably and beautifully accomplish achievements that place them higher in a hierarchy of human excellence than their competition." The problem with gene doping, Juengst then concludes, is that tinkering with one's genetically based talents "threatens sport's commitment to the creation and promotion of human genetic stratification." He worries about the broader social implications of such a focus on genetic hierarchies: "As a human project, what differentiates the hierarchical ranking of genetic talents by sports institutions from the reciprocal devaluing of genetic defects by insurance risk underwriters? In both cases, the internal logic of the practice is clear, but their use of inherited genetic identity as a social ranking criterion raises large questions about the fairness of the enterprise as a whole."

Look more closely at two elements of Juengst's argument: that sport is about establishing a hierarchy, and that the hierarchy is best described as "genetic." I will take the latter claim first. Are whatever hierarchies sport creates genetic? It would be foolish to deny that genetics can affect an individual's prospects for success in a particular sport. Leaving aside genetically caused disease and physical disability, there is an undeniable raw physical component to excellence in sport. Some portion of this raw physical component is genetic, but it is also shaped by other factors: epigenetic programming, the prenatal environment, nutrition, and the good fortune to escape injuries and diseases that would hamper the ripening of those physical capacities. Still, it seems more accurate to speak of "physical" capacities or talents rather than narrowly "genetic" ones. I explain later why this is a distinction that makes a difference.

The "genetic hierarchy" conception of sport also faces difficulties in grappling with whatever it is that transforms raw physical talent into excellent performance. Athletes need to hone their talents through dedication, hard work, sacrifice, practice—the set of character traits and activities I earlier called "virtuous perfection." It is important not to fall into the error of genetic reductionism: there is no gene for dedication—at least, no one is claiming they've found such a gene. But neither is it a crazy idea to assume that some genetic bases may be found that correlate, at least a little, with those character traits and activities. To cite an earlier example, people experience pain differently, and it seems reasonable to believe that some of that difference might be accounted for by the physiological systems that send and receive pain signals. Of two otherwise identical would-be athletes, one may be able to train much harder than the other before the pain becomes unbearable. So dedication and sacrifice may have a subtle but undeniable genetic component. If there is some sort of genetic hierarchy that sport aims to identify, it's a complex one shaped, not just by our genes, but by the many things that affect our physical development; and it reaches at least a little into the nonphysical realm, into those aspects of persons that we usually deem to be worthy of moral praise. (This poses a problem for Mehlman's proposal, as discussed above.)

Whatever hierarchies competitive sport creates, genetics is likely to play some role, but a highly mediated one. The impact of genes is filtered through and diluted by all of the forces that affect the wondrously complex ecosystem that is our genome, and then again by the interactions of our modified and expressed genomes with the world external to the body. Those raw physical capacities are then further perfected (or neglected) according to one's character, opportunities, horizons, parental encouragement or discouragement, coaching—in short, the myriad factors that shape our raw capacities into living actualities.

If sport were truly all about selecting for genetic hierarchies, we could do much better than resort to the complicated, prolonged systems we use in sport. We could dispense with teams, coaches, leagues, rulebooks, officials, and all those distractions. What more direct expression of a genetic hierarchy exists in sport than basketball and height? All other things being equal, being taller is a clear advantage. Why not just hold a contest for the tallest person? It's so much cleaner and simpler than making someone bounce a ball, throw it through a hoop, and cooperate with teammates. Of course, if you know anything about basketball you will recognize immediately what a dumb idea this is. Sure, height is advantageous in basketball, and height is largely heritable (although also much influenced by nutrition, health, and other factors); but good basketball is about so much more than merely being tall. It rewards speed, grace, leaping ability, coordination, clever team play, and the capacity to block out everything except the rim when releasing a jump shot. Genes probably play some role in shaping this mix of talents in each person, and genes account for some share of the differences among persons. But describing this as mostly a "genetic hierarchy" seems a gross oversimplification.

The notion of a genetic hierarchy also evokes inauspicious associations. Hereditary monarchies, inherited peerages, and the like—at least those that carry political power—are, fortunately, out of fashion. It may take a run of doltish, narcissistic, lazy, and stupid monarchs before people disenchant themselves of the notion that hereditary rule is a good way to run a country. But most people now recognize the folly of assuming either that their rulers are inherently superior people or that whatever makes wise, strong, and just leaders is passed down through their genes. And the obscene myth that entire groups of people are genetically superior to other groups, most monstrously given expression in the Nazi racial hygiene ideology, further consigns the belief in genetic hierarchy to the darkened territory of suspicious and dangerous ideas.

Whatever hierarchies sport establishes are worlds apart from heredity monarchies or racist ideologies. Sport is relentlessly meritocratic, for one thing. You don't get to be a champion athlete just because your parent once was. And you can be knocked off your perch at any time by a challenger who is hungrier, more dedicated, or more talented than you. Belonging to a particular group doesn't take you very far either. You succeed or fail based on your talents and what you do with them. In any event, why should we believe that sport, at its heart, is primarily about establishing hierarchies?

As Juengst acknowledges, there are many different kinds of hierarchies in competitive sport. Different sports call on a vast range of different abilities. In any team sport, on any given team, a diverse array of talents are usually represented. A basketball team composed exclusively of massive seven-footers would not be able to compete with a more balanced opponent. Who would bring the ball up? Who would distribute it? Who would shoot accurately beyond the three-point line? Who would execute swift drives to the basket? Nor is success in one sport any guarantee of success in another. A lean marathoner has the wrong body to be a successful weightlifter; and woe betide the muscular weightlifter who tries to keep up with the lithe marathoner over 26-plus miles. The story is the same across sports. Remember that Michael Jordan, the dominant basketball player of his era, tried and failed at baseball.

The hierarchies that competitive sport establishes are, in any case, radically unstable. You are at the pinnacle of your particular sport hierarchy only until the next race, game, match, or season. Rare is the champion athlete or team that repeats its wins year after year. Edwin Moses may be the most notable exception. From 1977 until 1987, he won 107 consecutive finals in the 400-meter hurdles, winning 122 races in all, including two Olympic gold medals, while breaking the world record several times along the way. (Moses is also an exception to the rule against excelling in more than one sport. In 1990, after retiring from track, he won a medal for the two-man bobsled at a world cup event; it was a bronze medal, but impressive nevertheless.)

Is the meaning of sport better understood as setting up hierarchies or as finding out how well an individual can perform? Competitive sports do create hierarchies in the form of league tables, rankings, and statistical comparisons. And much of the interest in sport is in how well your team—the one you root or play for—is doing. But is climbing to the top of the hierarchy the primary reason people play or watch sports? It may be for some. But I don't believe this explains the baseball player who toils away for years in the minor leagues, or the college basketball player at a so-called mid-major school who is thrilled merely to qualify for the National Collegiate Athletic Association tournament. These athletes can derive deep satisfaction from drawing out every last bit of natural talent they have, even though they have no hope of competing successfully against the very best.

What explains the motivation of Division III college athletes who receive no athletic scholarships and who will never have the opportunity to climb anywhere near the top of their sport's hierarchy? What about the intramural sports participants, not talented enough to make the school's team but eager to test themselves against others of roughly similar talent? Or the ballplayers that gather in parks, schoolyards, or playgrounds? Finally, what about the largest category of all, noncompeting athletes?

For every athlete with a realistic hope of reaching the top of the hierarchy, there are thousands, perhaps millions of people participating in the same sport, the vast majority of whom have no illusions of attaining the pinnacle. There are multitudes pushing themselves to run, cycle, swim, or do other sports who do not participate in formal or even informal competitions. Why do they do it? For many reasons, certainly, including health and fitness, the pleasure of companionship, perhaps to enjoy fresh air and scenery. But it would be a mistake to think that just because there is no explicit competition, there are no challenges being confronted.

Here is where a distinction may be helpful: between sports *participation* and sports *competition*. Loland's claim that the "characteristic, structural goal of sports competitions is to measure, compare, and rank competitors" is plausible on its face. Yet, again, the overwhelming majority of sports participation is not in competition per se; it does not directly pit one person or team against another: think of the bike rides for charity that can pose significant physical challenges to riders but don't award prizes—except for who raises the most money for the charity. Or whatever competition exists may be friendly and informal—the pickup basketball game, a neighborhood softball or soccer game. Such contests can be intense; but, typically, little hangs on the outcome beyond a sense that one played well or poorly.

## What's Fair?

Loland wants to link his articulation of a fair opportunity principle to John Rawls's concept of justice as fairness. To reiterate FOP: "we should eliminate or compensate for essential inequalities between persons that cannot be controlled or influenced by individuals in any significant way and for which individuals cannot be deemed responsible." The problem with invoking Rawls in support of

FOP is that what Rawls calls the *principle of redress*, which Loland's statement articulates, is not in fact Rawls's position, although more than a few philosophers have tried to attribute such a view to him.

In effect, the proposed linkage confuses three questions. First, what role should differences in social position or natural talents play in evaluating the basic structures of society? Second, how should those social positions or talents affect the distribution of social resources? And third, what views of human nature and the natural talents that underlie sport are permissible once the basic structure has been established?

With respect to the first question, neither social position nor natural talent should be permitted to influence the deliberations that take place behind Rawls's famous "veil of ignorance." The veil serves to blind us to our individual advantages and disadvantages as we devise the principles and institutions that underlie the basic structure of our political community. If the veil were lifted, the wealthy, well-born, and talented might try to tilt the basic structure of society to their advantage. If no one knew what their actual situation would be outside the veil— rich or poor, connected or isolated, marvelously athletic or total klutz—then, Rawls argues, all would agree on a basic structure that includes equal rights and liberties for all, along with a concern that the least advantaged receive a decent share of social resources. It may be true that, on the internet, no one knows you're a dog; it's also the case that behind the veil of ignorance, no one knows whether they are a prince or a pauper. So, Rawls reasons, behind that veil people would choose a set of principles, basic political institutions and a constitution, and social, economic, and judicial institutions with certain characteristics. The second of the two principles that Rawls argues would be chosen behind the veil of ignorance is the famous "difference principle": "Social and economic inequalities are to be arranged so that they are both (a) to the greatest expected benefit of the least advantaged and (b) attached to offices and positions open to all under conditions of fair equality of opportunity."[2] But, as Rawls explains, the difference principle is not the principle of redress. He makes this clear in his analysis of how differences in social position or talent may be permitted to influence the distribution of resources once the basic structure is set.

Rawls describes the principle of redress this way: the principle "that undeserved inequalities call for redress; and because inequalities of birth and natural endowment are undeserved, these inequalities are to be somehow compensated for." It should now be clear that the principle of redress is what Loland draws on for his fair opportunity principle. The difference principle, in contrast, "does not require society to try to even out handicaps as if all were expected to compete on a fair basis in the same race." Instead, Rawls explains, it "represents, in effect, an agreement to regard the distribution of natural talents as a common asset and to share in the greater social and economic benefits made possible by the complementarities of this distribution. Those who have been favored by nature, whoever they are, may gain from their good fortune only on terms that improve the situation of those who have lost out . . . No one deserves his greater natural capacity nor merits a more favorable starting place in society. But, of course, this is no reason to ignore, much less to eliminate these distinctions. Instead, the basic structure can be arranged so that these contingencies work for the good of the least fortunate."[3] A society that refuses to recognize that individuals vary greatly in talents and that fails to provide opportunities for those talents to be developed and to contribute to the flourishing of individuals and to the overall stock of public good is, for that reason, not a more just society. It is almost certainly a poorer one, in both material goods and spirit.

Rawls's view of how we should regard individual differences in talents is subtle and sensible. We do not deserve our natural talents in the sense of moral desert, any more than we deserve whatever advantages we may gain through being born in favorable circumstances—say, to wealthy and sophisticated parents. But these are two starkly different sorts of undeserved advantages. Social positions that stem from wealth, class, or aristocracy provide advantages to the individual with no compensating benefit to the disadvantaged. In contrast, differences in natural talents—special abilities, dispositions to work hard or long, and the like—can serve to improve the lot even of the disadvantaged. Rawls does not want to level differences in talents, not at all. But neither does he confuse talent with moral desert. Differences in talent, unlike differences in social position, may lead to different allotments of social resources against a background of fair basic institutions and through pure procedural justice.

Finally, what views of human nature and the natural talents that underlie sport are permissible once the basic structure has been established? In his later work, *Political Liberalism*, Rawls further develops his account of the relationship of justice to human flourishing. People are more than merely political creatures. From his conception of the person as citizen, Rawls derives an account of the two moral powers such persons must have. Consider Rawls's description of the second of those powers: "The capacity for a conception of the good is the capacity to form, to revise, and rationally to pursue a conception of one's rational advantage or good." In addition to these moral powers:

Persons also have at any given time a determinate conception of the good that they try to achieve. Such a conception must not be understood narrowly but rather as including a conception of what is valuable in human life. Thus, a conception of the good normally consists of a more or less determinate scheme of final ends, that is, ends we want to realize for their own sake, as well as attachments to other persons and loyalties to various groups and associations. These attachments and loyalties give rise to devotions and affections, and so the flourishing of the persons and associations who are the objects of these sentiments is also part of our conception of the good. We also connect with such a conception a view of our relation to the world—religious, philosophical, and moral—by reference to which the value and significance of our ends and attachments are understood.[4]

In our determinate conception of the good, in our quest for flourishing, in our view of our relation to the world, we are entitled to a conception of sport in our lives and our communities in which we pursue flourishing, in part, by embracing our physical embodiment and perfecting our talents. Other physical talents can be equally central to a person's flourishing—the ability to sing or play a musical instrument, to dance, to draw, paint, or sculpt. These are different practices from sport, with different institutional contexts and different intrinsic values. But they share with sport a vast distribution of individual talents. We would be a poorer world if we insisted on handicapping great sopranos or painters because it was somehow "unfair" that they possess a rare and special talent. It would also be odd for us to describe what art critics and lovers of great art or music do as an attempt to establish a genetic hierarchy. The fundamental point is that sport may become a component of a person's determinate conception of the good, of his or her flourishing. Sport, like art, like music, can be one way of accomplishing something that Rawls argues we must do: to connect our view of our relation with the world with "the value and significance of our ends and attachments."[5]

## Conclusion

Perhaps there is a deeper account of sport to be given than one that relies on hierarchies, genetic or otherwise. Why do amateur athletes give the hours, sweat, and suffering that they do to their sports? In the first instance, performance in sport is both a celebration of and a challenge posed by our embodiment. The challenge is ever present. Have I prepared myself to give my best? Do I have the courage and the will to perform up to the limits of my capacities? This element of the experience of sport—the drive to explore the limits of my physical talents, to test my determination and self-discipline—doesn't diminish in importance merely because I am not competing against others. If anything, it enlivens my appreciation for what elite athletes, those at the top of the sport hierarchy, can do. When I struggle up the four-mile hill into Fahnestock Park before the descent to Canopus Lake, my respect for the cyclists in the Tour de France who ascend the long and steep climb to the top of l'Alpe d'Huez deepens (though my admiration is tempered by reports of rampant doping in that event). Even amateur athletes can experience moments of grace. The weekend duffer hitting a perfect drive down the middle of the fairway or making a long, sinuous putt gets a brief glimpse of what it must be like to be a pro at the top of his or her game. With every stroke of the club or pedal, the noncompeting athlete can concentrate on improving technique and focus. So our golfer will never play in the Masters, so what? So I will never compete in any cycling event, who cares? Golfers work at improving their game; I work at increasing my speed and endurance.

These amateur athletes are not competing against anyone else, and they are not exactly, or exclusively, competing with themselves. I think it may be more true to the experience of amateur athletes to say that they are embracing their embodiment and, at the same time, pushing and testing themselves to see what, as an inextricable mix of body and mind, they are capable of. We all have bodies. Sports provide an opportunity to live fully in those bodies, to test their capabilities and limits, and to integrate them with our will, intellect, and character.

Describing sport as all about creating genetic hierarchies may be getting it backward. Yes, people come into this world embodying complex combinations of physical attributes. And the variations among persons are immense. Genes play a role in deciding what sorts of physical talent, and in what measure, you will have. Those raw talents are at best aptitudes for success in particular sports, never a guarantee. Those capacities must be honed, polished, practiced, and performed before they translate into excellence in any sport. Sports competitions at all levels, from the spontaneous pickup basketball game to Little League to the Super Bowl, spur participants to do their best at the same time that they provide examples of excellence in athletic performance. The rankings, hierarchies, and such grow out of the engagement of body and mind in the quest for excellence—including *your* level of excellence—that sport represents. They are followed avidly, but they are a consequence, not the underlying meaning, of sport. That meaning is to be found in our engagement with our finite but often surprisingly capable bodies, in our perseverance, our courage, and, when we hit the perfect drive, take the ideal line on our skis, release a beautiful jump shot, or reach the crest of the hill after that miserable, lung-aching climb, exhilaration.

NOTES

1. T. Murray, "Enhancement," in *The Oxford Handbook of Bioethics,* ed. B. Steinbock (Oxford: Oxford University Press, 2008).

2. J. Rawls, *A Theory of Justice,* rev. ed. (Cambridge, MA: Harvard University Press, 1999 [1971]), 72.

3. Ibid., 86–87.

4. J. Rawls, *Political Liberalism,* expanded ed. (New York: Columbia University Press, 2005 [1993]), 19–20.

5. Ibid.

# PART III

# CURRENT AND FUTURE SCIENCE

# CHAPTER TWELVE

# Genetic Doping in Sport

## Applying the Concepts and Tools of Gene Therapy

THEODORE FRIEDMANN, M.D., AND
ERIC P. HOFFMAN, PH.D.

The use of drugs in sport to enhance athletic performance is widespread. Some athletes, trainers, and handlers, even some sports organizations and federations, either condone the practice or take ineffective steps to control it. Parts of the sports community, however—some athletes, trainers, and sports organizations, including the International Olympic Committee, the World Anti-Doping Agency, the U.S. Anti-Doping Agency, and others—have mounted serious efforts, through random or scheduled testing programs, to counteract the practice. But the pressures of athletic performance and the risk-taking nature of athletics, combined with the enormous political and financial influences in sport, have helped to perpetuate the problem and led to ever more sophisticated approaches to performance enhancement that are alluring to some in the sports community who are intent on illicit use. Moreover, as a society, we applaud, reward, and even demand ever more stunning feats in sport—*citius, altius, fortius*—and thereby, at least indirectly, encourage the use of any means, licit or illicit, toward the ultimate goal of athletic victory at all costs.

Potential application of the powerful emerging technologies of gene transfer and gene therapy to inserting performance-enhancing genes into athletes has raised the specter of the genetically engineered athlete and indicates the need for increasingly sophisticated methods of screening and monitoring—to counter a perception that gene-based doping will be even more difficult to detect than drug-based doping. In this chapter we discuss the current status of gene-transfer technology, with an emphasis on the introduction of genetic material into humans and animal models, current experience in human gene therapy clinical trials, and general methods for detecting and monitoring such genetic changes.

We conclude that gene-transfer technology, even in applications to life-threatening disease, is still immature and potentially hazardous. And the physiological complexities and still unrecognized immune and other responses of the human body to genetic modification make the use of such methods in healthy young athletes not only of unproven efficacy but also, potentially, of far greater risk than benefit. We further conclude that the use of current gene-transfer technology in humans by licensed professionals, using procedures that circumvent established local and federal regulatory and review processes, constitutes professional misconduct or malpractice.

## Introduction to Gene-Transfer Technology

One emerging potential approach to performance enhancement in sport is a direct outgrowth of the gene-transfer technology underlying the field of gene therapy—the use of genes to treat dire human diseases. That technology is built on the knowledge that most human disease is associated with abnormal gene functions, abnormalities either inherited or acquired, and that such genetic aberrations might be corrected by restoring normal genetic functions or by interfering with disease-causing genetic mechanisms. The scientific discipline of "gene therapy" has emerged and evolved over the past 30 years, and while straightforward in concept, application to human patients has proved extremely difficult. Indeed, gene therapy has been epitomized as a scientific discipline full of unanticipated risks and adverse events—some even lethal.[1] Stringent review and regulatory structures have been put in place to oversee human studies in this area, including federally mandated local institutional committees (institutional review boards, institutional biosafety committees, etc.) and federal oversight bodies such as the Recombinant DNA Advisory Committee at the National Institutes of Health (NIH) and the Food and Drug Administration (FDA). Similar structures have also been developed in most other countries where gene-therapy studies are being carried out. To underscore further the difficulty and dangers inherent in this area of clinical research, after more than three decades of basic research studies and 15 years of rigorous and controlled clinical application to thousands of human subjects in more than 600 studies worldwide, and at least one study-related death, only in the past several years has the first rigorous evidence emerged for effective therapy of a human disease by gene-transfer methods. The lesson to be drawn from this relatively extensive human clinical trial experience is that gene-transfer technology in human beings is immature and filled with many potential and recognized dangers. These facts suggest that gene transfer is justifiable only for serious and usually life-threatening disease, and certainly is not ready for nondisease, enhancement purposes.

Interestingly, the same techniques being developed for the treatment of human disease are being, and will be, applied to modify many other nondisease human traits, and early among these are likely to be traits that affect athletic performance—genetic doping. Success in sport is a combined result of extensive physical training and psychological preparation, on top of talent and genetic predispositions. Most current attention to genetic doping in sport involves manipulations designed to enhance the structure or physiology of muscle, improve repair mechanisms after injury, enhance circulation and oxygen delivery to and waste removal from exercising muscle, and alter the muscle's use of energy. At its present immature and risk-laden stage of development, any application of human clinical gene-transfer technology, whether for therapy of disease or, eventually, for enhancement, must certainly be considered experimental clinical research. As such, it must conform to worldwide ethical norms and to all local and federal standards of oversight implemented to ensure ethical conduct and maximal protection for human research participants. Below, we examine the current technologies used for gene transfer and the potential applications to sport. In this context we emphasize gene delivery to skeletal muscle, because it is the most well-developed of the direct, in vivo, gene-transfer approaches that are potentially applicable to sport, but arguments related to other target tissues and organs are likely to be similar.

Two general technical approaches have been developed to introduce foreign genetic material into human tissues and into human patients: (1) physical methods to drive purified genes (DNA) into cells (e.g., electricity or simple, direct, and at times forceful injection), typically called *nonviral gene transfer*; (2) biological systems such as modified and nonpathogenic viruses to deliver foreign therapeutic genes instead of their own, potentially disease-causing genes, systems often referred to by the type of carrier (vector)—*viral gene-transfer vectors*. Both of these approaches have been studied extensively in a range of target cells and tissues in laboratory in vitro systems and, of course, in preclinical studies with animal models before being applied to human clinical studies. Because of its importance to many human diseases and its potential use for producing systemically useful gene products, skeletal muscle is a well-studied target organ in many of these preliminary studies and remains one of the most important potential target organs in approaches to doping in sport.

## Nonviral Gene Transfer

The simplest approach for genetic modification of muscle function is the injection of a preparation of a gene as a purified plasmid directly into the target tissue, such as skeletal muscle (intramuscular injection, IM). The first publication reporting that purified DNA could be successfully delivered to mouse skeletal muscle was by Wolff and colleagues, who demonstrated delivery of a "marker" bacterial gene (the enzyme beta-galactosidase) into muscle, followed by detection of gene expression by color change in the cells after their exposure to a substrate for the enzyme.[2] This method quickly expanded in three directions: IM injection of DNA for treating muscle disease (e.g., muscular dystrophy), IM injection of DNA for immunization, and IM injection of DNA for enhancement of muscle function.[3] Gene-transfer studies in rodents and nonhuman primates with a muscle disorder similar to human muscular dystrophy have shown varying efficiencies of expression of the wild-type copy of the defective dystrophin gene. Human clinical trials have been undertaken in patients with muscular dystrophy, using IM injection of the dystrophin (Duchenne muscular dystrophy) gene.[4] These human trials have shown only limited success in delivery and expression of the therapeutic gene to some muscle fibers. Several methods have also been developed to increase the uptake of foreign genes into cells through the use of physical forces such as electrical stimulation (electroporation) or chemicals such as lipids and lipid vesicles. These methods are sufficiently effective in some tissue culture systems in the laboratory to allow basic studies of gene transfer and to permit detectable but low-level gene delivery by direct injection to some tissues in vivo, such as the skin, the liver, and even the brain. Unfortunately, the expression of foreign genes achieved by these methods is almost always transient or unstable and thus inadequate for situations in which prolonged expression of a newly introduced gene is required. These methods are therefore not ideal or even suitable in their present form for studies that require stable genetic alteration in a large number of cells in a target tissue in vivo.

In some different settings, gene transfer by such nonviral methods has been somewhat more promising. DNA injection has been more consistently successful for immunization studies in which the product of the injected gene acts as an immunogen to induce a protective response—for instance, to infectious agents. Success in this application has come more readily because the induction of an effective immune response requires shorter duration and lower levels of gene expression than those required to replace a disease-related genetic function, such as dystrophin deficiency in muscular dystrophy. This IM DNA immunization is in widespread use, both as a research tool and in many clinical infectious disease and cancer studies. The efficiency of this kind of immune response to the product of injected genes illustrates one of the inherent technical difficulties of gene transfer into tissues, because the technique seems to be better suited to making antibodies against the delivered protein than to supplying protein to correct or enhance muscle function. Indeed, as recently recognized, if the product of the therapeutic gene is not made in its normal tissue of origin, in correct amounts, and at correct times in the development of the organism, biochemical and immunological mechanisms can cause the product of even sequence-correct endogenous genes to be recognized as "foreign" and therefore lead to immune destruction of the genetically corrected cells and even life-threatening autoimmune disease.[5]

## Viral Gene-Transfer Vectors

There are agents in nature that carry out stable and highly efficient gene transfer into mammalian cells and into living animals. Viruses have evolved to perform exactly this task, and the tools of molecular biology and recombinant DNA technology have been used to convert pathogenic viruses into therapeutic tools by removing their genetic material and replacing it with potentially therapeutic genes for efficient and potentially safe gene delivery—swords into plowshares. The first of these engineered viral vectors for gene transfer were the derivatives of the retrovirus Moloney murine leukemia virus, early in the 1980s; since then, many other viruses have been adapted to function as gene-transfer vectors.[6] These disarmed viruses provide an enormous increase in efficiency and ease in carrying out gene-transfer studies, and some, such as the retroviruses, provide a mechanism for potentially prolonged expression through integration into the host cell's genome. The availability of multiple gene-transfer vectors, both viral and nonviral, allowed many proof-of-principle studies to be carried out that give experimental support to the concepts of gene therapy and led to the initiation of human clinical trials in 1989–90.[7]

None of the viral vector systems is ideal, and all have disadvantages, weaknesses, and even hazards. The most commonly used viral vector systems, using retroviruses, are no exception. Their strengths include ease of manipulation and their ability to provide long-term gene expression by integrating themselves into the genetic material of the host cell, thereby becoming a permanent part of its genome. Integration is not a cost-free event, however, and in an occasional cell the integrated virus will activate or otherwise interfere with the function of endogenous normal genes, thereby bringing about incorrect gene regulation in those functions and possible new genetic defects, such as cancer. Indeed, there are recent reports of patients that were given therapeutic retroviruses to cure blood disorders but later developed blood cancer due to the retrovirus insertions.[8] Retroviruses and their vectors generally do not infect nondividing cells, such as the mature myofibers of muscle, and this limits their potential use for therapeutic goals in muscle and also in athletic doping settings. However, retroviral vectors derived from the class of viruses known as lentiviruses, the class that includes HIV (human immunodeficiency virus), are able to infect nonreplicating cells and are potentially applicable to gene therapy of muscle disease, as well as use in athletic enhancement.

Because of the inadequacies and deficiencies of the retroviral vectors, engineered forms of other viruses, such as adenoviruses, adeno-associated viruses, and herpesviruses, have found important uses. Adenoviruses, often incorrectly referred to as the cause of the common cold, readily infect humans and often cause moderate to severe respiratory disease. Modified adenoviruses are non-integrating vectors and induce a brisk but usually short-lived expression of a foreign gene. They have shown promise in gene delivery to a variety of target tissues including, to a limited extent, skeletal muscle.[9] Adenoviral vectors have a relatively large capacity for foreign genes and thus can transfer large genes, such as the dystrophin gene. However, adenoviruses and their derived vectors are efficient at provoking a host immune response that can be aimed both at the foreign gene being transferred by the vector and at the vector itself. In some settings, this response is a useful property, as in approaches to immunotherapy for cancer. In other settings, the immune response is a major disadvantage because it can lead to destruction of the genetically corrected cells and even produce an explosive generalized immune response that can be lethal.[10]

The adeno-associated virus (AAV) vector system has emerged recently as a popular and important system for gene delivery to many target organs, including muscle.[11] AAV vectors are generally considered to be nonpathogenic and are not known to be associated with any human disease. AAV is a small virus with capacity for a concomitantly small foreign gene "payload." Vectors derived from AAV can infect a broad range of cells in many target tissues, including muscle cells and neurons. Recombinant AAV has been shown, by several groups, to achieve widespread gene delivery and expression in skeletal muscle, for "marker" genes, for prevention of muscular dystrophy, and for compounds that could enhance muscle function or blood function.[12] Of particular interest to athletic enhancement are studies by Sweeney and colleagues demonstrating partial correction of the muscle defect in a mouse model for Duchenne muscular dystrophy after IM injection of AAV vector expressing the muscle growth factor IGF-1, as well as increased muscle strength and function in similarly injected rats.[13] Early conventional wisdom was that given the nonpathogenicity of adeno-associated viruses, AAV vectors would likewise be spared from immune response by the host. But recent human clinical gene-transfer studies of the antihemophilia factor IX have demonstrated severe enough clinical toxicity resulting from an immune response to AAV vectors to cause the study to be abandoned. It is therefore clear that the AAV system, while promising, is not yet fully understood and at its present state of development does not constitute a magic bullet for gene transfer in any gene-therapy model. Like all other systems, then, it is clearly not ready for use in enhancement settings, such as in athletics.

## Genetic Modulation Using Small-Molecule Antisense Drugs

Both the nonviral gene delivery and viral gene-vector approaches described above add a new exogenous gene into the cells (muscle). Typically, the gene then drives the production of a new protein or an overproduced protein, and the protein mediates a change in the muscle tissue (e.g., increased strength or endurance). As noted above, it has been difficult to transition these approaches into routine clinical use in sick patients, and it is highly unlikely that the same methods could be successfully used for routine doping in sport.

An alternative method of gene doping involves delivery of small sequences of genetic material into the bloodstream, whereupon they enter cells and modulate genes already in the cell. This approach, typically termed *antisense*, is more likely to enter routine clinical use and may be applied to doping in sport. The key advantages of antisense compared with gene delivery are that antisense drugs are much smaller than viral vectors and seem able to diffuse into muscle cells, and these small nucleic acid drugs do not invoke toxicity and immune responses, as do viral vectors.[14]

Antisense nucleic acid drugs generally work by "knock-down" of endogenous mRNAs, and thus of protein production. The loss of target protein is in direct contrast to gene-delivery methods, in which the target protein is added or increased. This difference of loss (antisense) versus gain (gene delivery) has major consequences for possible applications to genetic doping in sport: for antisense to confer an advantage in either strength or endurance, a target protein must be identified for which knock-down of that target leads to better muscle. To date, there is a single, relatively well-documented example of such a target:

myostatin.[15] Loss-of-function mutations in the myostatin (TGFB8) gene result in double-muscled cattle, mighty mice, and a single report of a highly muscled human infant. Given the impressive muscle hypertrophy known to result from inborn gene mutations of myostatin, there have been many efforts to knock down myostatin as a novel approach to experimental therapeutics for muscular dystrophies. However, the results so far have been variable in both mouse models and human trials, with some studies showing a beneficial effect, some a deleterious effect, and some no change.[16] Using antisense to knock down myostatin as a form of drug doping is unlikely to provide a competitive advantage, based on the available data.

## Can Gene Transfer Enhance Athletic Performance?

The lessons being learned in the world of disease treatment and gene therapy are not unknown in the world of sport. There are several obvious ways in which gene-transfer technology might be envisioned to enhance athletic performance. Most forms of competitive sport require optimized force and speed of muscle contraction, efficient delivery of oxygen and other metabolic fuels to exercising muscle, and rapid recovery from muscular work and efficient removal of metabolic wastes. Some of the genes involved in these processes are known, and the products of these genes have already been used in athletic settings to improve performance. The most common one is erythropoietin (EPO), a hormone heavily used for treatment of anemias associated with cancer and kidney disease and, unfortunately, also heavily used and abused in endurance sport to increase erythrocyte (red blood cell) production in the bone marrow and thereby maximize oxygen delivery and waste removal in tissues such as exercising muscle. Mouse studies have shown that expression of a foreign EPO gene in a variety of tissues, including liver, muscle, and even skin, can produce elevated erythrocyte levels and therefore enhanced oxygenation of muscle and other tissues and more efficient removal of toxic metabolites from exercising muscle. If well controlled, such a manipulation could be relatively safe, but, of course, unregulated elevation of erythrocyte numbers could be, and has proved to be, catastrophic—even fatal—in both athletes and nonathletes through the induction of strokes and other cardiovascular calamities. But it is clear that the production of a circulating factor such as EPO in a small tissue "factory" anywhere in the body could be an effective method of regulating red blood cell production, and AAV has already been shown to stimulate EPO expression from a single IM injection. That said, EPO in the injected-protein form is already extensively used by many athletes, and its use has led to extensive rulings on the maximum permissible hematocrit in cyclists and other athletes. Indeed, there is a good and widely disseminated ability to precisely monitor hematocrit and then regulate one's hematocrit through injections of EPO. This same degree of regulation is impossible through gene delivery; the technology to precisely adjust the expression levels of delivered genes is simply "not there." Thus, while gene delivery of EPO may sound attractive, it is technically inferior.

Muscle function itself is an attractive target for pharmacological and even genetic modification. Several factors that control muscle growth, strength, contractility, and repair are well known and their mechanisms of action are coming to be understood in detail. One of the most well studied of these functions is insulin-like growth factor (IGF-1), which has been shown through both in vitro studies and in vivo studies in rodents to cause muscle growth and hypertrophy, to increase the power and strength of contraction, and to increase the risk of some kinds of neuromuscular and orthopedic injuries. Transgenic mice expressing IGF-1 develop markedly larger and more powerful muscles. Furthermore, from the potential therapeutic point of view, expression of a foreign IGF-1 gene in mice, from an AAV vector injected into muscle, prevents the loss of muscle mass during the normal aging process, enhances the healing process of injured muscle, and prevents muscle degeneration in the mouse model of Duchenne muscular dystrophy. One of the most impressive demonstrations of the action of IGF-1 on muscle and its potential application in sport comes from studies of the effects of IGF-1 injection into limb muscles of rats engaged in a program of weight training. Such rats demonstrate a level of increased muscle mass and contractile power much greater than that achieved by IGF-1 without weight training.

## The Apparent Allure of Gene-Based Doping Rather than Pharmacological Doping: Impaired Detection?

Accurate and sensitive detection methods are a potent deterrent against the use of drugs for enhancement of sports performance. Effective assays and screening programs are available for many, but not all, of the drugs and other agents generally abused in sport. Such methods are aimed either at detecting the offending substance itself (direct test) or at detecting the physiological consequences of drug exposure (indirect test). Some substances used for drug doping, such as EPO, are so similar in structure to the normal circulating substance that direct detection of doping can become impossible. In these instances, it can be more sensitive and specific to measure the downstream consequences of supraphysi-ological doses (e.g., elevated hematocrit in EPO doping). A conventional wisdom has evolved around the notion that gene-based doping would be more difficult to detect and therefore would be attractive to those engaged in illicit gene-transfer techniques for athletes. Indirect tests for the action of foreign genes introduced into athletes' body tissues would, of course, be susceptible to the same meth-ods used in drug-based doping (e.g., detecting an elevated hematocrit in EPO doping). But some kinds of direct detection would certainly be more difficult in gene-based than in drug-based doping. For instance, detection of a foreign IGF-1 gene in muscle or other tissues would not be readily feasible without specific knowledge of the site into which the gene was injected. In that case, detection, at least by today's technology, would require the invasive step of muscle biopsy, a procedure to which no athlete is likely to agree.

However, just as molecular genetic techniques are developing rapidly to per-mit gene-transfer approaches, not only for gene therapy of disease but for the modification of human traits for "enhancement" purposes, molecular genetic methods are also permitting the development of ever more effective methods for detecting foreign gene expression. The concepts and tools used so effectively for determination of the full nucleotide sequences of so many mammalian and nonmammalian genomes are being applied to detection of the complex genetic and proteomic interactions that are likely to provide at least some molecular evidence, and possibly diagnostic molecular signatures, for the presence and ex-pression of exogenous genes in the wrong tissue, in nonphysiological amounts, at inappropriate times during development. The World Anti-Doping Agency, the U.S. Anti-Doping Agency, and other antidoping organizations have growing re-search and development programs aimed at the identification of these molecular signatures in tissues such as blood, urine, saliva, and buccal (cheek) scrapings—tissues available by noninvasive procedures that are accepted by the athletic world and that serve as the basis for today's drug-based screening and detection testing programs. It seems likely that tests for expression of major genes whose products are commonly used in drug-based doping (growth hormones includ-ing IGF-1, EPO, and others) will begin to appear as the pressures for, and the likelihood of, illicit gene-based doping increase and as attempts at gene doping become reality.

In addition to molecular detection and monitoring tools, noninvasive imag-ing methods may also eventually be developed to identify sites of foreign gene expression and to detect genetically modified tissues. Such tests are somewhat more difficult to conceive at the moment than the molecular methods, and while no such tests are currently available, imaging research is advancing rapidly and these methods are probably going to become available in time. And so, while gene-based doping, under current conditions, could well offer a greater degree of stealthiness than drug doping, the constant race between rogue abusers and the detection machinery in sport will continue, with neither side standing still.

## Review and Regulation of Human Gene-Transfer Experiments

The techniques for gene transfer in human subjects for the purpose of developing gene therapy for human disease are immature, highly experimental, and filled with many known and unknown risks. The seriousness of these risks is underscored by the fact that one research subject—an 18-year-old man with a chronic liver disorder—died in 1999, and five young boys enrolled in what had been a therapeutically successful gene-therapy study of an immune defect developed the life-threatening complication of acute leukemia as a direct result of the gene-transfer procedure, one of whom has died.[17] In both of these instances, there was little reason to anticipate such severe adverse events. There was, to be sure, always the presumption that things can and will go awry, but such potential dangers are generally acceptable to patients, doctors, and society if the goal is the overriding good of treating an otherwise life-threatening and intractable disease. In the United States, extensive review and regulatory structures are now in place to ensure that studies of gene transfer in human beings are carried out under conditions that maximally protect the welfare of research subjects and patients. Several levels of careful review and regulation exist at the local level— universities, hospitals, research institutes, and so on—and at the federal level in the form of rigorous study evaluation of proposed gene-transfer studies by the FDA and by the NIH through its Recombinant DNA Advisory Committee. Other countries carrying out gene-transfer studies have instituted similar rigorous levels of regulation and oversight to prevent misapplication of the powerful, but still inadequately understood, gene-transfer methods for purposes other than treatment of serious disease. In no case has any proposal dealing with enhancement goals been approved at any of the oversight levels.

## Conclusion

A clear principle emerges from the extension of risky but potentially beneficial gene-transfer technology to human beings: the methods of gene transfer in humans are not yet sufficiently developed to be appropriate for any purposes other than disease correction. Application to the enhancement of athletic capability, or any enhancement goal for that matter, would circumvent these careful review procedures and would therefore constitute a clear breach of the standards of full disclosure, informed consent, and experimental subject protection that constitute the bedrock principles of all acceptable forms of human clinical experimentation. Illicit application of these hazardous and immature gene-transfer methods without approval from the existing local and federal oversight bodies would be medically unjustified and unethical. If carried out by medical personnel, it would seem to constitute medical malpractice. If carried out by nonmedical figures such as athletic trainers, drug manufacturers, sports federation officials, or national sports agencies, the procedure would be foolhardy, in violation of the safety interests of the athletes, and therefore reprehensible, possibly in violation of licensing requirements, and potentially illegal. If carried out in the United States in an institution that receives federal funding, such an action would almost certainly trigger cut-off of federal funds to the investigator and institution.

NOTES

1. S. Hacein-Bey-Abina, C. Von Kalle, M. Schmidt, M. P. McCormack, N. Wulffraat, P. Leboulch, A. Lim, et al., "LMO2-Associated Clonal T Cell Proliferation in Two Patients after Gene Therapy for SCID-X1," *Science* 302 (2003): 415–19, erratum in *Science* 302 (2003): 568; E. Raper, N. Chirmule, F. S. Lee, N. A. Wivel, A. Bagg, G. P. Gao, J. M. Wilson, and M. L. Batshaw, "Fatal Systemic Inflammatory Response Syndrome in an Ornithine Transcarbamylase Deficient Patient following Adenoviral Gene Transfer," *Molecular Genetics and Metabolism* 80 (2003): 148–58.

2. J. A. Wolff, R. W. Malone, P. Williams, W. Chong, G. Acsadi, A. Jani, and P. L. Felgner, "Direct Gene Transfer into Mouse Muscle in Vivo," *Science* 247 (1990): 1465–68.

3. H. Herweijer and J. A. Wolff, "Progress and Prospects: Naked DNA Gene Transfer and Therapy," *Human Molecular Genetics* 2, no. 12 (1993): 2055–61.

4. I. Danko, J. D. Fritz, J. S. Latendresse, H. Herweijer, E. Schultz, and J. A. Wolff, "Dystrophin Expression Improves Myofiber Survival in MDX Muscle following Intramuscular Plasmid DNA Injection," *Gene Therapy* 10, no. 6 (2003): 453–58; G. Zhang, V. Budker, P. Williams, V. Subbotin, and J. A. Wolff, "Efficient Expression of Naked DNA Delivered Intraarterially to Limb Muscles of Nonhuman Primates," *Human Gene Therapy* 12, no. 4 (2001): 427–38; N. B. Romero, "Current Protocol of a Research Phase I Clinical Trial of Full-Length Dystrophin Plasmid DNA in Duchenne/Becker Muscular Dystrophies. Part II: Clinical Protocol," *Neuromuscular Disorders* 12, suppl. (2002): S45–48.

5. G. Gao, C. Lebherz, D. J. Weiner, R. Grant, R. Calcedo, B. McCullough, A. Bagg,

Y. Zhang, and J. M. Wilson, "Erythropoietin Gene Therapy Leads to Autoimmune Anemia in Macaques," *Blood* 103 (2004): 3300–3302.

6. T. Friedmann, *The Development of Human Gene Therapy* (Woodbury, NY: Cold Spring Harbor Laboratory Press, 1999).

7. Ibid.

8. Hacein-Bey-Abina et al., "LMO2-Associated Clonal T Cell Proliferation."

9. C. DelloRusso, J. M. Scott, D. Hartigan-O'Connor, G. Salvatori, C. Barjot, A. S. Robinson, and R. W. Crawford, "Functional Correction of Adult MDX Mouse Muscle Using Gutted Adenoviral Vectors Expressing Full-Length Dystrophin," *Proceedings of the National Academy of Sciences* 99, no. 20 (2002): 12979–84.

10. Raper et al., "Fatal Systemic Inflammatory Response Syndrome."

11. T. M. Daly, "Overview of Adeno-Associated Viral Vectors," *Methods in Molecular Biology* 246 (2004): 157–65.

12. K. J. Fisher, K. Jooss, J. Alston, Y. Yang, S. E. Haecker, K. High, R. Pathak, S. E. Raper, and J. M. Wilson, "Recombinant Adeno-Associated Virus for Muscle Directed Gene Therapy," *Nature Medicine* 3, no. 3 (1997): 306–12; R. O. Snyder, S. K. Spratt, C. Lagarde, D. Hohl, B. Kaspar, B. Sloan, L. K. Cohen, and O. Danos, "Efficient and Stable Adeno-Associated Virus-Mediated Transduction in the Skeletal Muscle of Adult Immunocompetent Mice," *Human Gene Therapy* 8, no. 16 (1997): 1891–1900; J. Li, D. Dressman, Y. P. Tsao, A. Sakamoto, E. P. Hoffman, and X. Xiao, "rAAV Vector-Mediated Sarcoglycan Gene Transfer in a Hamster Model for Limb Girdle Muscular Dystrophy," *Gene Therapy* 6, no. 1 (1999): 74–82; X. Xiao, J. Li, Y. P. Tsao, D. Dressman, E. P. Hoffman, and J. F. Watchko, "Full Functional Rescue of a Complete Muscle (TA) in Dystrophic Hamsters by Adeno-Associated Virus Vector-Directed Gene Therapy," *Journal of Virology* 74, no. 3 (2000): 1436–42; B. Wang, J. Li, and X. Xiao, "Adeno-Associated Virus Vector Carrying Human Minidystrophin Genes Effectively Ameliorates Muscular Dystrophy in MDX Mouse Model," *Proceedings of the National Academy of Sciences* 97, no. 25 (2000): 13714–19; D. Dressman, K. Araishi, M. Imamura, T. Sasaoka, L. A. Liu, E. Engvall, and E. P. Hoffman, "Delivery of Alpha- and Beta-Sarcoglycan by Recombinant Adeno-Associated Virus: Efficient Rescue of Muscle, but Differential Toxicity," *Human Gene Therapy* 13, no. 13 (2002): 1631–46; D. S. Chang, M. Kapturczak, S. A. Liler, S. Zolotukhin, O. Y. Glushakova, K. M. Madsen, R. J. Smulski, et al., "Adeno-Associated Viral Vector-Mediated Gene Transfer of VEGF Normalizes Skeletal Muscle Oxygen Tension and Induces Arteriogenesis in Ischemic Rat Hindlimb," *Molecular Therapy* 7, no. 1 (2003): 44–51; P. D. Kessler, G. M. Podsakoff, X. Chen, S. A. McQuiston, P. C. Colosi, L. A. Matelis, G. J. Kurzman, and B. J. Byrne, "Gene Delivery to Skeletal Muscle Results in Sustained Expression and Systemic Delivery of a Therapeutic Protein," *Proceedings of the National Academy of Sciences* 93, no. 24 (1996): 14082–87; V. R. Arruda, J. Schuettrumpf, R. W. Herzog, T. C. Nichols, N. Robinson, Y. Lotfi, F. Mingozzi, W. Xiao, L. B. Couto, and K. A. High, "Safety and Efficacy of Factor IX Gene Transfer to Skeletal Muscle in Murine and Canine Hemophilia B Models by Adeno-Associated Viral Vector Serotype 1," *Blood* 103, no. 1 (2004): 85–92.

13. E. R. Barton, L. Morris, A. Musaro, N. Rosenthal, and H. L. Sweeney, "Muscle-Specific Expression of Insulin-Like Growth Factor I Counters Muscle Decline in MDX

Mice," *Journal of Cell Biology* 157, no. 1 (2002): 137–48; H. L. Sweeney, "Gene Doping," *Scientific American* 291 (2004): 62–69.

14. E. P. Hoffman "Skipping toward Personalized Molecular Medicine," *New England Journal of Medicine* 357 (2007): 2719–22; B. Wu, H. M. Moulton, P. L. Ibersen, J. Jiang, J. Li, J. Li, C. F. Spurney, A. Sali, A. D. Guerron, K. Nagaraju, T. Doran, P. Lu, X. Xiao, and Q. L. Lu, "Effective Rescue of Dystrophin Improves Cardiac Function in Dystrophin-Deficient Mice by a Modified Morpholino Oligomer," *Proceedings of the National Academy of Sciences* 105, no. 39 (2008): 14814–19; T. Yokota, Q.-L. Lu, T. Partridge, M. Kobayashi, A. Nakamura, S. Takeda, and E. Hoffman, "Efficacy of Systemic Morpholino Exon-Skipping in Duchenne Dystrophy Dogs," *Annals of Neurology* 65 (2009), in press.

15. K. R. Wagner, "Muscle Regeneration through Myostatin Inhibition," *Current Opinion in Rheumatology* 7 (2005): 720–24.

16. E. P. Hoffman and D. Escolar, "Translating Mighty Mice into Neuromuscular Therapeutics: Is Bigger Muscle Better?" *American Journal of Pathology* 168 (2006): 1775–78; K. R. Wagner, J. L. Fleckenstein, A. A. Amato, R. J. Barohn, K. Bushby, D. M. Escolar, and K. M. Flanigan, "A Phase I/II Trial of MYO-029 in Adult Subjects with Muscular Dystrophy," *Annals of Neurology* 63 (2008): 561–71.

17. J. M. Wilson, "Lessons Learned from the Gene Therapy Trial for Ornithine Transcarbamylase Deficiency," *Molecular Genetics and Metabolism* 96, no. 4 (2009): 151–57; D. B. Kohn, "Gene Therapy for Childhood Diseases," *Bone Marrow Transplantation* 41 (2008): 199–205.

# CHAPTER THIRTEEN

# Technologies to Enhance Oxygen Delivery and Methods to Detect the Use of These Technologies

LARRY D. BOWERS, PH.D.

All cells in the body use oxygen to produce energy. In the process called glycolysis, one molecule of glucose can be converted into two molecules of pyruvate with a net production of two molecules of adenosine-5'-triphosphate (ATP), which is the energy provider for the cell. In the absence of sufficient $O_2$ (anaerobic conditions), cells produce excess lactate (lactic acid) from the pyruvate produced during glycolysis. In addition to glycolysis being a relatively inefficient process, the lactic acid produced results in the "burning" sensation associated with muscular effort. In the presence of sufficient $O_2$ (aerobic conditions), the pyruvate can be transported to subcellular units called mitochondria, where an additional 36 molecules of ATP (per molecule of glucose) can be generated by oxidative phosphorylation. In addition to the pyruvate from carbohydrates, the products of amino acid and fatty acid metabolism can also be oxidized in the mitochondria, the energy "factories" in the cell, to provide ATP. Unlike other subcellular components, mitochondria have their own DNA specifically for producing some of the machinery necessary for energy production. Mitochondria are also unique in that they are inherited from the oocyte (i.e., from the mother) only and do not divide evenly between the cells during cell division.

In complex, multicellular organisms such as humans, oxygen must be delivered to the tissues throughout the body. Oxygen is taken up in the lungs and transferred to hemoglobin (Hb), a specialized oxygen-transport protein found in the red blood cells (RBCs; also called erythrocytes). The blood then moves the RBCs to the tissues, where physiological conditions favor off-loading of the $O_2$ and pickup of the $CO_2$ produced as a waste product. Tissue hypoxia (insufficient $O_2$), due to any cause, is detected primarily by the peritubular interstitial cells of the kidney, which in turn results in increased production of erythropoietin (EPO). EPO causes hematopoietic stem cells in the bone marrow to commit to becoming reticulocytes, which mature into RBCs, thus increasing the RBC mass and the amount of Hb available to transport oxygen to the tissue.

The most efficient generation of energy for exercise, then, would involve a large maximal stroke volume in the heart to deliver blood at a high flow rate; a high Hb concentration to facilitate transport of oxygen from the lungs to the muscle; large muscle capillary volume and high vascular conductance in the skeletal muscle to ensure rapid delivery and diffusion of oxygen to the muscle; and a large number of efficient mitochondria in each cell to generate energy. Therapeutic or molecular biological intervention in each of these systems has been investigated (see table 13.1). In addition, training affects each of these systems to improve efficient energy production, making detection of doping more complex. For the past two decades, increasing the transport of oxygen to tissues by artificially increasing the RBC mass was the most easily modified parameter for increasing sports performance.

Increased RBC mass, termed *polycythemia*, is not without risk. Several inherited diseases are characterized by polycythemia. In the condition polycythemia vera, usually identified in the fifth decade, there is significantly increased RBC mass. The primary morbidity associated with polycythemia vera is thrombosis and bleeding, which are thought to be the result of both increased RBC mass and other unidentified disease-related events. The risk of thrombosis is related to age in patients with polycythemia vera, and they also display symptoms related to blood hyperviscosity, such as headache, dizziness, visual symptoms, parasthesias, and fatigue. Blood viscosity is affected by plasma viscosity and by the number, deformability, and aggregability or "stickiness" of the RBCs. Plasma viscosity is determined by the content of proteins such as fibrinogen, immunoglobulins, and albumin in the plasma. Increased blood viscosity decreases blood flow in the microcirculation and could impede oxygen transfer to tissues. Treatment of polycythemia vera is phlebotomy—blood-letting—to bring the hematocrit (the volume percentage of RBCs in the blood) down to 45 percent in men and 42 percent in women. There are other genetic diseases, such as Chuvash polycythemia, in which the increased RBC mass is due to augmentation of hypoxic sensing. Understanding the molecular mechanism of this disease could be used to genetically alter RBC production in healthy athletes.

TABLE 13.1
## Potential Approaches for Enhancing the Use of $O_2$

| Biological System, Substance, or Method Targeted | Potential Effect | Approach | Reference(s) |
|---|---|---|---|
| HIF $O_2$-sensing pathway | Increased tissue response to $O_2$ | Genetic intervention; inhibitors of HIF-deactivating enzymes | Hewitson and Schofield 2004 |
| Capillary bed in the muscle | Increased blood supply to the muscle, increasing $O_2$ delivery | Vascular endothelial growth factor, either local gene insertion or recombinant protein | |
| Mitochondria | Increased efficiency of energy production | Increased numbers of mitochondria; mitochondrial DNA alterations | Wallace 2005 |
| Hypoxia | Increased $O_2$ transport | "Live high, train low"; normobaric, hypoxic tents, apartments, etc. | Levine and Stray-Gundersen 1997; Rusko, Tikkanen, and Peltonen 2004 |
| Blood transfusion | Increased $O_2$ transport | Introduction of RBCs from self or a cross-matched donor | See text |
| EPO | Increased $O_2$ transport | Genetic intervention; injection of rHuEPO | See text |
| EPO mimetics | Increased $O_2$ transport | Injection of EPO mimetics, resulting in increased RBC production | Johnson and Jolliffe 2000 |
| Blood substitutes (HBOCs, perfluorocarbons) | Increased $O_2$ transport | Intravenous administration of substitute $O_2$ carriers | Gaudard et al. 2003; Chang et al. 2000 |
| Allosteric modifiers of Hb | Increased $O_2$ off-loading at the tissue | Intravenous administration of agents that cause off-loading of $O_2$ | Youssef et al. 2002 |

*Abbreviations:* HIF, hypoxia-inducible factor; EPO, erythropoietin; rHuEPO, recombinant erythropoietin; RBC, red blood cell; HBOCs, hemoglobin-based oxygen carriers; Hb, hemoglobin.

*References*
Chang, T. M. S., F. D'Agnillo, W. P. Yu, and S. Razack. 2000. Two Future Generations of Blood Substitutes Based on Polyhemoglobin-SOD-Catalase and Nanoencapsulation. *Advanced Drug Delivery Review* 40:213–28.
Gaudard, A., E. Varlet-Marie, F. Bressolle, and M. Audran. 2003. Drugs for Increasing Oxygen and Their Potential Use in Doping: A Review. *Sports Medicine* 33:187–212.
Hewitson, K. S., and C. J. Schofield. 2004. The HIF Pathway as a Therapeutic Target. *Drug Discovery Today* 9:704–11.
Johnson, D. L., and L. K. Jolliffe. 2000. Erythropoietin Mimetic Peptides and the Future. *Nephrology Dialysis Transplantation* 15:1274–77.
Levine, B. D., and J. Stray-Gundersen. 1997. "Living High Training Low": Effect of Moderate-Altitude Acclimatization with Low-Altitude Training on Performance. *Journal of Applied Physiology* 83:102–12.
Rusko, H. R., H. O. Tikkanen, and J. E. Peltonen. 2004. Altitude and Endurance Training. *Journal of Sports Sciences* 22:928–44.
Wallace, D. C. 2005. The Mitochondrial Genome in Human Adaptive Radiation and Disease: On the Road to Therapeutics and Performance Enhancement. *Gene* 354:169–80.
Youssef, A. M., M. K. Safo, R. Danso-Danquah, G. S. Joshi, J. Kister, M. C. Marden, and D. J. Abraham. 2002. Synthesis and X-Ray Studies of Chiral Allosteric Modifiers of Hemoglobin. *Journal of Medical Chemistry* 45:1184–95.

## Enhancement of Oxygen Transport and Sport

Eero Mäntyranta, a Finnish cross-country skier who competed in the 1960, 1964, and 1968 Winter Olympic Games, won three gold medals and eight medals in all. Impressively, at the Innsbruck Olympics (1964) he won the 15-kilometer race by 40.7 seconds and the 30-kilometer race by 71.6 seconds. He was later found to have autosomal dominant benign erythrocytosis, a rare genetic condition caused by a mutation in the EPO receptor. In this condition, the hematocrit (Hct) is 25 to 50 percent higher than normal.

Lasse Virén, a Finnish runner who won gold medals in both the 5000 and 10,000 meters at the 1972, 1976, and 1980 Olympics, was suspected of blood doping, due to his unusually good Olympic performances. Although he never admitted to this practice, a teammate, Kaarlo Maaninka, did admit to injecting blood. The U.S. cycling team, unheralded before the 1984 Olympic Games in Los Angeles, won the team gold medal and later admitted to blood doping. In 1986, the International Olympic Committee declared "blood doping" against the rules. In 1990, the use of biosynthetic EPO was prohibited, although there was no test for this substance. The American College of Sports Medicine issued a position paper on blood doping, stating: "It is the position of the American College of Sports Medicine that any blood doping procedure used in an attempt to improve athletic performance is unethical, unfair, and exposes the athlete to unwarranted and potentially serious health risks."[1] In 2000, the International Olympic Committee included "administering artificial oxygen carriers or plasma expanders" on the "Prohibited List."

Videman and colleagues found that the mean Hb concentrations among male elite cross-country skiers at the 1989 world championships were 8 g/L below the reference population mean, whereas the mean concentrations observed since 1997 are 5 to 8 g/L above the reference population mean. The institution of a rule in 1997 that Hb concentrations should be less than 185 g/L for an athlete to compete has eliminated the extreme values seen earlier, but gives the impression that the athletes are titrating up to the legal limit. After several incorrect public statements that there was no test for Darbepoetin, a therapeutic agent for treating anemia, three cross-country skiers (Johann Muehlegg, Larissa Lazutina, and Olga Danilova) tested positive for this agent at the 2002 Winter Olympics. As an exclamation point to this finding, Stray-Gundersen and colleagues concluded, based on the highly abnormal hematological profiles of the winners of cross-country skiing events, that "blood doping is both prevalent and highly effective in cross-country ski racing."[2]

In October 2002, the U.S. Anti-Doping Agency had its first Annual Symposium on Anti-Doping Science, with the topic "Oxygen Transport Enhancing Agents and Methods," focused on all the technologies for artificially increasing $O_2$ transport. When the World Anti-Doping Agency (WADA) took responsibility for the "Prohibited List" in 2003, more methods of enhancing $O_2$ transport were included, such as infused homologous or autologous blood or red blood cells, modified hemoglobin products, perfluorocarbons, and 2,3-diphosphoglycerate mimetics.[3]

In addition to tests carried out under the rules of doping control, several sports have adopted a "health test" philosophy in which the athlete is tested before the competition and, if the Hct, Hb, or other parameters are not below a specified value, the athlete is not allowed to start the competition and must not compete for some period of time. There are limitations to this approach, including the fact that "dilution" with an intravenous infusion of saline before the test can temporarily bring the Hct or Hb below the threshold. Also, because the increase in maximal aerobic power per gram change in Hb is consistent up to about 210 g/L, a "threshold" concentration for Hb or Hct provides an advantage to those athletes with a lower "natural" Hb or Hct. The argument has been made that the health test does not result in a sanction as imposed under doping-control rules and is done out of concern for athletes' health. But this approach does impose a period of ineligibility, and the ineligibility was challenged at the Court of Arbitration for Sport, for the first time, before the cross-country skiing events at the 2006 Winter Olympics.

## Exercise Performance and Maximal Aerobic Power

The $VO_2$ max is defined as the maximal rate of oxygen use by body tissues during exercise. The $VO_2$ max is determined by both oxygen-delivery and oxygen-extraction factors. Hemoglobin is the main component in $O_2$ pickup in the lung, transport through the blood, and off-loading at the tissue. A direct relationship between the Hb concentration and RBC mass and the $VO_2$ max has been shown. Because of the dynamic exchange between the plasma and extracellular water, however, it is impossible to obtain an accurate measure of RBC mass from measurement of the Hct. Intense physical training results in an increase in plasma and RBC volume, but the net result is a decrease in the Hct as the increased liquid volume reduces the concentration of RBCs in a given unit of plasma.[4]

Infusion of RBCs and the resulting increase in Hb result in increased $VO_2$ max and aerobic physical performance.[5] Gledhill concluded from a review of the literature that infusion of 900 to 1350 milliliters of blood results in a 4 to 9 percent increase in $VO_2$ max.[6] RBC infusion decreased 1500-meter run time by about 5 seconds, which corresponds to the time between first and eleventh place in the 2004 Olympic Games.[7] Increasing the RBC mass by injection of EPO has a similar effect on performance.[8]

Although most commentators associate the benefits of increased oxygen transport with distance events, high-intensity intermittent exercise also benefits from increased maximal aerobic power.[9] It is also clear from the documentation garnered from the BALCO (Bay Area Laboratory Cooperative) scandal that track-and-field sprinters were using recombinant human EPO (rHuEPO) to train harder and recover faster.

## The Use of Oxygen Content of Air to Alter the Hematological System

One of the earliest approaches to increasing oxygen-transport capacity was to live and train at high altitude. The physiological principle of high-altitude training is that the body detects the decreased arterial $O_2$ content that results from the lower amount of $O_2$ per unit volume of atmosphere. A hypoxia-regulated gene transcription factor, hypoxia-inducible factor 1 (HIF-1α), is not degraded as rapidly under hypoxic conditions and is able to combine with an oxygen-independent subunit, HIF-2α, in the nucleus. This dimeric transcription factor is then recognized by hypoxia response elements (HREs) in the regulatory DNA sequences of several proteins. The response to HIF-1α transcription factor is tissue specific: renal cells make EPO, whereas skeletal muscle cells increase the amount of the enzymes involved in glycolysis, and the vascular endothelium produces vascular endothelial growth factor (VEGF) to increase blood vessel formation. EPO facilitates commitment of stem cells in the bone marrow to form reticulocytes, which are the nucleated precursors of RBCs.

There are limitations to living and training at high altitude. Above 2000 meters, there is a 10 percent decrement in $VO_2$ max for each 1000-meter increase in altitude. Training intensity is negatively affected by increasing altitude, and thus it is possible to suffer from de-training after prolonged periods at high altitude. The EPO concentration peaks after about 48 hours at high altitude, and after 5 to 10 days of altitude acclimatization, EPO concentrations have returned to baseline. Not surprisingly, the erythopoietic system is down-regulated over the same time frame on return to low altitude. The degree of erythropoietic response is variable at 2200 to 2800 meters, with slightly more than 50 percent of individuals being robust responders.

One approach developed by Levine and Stray-Gundersen, called "living high, training low," has been shown to improve sea-level performance over events lasting 8 to 20 minutes.[10] This strategy combines high-altitude (2500 m) acclimatization with low-altitude (1200 m) training to achieve the optimal effect. A 1.4 percent improvement in performance in the 5000-meter run accompanied the 1.1 g/dL increase in Hb and 3 percent increase in $VO_2$ max. Similar results were obtained in elite athletes.[11] Perhaps of greater significance to the athlete, one-third of the runners achieved their personal best times after four weeks of acclimatization at 2500 meters. The drawback to this approach is the need for access to mountains and valleys that allow physically moving from high to low altitude.

In the early 1990s, artificial devices called "altitude houses" or "hypoxic houses" began to appear.[12] Subsequently, altitude devices that can be installed around a bed or that control the air in a single room have also been marketed. In contrast to high-altitude training, hypoxic houses either add nitrogen to ambient air to decrease the partial pressure of $O_2$ or remove $O_2$ from the air relative to the other gases, such as nitrogen, to create an artificial situation in which the amount of $O_2$ per volume of air is similar to that at high altitude. These devices can be programmed to simulate altitudes up to 4000 meters. An important distinction between the normobaric hypoxic house and high-altitude training is that above a critical altitude of about 2500 meters, the increase in RBC mass seems to be directly related to the increase in altitude. In theory, the altitude house provides the athlete with maximum RBC generation without the decrement in $VO_2$ max that accompanies training at high altitude. In addition, marginal responders at 2500 meters could in theory achieve a better response at higher altitude. In summary, the argument that a normobaric, hypoxic chamber is equivalent to high-altitude training does not withstand critical review.

The efficacy of the altitude tents has been a topic of controversy. Study design differences (e.g., length of daily hypoxic exposure, total length of hypoxic exposure, choice of biomarker of effect, effect of training) have significantly complicated the attempt to understand the effects of short-term exposure to normobaric hypoxia. Studies that use serum EPO concentrations as an indicator of response have universally demonstrated that EPO production is modestly increased. When increases in reticulocyte numbers or Hb concentration were measured, the results were not consistent across studies. For example, Piehl Aulin and colleagues showed that after an initial increase in Hb and Hct during the first two days, the concentrations returned to prestudy levels.[13] Two groups that measured $VO_2$ max in trained athletes found no significant increase.[14] It appears that the necessary acclimatization requires at least 12 hours per day of hypoxic exposure at an altitude of about 2500 meters for a period of at least three weeks.[15]

## Blood Transfusions

Increasing the RBC mass by transfusion is also an effective doping method. Although, in principle, blood from another species could be used (heterologous transfusion), this presents many risks to the recipient. Transfusion of blood from another person, or allogeneic (or homologous) transfusion, can also be used to increase RBC mass, but there is a risk of a potentially fatal transfusion reaction for the recipient if the blood is not properly cross-matched. Collecting a portion of one's own RBCs for reinfusion at a later time, or autologous transfusion, can also be used to increase RBC mass. The main limitation for blood storage is the length of time the blood can be stored. RBCs can be stored at 4°C for up to four weeks and maintain essentially full functionality. Storage for a longer period requires stabilization of the RBCs with glycerol and specialized cell-washing equipment before reinfusion. This process could be accomplished only with the assistance of health care professionals. One argument against athletes using autologous transfusion is the anemia associated with the removal of RBCs for storage and its negative impact on training. The use of rHuEPO to enhance RBC mass before phlebotomy has been thoroughly studied in conjunction with autologous blood donation programs developed for elective surgery in the 1990s. There is a linear relationship between EPO dose and increase in RBC volume. It is thus possible to use rHuEPO to allow collection of RBCs for autologous transfusion with minimal effect on the hematocrit and thus on training intensity.

## Potential Pharmacological Approaches for Enhancing Oxygen Delivery

The introduction of recombinant human EPO in the mid-1980s ushered in a new era in doping practices. Amgen pioneered the production of rHuEPO (EPO α; trade name Epogen or Procrit) by expressing the human gene in a Chinese hamster ovary cell. This approach was necessary because EPO contains four sugar chains at various locations along the amino acid sequence that are integral to its function and clearance from the circulation; mammalian cells are necessary to accurately glycosylate the EPO protein. Other commercial entities have produced other forms of rHuEPO, using either Chinese hamster ovary cells (EPO β; Neo-Recormon) or baby hamster kidney cells (EPO ω; Epomax). EPO δ (Dynepo) is produced from engineered human cells and, as explained below, may present the most difficult detection problem. With the increased availability of rHuEPO, its use to increase RBC mass became relatively easy.

Novel erythropoiesis stimulating protein (NESP; Darbepoetin alfa) is a genetically engineered EPO protein sequence that was developed to increase the length of time the drug could be effective in the circulation.[16] It has five N-linked carbohydrate chains, compared with three on native EPO. The increased number of sialic acid residues increases the half-life in serum by a factor of three and decreases the pI (isoelectric pH) from about 4.0 to about 3.3. These two factors make detection of NESP in doping-control samples relatively easy. EPO mimetics are under development, and their detection can be expected to challenge the antidoping laboratories.[17]

Berglund and colleagues demonstrated the performance-enhancing potential of rHuEPO. With administration of 20 or 40 U/kg three times per week for six weeks, the Hb and Hct increased 10 percent and $VO_2$ max rose. Casoni, using 30 U/kg doses, showed similar increases in Hb and Hct. Using a dose of 200 U/kg, Bressolle and co-workers studied the pharmacodynamic effects of rHuEPO on serum transferring receptor (sTfr) and ferritin over 10 days.[18] Doses of 20 IU/kg three times per week for five weeks were sufficient to maintain an elevated Hct and $VO_2$ max achieved by a more robust dose of 50 U/kg during the initial three weeks.[19] Whether any of these regimens was used by athletes is not clear.

The use of rHuEPO and Darbepoetin is not without risk. Berglund and Ekblom observed a marked increase in exercise-induced blood pressure response, probably due to increased viscosity.[20] A case of cerebral sinus thrombosis was reported in a professional cyclist.[21] The suspicious deaths of 18 Dutch and Belgian cyclists between 1987 and 1990 were also circumstantially linked to their EPO use, due to the close proximity in time to the introduction of rHuEPO and earlier admission to its use by some of the cyclists. It has recently been reported that long-term administration of either Epogen or Darbepoetin can elicit the development of anti-EPO antibodies and result in pure red cell aplasia, a condition in which RBC precursors in bone marrow are nearly absent, while other precursor cells made in the bone marrow are usually present at normal levels.[22]

Normally, Hb molecules circulating in the plasma (i.e., outside the RBCs) would be toxic to the kidneys. Several modified hemoglobin-based oxygen carriers (HBOCs) have been reported.[23] Oxyglobin, approved for animal use, and Hemopure, approved for human use in some countries, are the first generation of HBOCs. The basic approach to producing an HBOC has been to increase the size of the Hb molecule by cross-linking, polymerization, or nanoencapsulation so that it cannot pass through the kidney and into the urine. In addition, modified hemoglobins have been engineered to avoid problems associated with the binding of nitric oxide and removal of free radicals. Nanoencapsulation allows the inclusion of enzymes and Hb in a capsule much smaller than a red blood cell.[24] This artificial cell behaves more like a native RBC under physiological conditions. Due to its small size, it should be readily detectable in the plasma.

Another method of directly transporting oxygen to the tissues is through the use of perfluorocarbons (PFCs). The PFCs are not soluble in water and thus make finely dispersed particles in which $O_2$ can dissolve. Unlike Hb, PFCs dissolve and release $O_2$ based on the partial pressure of oxygen in the surrounding tissue. To function as a good $O_2$ transporter, PFCs require amounts of $O_2$ that can be achieved only by continuous inhalation of an oxygen-rich mixture. It is thus unclear whether any performance advantage can be conveyed with current technology. In addition, it is relatively easy to visually detect either HBOCs or PFCs in the plasma.

## Potential Abuse of Gene Therapy

Genetic modification of tissue to continuously deliver proteins to the circulation would be a serious problem for doping control. It should be pointed out, too, that selective modification/expression of a single gene has potentially unpredictable results. For example, delivery of the EPO gene is potentially hazardous because continuous production of EPO could result in deadly consequences due to the continuously increasing RBC mass. In addition, EPO is a member of a class of growth factors and its overexpression could have unexpected effects on other tissues. Thus this simplistic approach of continuous delivery of EPO is unlikely to be successful. Advances in molecular biological techniques, however, are providing control mechanisms for gene insertions. Constructing an adeno-associated viral vector in which an inducible promoter is inserted near the gene of interest allows that gene to be modulated in response to the inducer in drinking water, as demonstrated for EPO.[25] Repoxygen is a viral gene-delivery vector, designed for injection into muscle, carrying both the human EPO gene and an HRE control element. The HRE detects low $O_2$ concentrations and turns on the EPO gene.

While there is little chance that Repoxygen itself will pose a threat in sports doping, it does illustrate the routine nature of this technology.

# The Challenge for Testing

The goal for antidoping programs is deterrence of the abuse of performance-enhancing substances. Performance enhancement in sport goes beyond increases in strength and body mass to include improved concentration, improved eyesight, and pharmacologically shortened recovery time. To act as an effective deterrent, the testing program must have the capability to detect those athletes who choose to dope, and the adjudication program must be able to hold the athletes accountable for their behavior. The appropriate timing of sample collection as well as the development of new and better test technologies are important elements in the execution of an effective deterrence program.

## Blood Transfusions

As described above, RBC injection has been used in sport for at least two decades. Attempts have been made to develop biomarker tests for autologous and homologous transfusions, but they have been relatively ineffective in detecting a majority of individuals who are using transfusions.[26]

Every RBC in an individual has hundreds of different markers on its cell surface, predetermined by the individual's genetics as "nonexpressed" or "expressed" (homozygous or heterozygous expression). Major blood group markers such as A, B, O, and Rh(D) are important in ensuring that a transfusion reaction does not occur. There are also many minor surface markers, such as Kell, Duffy, and Kidd, that do not require determination for blood transfusion but nevertheless define the population of RBCs. The finding of a subpopulation of RBCs that express a particular surface marker in the presence of a majority of RBCs that are nonexpressors requires some explanation, as does a minor population of nonexpressing RBCs in the presence of predominantly expressing RBCs. Possible explanations are a homologous blood transfusion, bone marrow transplantation, blood group chimerism, and a few diseases such as paroxysmal nocturnal hemoglobinuria. As in the situation with measurement of the testosterone/epitestosterone ratio in testing for androgenic steroid abuse, the athlete should be able to provide medical documentation of a pathological reason for such a finding.

An agglutination test called the "mixed field reaction" was used at the Winter

Olympics in Lillehammer, Norway, in 1994 to detect homologous blood transfusion. The sensitivity of the test was such that a transfusion would be detected only if the athlete had been transfused within a few days before the sample collection. More recently, Nelson developed a test based on flow cytometry that, in principle, can be 20-fold more sensitive than the mixed field reaction. The potential for a blood donor to match the recipient in all 11 markers proposed by Nelson is 1.7 per thousand in Caucasians, 2 per thousand in Asians, and 3 per million in African Americans. This makes finding a completely matched donor significantly more difficult, and thus the test achieves the goal of deterrence.[27] In a recent case involving this technology, both an American Arbitration Association panel and a Court of Arbitration for Sport panel ruled, on appeal, that the test was valid and fit for its purpose.[28]

Another indicator of change in RBC mass is changes in the reticulocytes and young red blood cells. Studies have shown that physiological control of RBC mass is achieved by selective hemolysis of young red blood cells, a process called neocytolysis.[29] Thus, in the presence of a nonphysiological increase in RBC mass, through either transfusion or rHuEPO abuse, the body responds by selectively removing the youngest cells produced. This process creates a distribution of ages of red cells that is atypical of normal hematological control. An approach based on this atypical distribution has the potential for detecting any manipulation of the hematological system and is currently under development as an antidoping test.

The use of autologous transfusion is currently undetectable by a direct test, although active research is under way to identify potential biomarkers of this doping method.

## Pharmacological Agents

Indirect measurements of biomarkers to detect the use of rHuEPO have been reported for more than a decade.[30] Ethyroid cells require 5 to 9 days to mature under normal physiological conditions, so Hb concentration and Hct do not rise immediately after an rHuEPO dose. From about 4 to 17 days after an rHuEPO dose, the number of reticulocytes is increased. From 10 to 24 days after administration, the number of RBCs, Hb concentration, and Hct are increased. Given that iron is required for hemoglobin synthesis, rapid erthyropoiesis—red blood cell formation—is accompanied by changes in iron-storage parameters such as sTfr and ferritin. Co-administration of iron with the rHuEPO and the individual's rate of erythropoiesis affect the impact of rHuEPO administration on the biomarkers. Parisotto and co-workers did extensive studies and developed a logistic model for combining Hct, reticulocyte hematocrit, percentage macrocytes, serum EPO concentration, and sTfr concentration.[31] Models were developed for when EPO was being administered ("ON model") and after cessation of administration ("OFF model"). One of the limitations of this logistic model is the viability and detection of cellular parts of whole blood, which required rapid transport to the laboratory. The same team revised their testing scheme with a second-generation "ON" and "OFF" model score that incorporated Hb concentration (instead of Hct), serum EPO, sTfr, and percentage reticulocytes.[32] Measuring the amount of hemoglobin β-globin mRNA by the polymerase chain reaction seems to increase the sensitivity and specificity of the test, especially at early times postdose and with low doses of rHuEPO.[33] So far, these tests have been used in "health tests" and for identifying individuals whose abnormal erythropoietic profile requires further investigation.

The approach described above uses population reference ranges to identify individuals with unusual hematological profiles. As shown in clinical medicine, using an individual's historical data as his or her personal reference range is a much more sensitive approach to identifying changes due to disease. This has been used in the detection of prostate cancer based on an individual's prostate-specific antigen test results obtained over time. Sharpe and colleagues showed that this concept can also be applied to identify unusual patterns resulting from rHuEPO use.[34] The approach was more successful than comparison with population reference values at identifying rHuEPO use. Several sports have now adopted this approach to evaluating data.

Wide and coauthors reported that the isoform pattern of native EPO can be distinguished from the isoform pattern of recombinant EPO by electrophoresis.[35] Isoforms are proteins that have the same functionality but small differences in either amino acid sequence or, in this case, structure and charge of their carbohydrate side chains. While Wide and colleagues' work was an exciting development, a practical direct test for rHuEPO that uses isoelectric focusing (IEF) was not available until 2000.[36] The basis for the test is the difference in negative charge due to the difference in number of sialic acid residues in the branched carbohydrate side chains attached to the EPO protein. When the carbohydrate chains are made in a mammalian cell, certain types of branching may or may not occur in that particular species. Thus there are subtle differences between the carbohydrate side chains made by Chinese hamster ovary cells and by human cells. In addition, during purification, only a limited number of isoforms are isolated to prepare Epogen or Procrit. The IEF test is based on three steps: selective sample preparation, separation of the isoforms according to their charge, and a double immunoblotting technique that uses a fluorescent- or chemiluminescent-labeled antibody to rHuEPO.[37] The IEF-immunoblotting test is complex and requires significant expertise to obtain high-quality results. It is capable of detecting the difference between native EPO and both rHuEPO and NESP.[38]

Because EPO is a protein normally, or endogenously, produced in the human body, the interpretation of the IEF-immunoblotting test result is important. Several approaches have been proposed to characterize the pattern observed after rHuEPO use.[39] WADA approved a technical document that has specific criteria for interpreting a trace as an adverse analytical finding. Two important considerations are the existence of "active urines," in which the rHuEPO profile changes with time, and "atypical profiles," which appear rarely in certain individuals. While there have been recent criticisms, by some experts, of the specificity of the rHuEPO test in postexercise samples that show proteinuria, many of these critiques have not applied the interpretation criteria used by the WADA-accredited laboratories. Thus, the relevance of such critiques to the validity of test results is not clear.

## Conclusion

Manipulation of the body's oxygen-transport system is one of the simplest and most effective approaches to improving athletic performance. Exercise training alone causes changes in the delivery of $O_2$ to the tissues, so this makes detection of doping more complex. There are significant potential health risks to artificially increasing the RBC mass, however, and the coercive impact of the use of effective doping methods significantly affects the spirit of sport. The inclusion of these substances and methods on WADA's Prohibited List thus seems warranted. Deterrence, which is the primary goal of any antidoping program, requires education and effective testing. Since 2000, a variety of new testing strategies have been advanced to detect prohibited substances and methods used to enhance $O_2$ transport. Doping violations and sanctions for the use of biosynthetic EPO, NESP, and homologous blood transfusions emphasize the importance of continued vigilance and testing in this area. The potential for genetic enhancement of the oxygen-transport systems in healthy athletes poses a difficult and challenging problem for the future.

DISCLAIMER

The content of this publication does not necessarily reflect the views or policies of the United States Anti-Doping Agency.

NOTES

1. M. N. Sawka, M. J. Joyner, D. S. Miles, R. J. Robertson, L. L. Spriet, and A. J. Young, "American College of Sports Medicine Position Stand: The Use of Blood Doping as an Ergogenic Aid," *Medicine and Science in Sports and Exercise* 28, no. 6 (1996): i–viii.

2. T. Videman, I. Lereim, P. Hemmingsson, M. S. Turner, M. P. Rousseau-Bianchi, P. Jenoure, E. Raas, H. Schonhuber, H. Rusko, and J. Stray-Gundersen, "Changes in Hemoglobin Values in Elite Cross-Country Skiers from 1987–1999," *Scandinavian Journal of Medical Science and Sports* 10 (2000): 98–102; J. Stray-Gundersen, T. Videman, I. Penttila, and I. Lereim, "Abnormal Hematologic Profiles in Elite Cross-Country Skiers: Blood Doping or ?" *Clinical Journal of Sports Medicine* 13 (2003): 132–37.

3. www.wada-ama.org/en/prohibitedlist.ch2.

4. M. N. Sawka, A. J. Young, K. B. Pandolf, R. C. Dennis, and C. R. Valeri, "Erythrocyte, Plasma, and Blood Volume of Healthy Young Men," *Medical Science in Sports and Exercise* 24 (1992): 447–53.

5. B. Ekblom, A. N. Goldbarg, and B. Gullbring, "Response to Exercise after Blood Loss and Reinfusion," *Journal of Applied Physiology* 33 (1972): 175–80.

6. N. Gledhill, "The Influence of Altered Blood Volume and Oxygen Transport Capacity on Aerobic Performance," *Exercise and Sport Sciences Review* 13 (1985): 75–93.

7. A. J. Brien, R. J. Harris, and T. L. Simon, "The Effects of an Autologous Infusion of 400 mL Red Blood Cells on Selected Hematological Parameters and 1,500 m Race Time in Highly Trained Runners," *Bahrain Medical Bulletin* 11 (1989): 6–16.

8. B. Ekblom and B. Berglund, "Effect of Erythropoietin Administration on Maximal Aerobic Power," *Scandinavian Journal of Medical Science and Sports* 1 (1991): 88–93.

9. B. Balsom, B. Ekblom, and B. Sjodin, "Enhanced Oxygen Availability during High Intensity Intermittent Exercise Decreases Anaerobic Metabolite Concentrations in Blood," *Acta Physiologica Scandinavica* 1, no. 50 (1994): 455–56.

10. B. D. Levine and J. Stray-Gundersen, " 'Living High Training Low': Effect of Moderate-Altitude Acclimatization with Low-Altitude Training on Performance," *Journal of Applied Physiology* 83 (1997): 102–12.

11. B. D. Levine and J. Stray-Gundersen, "The Effects of Altitude Training Are Mediated Primarily by Acclimatization, Rather Than by Hypoxic Exercise," *Advances in Experimental Medicine and Biology* 502 (2001): 75–88.

12. H. R. Rusko, "New Aspects of Altitude Training," *American Journal of Sports Medicine* 24 (1996): S48–52.

13. K. Piehl Aulin, J. Svedenhag, L. Wide, B. Berglund, and B. Saltin, "Short-Term

Intermittent Normobaric Hypoxia: Haematological, Physiological, and Mental Effects," *Scandinavian Journal of Medical Science and Sports* 8 (1998): 132–37.

14. Ibid.; M. J. Ashenden, A. G. Hahn, D. T. Martin, P. Logan, R. Parisotto, and C. J. Gore, "A Comparison of the Physiological Response to Simulated Altitude Exposure and r-HuEPO Administration," *Journal of Sports Science* 19 (2001): 831–37.

15. Levine and Stray-Gundersen, "Effects of Altitude Training"; H. R. Rusko, H. O. Tikkanen, and J. E. Peltonen, "Altitude and Endurance Training," *Journal of Sports Sciences* 22 (2004): 928–44.

16. J. C. Egrie and J. K. Browne, "Development and Characterization of Novel Erythropoiesis Stimulating Protein (NESP)," *Nephrology Dialysis Transplantation* 16, suppl. 3 (2001): 3–13.

17. D. L. Johnson and L. K. Jolliffe, "Erythropoietin Mimetic Peptides and the Future," *Nephrology Dialysis Transplantation* 15 (2000): 1274–77.

18. B. Berglund, P. Hemmingsson, and G. Birgegard, "Detection of Autologous Blood Transfusions in Cross-Country Skiers," *International Journal of Sports Medicine* 8 (1987): 66–70; I. Casoni, "Hematological Indices of Erythropoietin Administration in Athletes," *International Journal of Sports Medicine* 14 (1993): 307–11; F. Bressolle, M. Audran, R. Gareau, R. D. Baynes, C. Guidicelli, and R. Gomeni, "Population Pharmacodynamics for Monitoring Epoetin in Athletes," *Clinical Drug Investigations* 14 (1997): 233–42.

19. G. Russell, C. J. Gore, M. J. Ashenden, R. Parisotto, and A. G. Hahn, "Effects of Prolonged Low Doses of Recombinant Human Erythropoietin during Submaximal and Maximal Exercise," *European Journal of Applied Physiology* 86 (2002): 442–49.

20. B. Berglund and B. Ekblom, "Effect of Recombinant Human Erythropoietin Administration on Blood Pressure and Some Hematological Parameters in Healthy Males," *Journal of Internal Medicine* 229 (1991): 125–30.

21. J. M. M. Lage, C. Panizo, J. Masdeu, and E. Rocha, "Cyclist's Doping Associated with Cerebral Sinus Thrombosis," *Neurology* 58 (2002): 655.

22. S. S. Prabhakar and T. Muhlfelder, "Antibodies to Recombinant Human Erythropoietin Causing Pure Red Dell Aplasia," *Clinical Nephrology* 47, no. 5 (1997): 331–35.

23. A. Gaudard, E. Varlet-Marie, F. Bressolle, and M. Audran, "Drugs for Increasing Oxygen and Their Potential Use in Doping: A Review," *Sports Medicine* 33 (2003): 187–212.

24. T. M. S. Chang, F. D'Agnillo, W. P. Yu, and S. Razack, "Two Future Generations of Blood Substitutes Based on Polyhemoglobin-SOD-catalase and Nanoencapsulation," *Advances in Drug Delivery Review* 40 (2000): 213–18.

25. D. Bohl, A. Salvetti, P. Moullier, and J. M. Heard, "Control of Erythropoietin Delivery by Doxycycline in Mice after Intra-Muscular Injection of Adeno-Associated Vector," *Blood* 92 (1998): 1512–17.

26. Bergland et al., "Detection of Autologous Blood Transfusions"; B. Berglund, "Development of Techniques for the Detection of Blood Doping in Sport," *Sports Medicine* 5 (1988): 127–35.

27. M. Nelson, H. Popp, K. Sharpe, and M. Ashenden, "Proof of Homologous Blood Transfusion through Quantification of Blood Group Antigens," *Hematologica* 88 (2003): 1284–95; M. Nelson, S. Cooper, S. Nakhla, S. Smith, M. King, and M. Ashenden, "Valida-

tion of a Test Designed to Detect Blood-Doping of Elite Athletes by Homologous Transfusion," *Australian Journal of Medical Sciences* 25 (2004): 27–33.

28. For cases in 2005 and 2006, see www.usantidoping.org/what/management/arbitration.aspx.

29. L. Rice and C. P. Alfrey, "The Negative Regulation of Red Cell Mass by Neocytolysis: Physiologic and Pathophysiologic Manifestations," *Cell Physiology and Biochemistry* 15 (2005): 245–50.

30. Berglund, "Development of Techniques"; Casoni, "Hematological Indices of Erythropoietin Administration"; M. Audran, R. Gareau, S. Matecki, F. Durand, C. Chenard, M. T. Sciart, B. Marion, and F. Bressolle, "Effects of Erythropoietin Administration in Training Athletes and Possible Indirect Detection in Doping Control," *Medical Sciences and Sports Exercise* 31 (1999): 639–45; R. Parisotto, C. J. Gore, K. Emslie, M. J. Ashenden, C. Brugnara, C. Howe, D. T. Martin, G. J. Trout, and A. G. Hahn, "A Novel Method for the Detection of Recombinant Erythropoietin Abuse in Athletes Utilizing Markers of Altered Erythropoiesis," *Haematologica* 85 (2000): 564–72.

31. Parisotto et al., "Novel Method for the Detection of Recombinant Erythropoietin Abuse"; R. Parisotto, M. Wu, M. J. Ashenden, K. R. Emslie, C. J. Gore, C. Howe, R. Kazlauskas, K. Sharpe, C. J. Trout, and M. Xie, "Detection of Recombinant Erythropoietin Abuse in Athletes Utilizing Markers of Altered Erythropoiesis," *Haematologica* 86 (2001): 128–37; R. Parisotto, M. J. Ashenden, C. J. Gore, K. Sharpe, W. Hopkins, and A. G. Hahn, "The Effect of Common Hematologic Abnormalities on the Ability of Blood Models to Detect Erythropoietin Abuse by Athletes," *Haematologica* 88 (2003): 931–40.

32. C. J. Gore, R. Parisotto, M. J. Ashenden, J. Stray-Gundersen, K. Sharpe, W. Hopkins, K. R. Emslie, C. Howe, G. J. Trout, R. Kazlauskas, and A. G. Hahn, "Second-Generation Blood Tests to Detect Erythropoietin Abuse by Athletes," *Haematologica* 88 (2003): 333–44; M. J. Ashenden, C. J. Gore, R. Parisotto, K. Sharpe, W. G. Hopkins, and A. G. Hahn, "Effect of Altitude on Second-Generation Blood Tests to Detect Erythropoietin Abuse by Athletes," *Haematologica* 88 (2003): 1053–62.

33. M. Magnani, D. Corsi, M. Bianchi, L. Paiardini, L. Galluzzi, E. Gargiullo, A. Parisi, and F. Pigozzi, "Identification of Blood Erythroid Markers Useful in Revealing Abuse in Athletes," *Blood Cells, Molecules and Diseases* 27 (2001): 559–71.

34. K. Sharpe, M. J. Ashenden, and Y. O. Schumacher, "A Third Generation Approach to Detect Erythropoietin Abuse in Athletes," *Haematologica* 91 (2006): 356–63.

35. L. Wide, C. Bengtsson, B. Berglund, and B. Ekblom, "Detection in Blood and Urine of Recombinant Erythropoietin Administered to Healthy Men," *Medical Sciences and Sports Exercise* 27 (1995): 1569–76.

36. F. Lasne and J. de Ceaurriz, "Recombinant Erythropoietin in Urine," *Nature* 405 (2000): 635; F. Lasne, L. Martin, N. Crepin, and J. de Ceaurriz, "Detection of Isoelectric Profiles of Erythropoietin in Urine: Differentiation of Natural and Administered Recombinant Hormones," *Annals of Biochemistry* 311 (2002): 119–26.

37. F. Lasne, "Double-Blotting: A Solution to the Problem of Non-Specific Binding of Secondary Antibodies in Immunoblotting Procedures," *Journal of Immunology Methods* 253 (2001): 125–31.

38. D. H. Catlin, A. Breidbach, S. Elliott, and J. Glaspy, "Comparison of the Isoelectric

Focusing Patterns of Darbepoetin Alfa, Recombinant Human Erythropoietin and Endogenous Erythropoietin in Urine," *Clinical Chemistry* 48 (2002): 2057–59.

39. A. Breidbach, D. H. Catlin, G. A. Green, I. Tregub, H. Truong, and J. Gorzek, "Detection of Recombinant Human Erythropoietin in Urine by Isoelectric Focusing," *Clinical Chemistry* 49 (2003): 901–7.

Page numbers in *italics* indicate figures and tables.